T0325464

PHARMACEUTICAL TOXICOLOGY IN PRACTICE

PHARMACEUTICAL TOXICOLOGY IN PRACTICE

A Guide for Non-Clinical Development

Edited by

Alberto Lodola
Jeanne Stadler

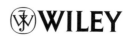

A JOHN WILEY & SONS, INC., PUBLICATION

Published by John Wiley & Sons, Inc., Hoboken, New Jersey.
Published simultaneously in Canada.

For general information on our other products and services or for technical support, please
contact our Customer Care Department within the United States at (800) 762-2974, outside the
United States at (317) 572-3993 or fax (317) 572-4002.

Wiley also publishes its books in a variety of electronic formats. Some content that appears in
print may not be available in electronic formats. For more information about Wiley products,
visit our web site at www.wiley.com.

Library of Congress Cataloging-in-Publication Data:

Pharmaceutical toxicology in practice : a guide for non-clinical development /
edited by Alberto Lodola, Jeanne Stadler.
    p. ; cm.
  Includes bibliographical references and index.
  ISBN 978-0-470-37137-4 (cloth)
1. Drugs–Toxicity testing.   I. Lodola, Alberto.   II. Stadler, Jeanne.
  [DNLM: 1. Drug Evaluation, Preclinical–standards. 2. Drug Toxicity. 3. Toxicity
Tests–standards. QV 600 P5356 2011]
  RA1238.P44 2011
  615′.7040724–dc22   2010019509

Printed in Singapore

10 9 8 7 6 5 4 3 2 1

CONTENTS

CONTRIBUTORS

Claudio Arrigoni   Accelera S.r.l. 20014 Nerviano (MI), Italy

Claudio Bernardi   Accelera S.r.l. 20014 Nerviano (MI), Italy

Marco Brughera   Accelera S.r.l. 20014 Nerviano (MI), Italy

Maurice G. Cary   Pathology Experts GmbH, Sundgauerstrasse 61, CH-4106 Therwil Switzerland

Claude Charuel   SARL CHARUEL 37270 St Martin le Beau, France

Franck Chuzel   Galderma Research & Development, Snc. 06902, BP87, Sophia Antipolis Cedex, France

Alberto Lodola   ToxAdvantage 37210 Noizay, France

Peggy Guzzie-Peck   Johnson & Johnson Pharmaceutical Research and Development, LLC; Raritan, NJ, 08869 USA

Valeria Perego   Accelera S.r.l. 20014 Nerviano (MI), Italy

Bernard Ruty   Galderma Research & Development, SNC. 06902, BP87, Sophia Antipolis Cedex, France

Jennifer C. Sasaki   Johnson & Johnson Pharmaceutical Research and Development, LLC; Raritan, NJ 08869 USA

Jeanne Stadler   EURL Jeanne STADLER 37000 Tours, France

Sandy K. Weiner   Johnson & Johnson Pharmaceutical Research and Development, LLC; Raritan, NJ 08869 USA

Monique Y. Wells   Toxicology/Pathology Services Inc. 75005 Paris, France

1

INTRODUCTION

Alberto Lodola and Jeanne Stadler

Toxicology is defined variously as: *"a science that deals with poisons and their effect"* and *"the scientific study of the characteristics and effects of poisons"* [1, 2]. Rather dramatically, the emphasis is on "poisons"; a more inclusive definition of toxicology is, in our view, *"the study of symptoms, mechanisms, treatments, and detection of poisoning, especially the poisoning of people."* Within this context, toxicology has a long, checkered history, which is described in an interactive online poster, which has been produced by Gilbert and Hayes [3]. This poster describes the principal milestones in the evolution of toxicology and effectively illustrates the point that, for many years, toxicology was indeed principally concerned with the use of and protection from, exposure to poisons. It was not until the sixteenth century that Paracelsus highlighted the link between poisons and "remedies" [3]. With the passage of time, this "preindustrial" view of toxicology gave way to the modern "postindustrial" era of toxicology. As a result, the toxicological sciences have matured and expanded to include a range of specific subdisciplines of toxicology as follows:

- *Clinical toxicology,* the diagnosis and treatment of poisonings,
- *Forensic toxicology,* the use of analytical chemistry, pharmacology, and clinical chemistry to aid medicolegal investigation of death, poisoning, and drug use,
- *Industrial or occupational toxicology,* which deals with potential harmful effects of materials, products, and wastes on health and working environments,

Pharmaceutical Toxicology in Practice: A Guide for Non-Clinical Development, Edited by Alberto Lodola and Jeanne Stadler
© 2011 John Wiley & Sons, Inc.

- *Environmental toxicology,* the study of the potential effects upon organisms of the release of materials derived from human activities into the natural environment and
- *Pharmaceutical toxicology,* the study of the potential effects on organisms of novel or established pharmaceuticals.

This book focuses on pharmaceutical toxicology and, in particular, nonclinical toxicology. Traditionally, nonclinical toxicology has had a bad image within pharmaceutical companies. This is often due to a poor understanding of the role of nonclinical toxicology in drug development. The regulatory guidelines that govern the design and conduct of toxicity studies still require, in most cases, that adverse events are produced in studies, or at a minimum, that very high doses (relative to clinical doses) be tested. As a result, toxicologists were/are seen as "drug killers," or colleagues who conduct animal studies at unrealistically high doses of the test compound. In recent years, reforms within pharmaceutical companies, driven by changing scientific, regulatory, and economic environments, have meant that there is a greater interaction between different areas of a drug development organization. Consequently, there is increased understanding of the role of toxicology studies within drug development. Not only is toxicology, and the toxicological scientist, an integral part of the identification of drug candidates, structural optimization, and lead candidate selection, but it is a cornerstone of managing attrition. Yes, toxicology can "kill" a compound, but ideally, they will be compounds with unacceptable and/or unmanageable toxicities, and this attrition will occur as early in the development cycle as possible. This is good for the patient and is good economics. Nevertheless, on occasion, despite the best efforts of all those involved, a drug has to be withdrawn from use. Consider the case of Vioxx (rofecoxib), a COX-2 selective nonsteroidal anti-inflammatory drug (NSAID). This class of drugs was developed as a safer alternative to mixed COX-1/COX-2 NSAIDs such as aspirin, ibuprofen, and naproxen. It is now believed that all NSAIDs, when taken chronically, produce an increased risk of gastrointestinal bleeding and liver and kidney toxicity. In addition to problems typically associated with NSAIDs, several studies questioned the cardiovascular safety of Vioxx. In 2000, the Vioxx Gastrointestinal Outcomes Research (VIGOR) study, which compared Vioxx and naproxen, found that the risk of cardiovascular problems, including heart attack, chest pain, stroke, blood clots, and sudden death, was more than two times higher in the Vioxx group than in the control group and five times the risk of heart attack when compared to patients taking naproxen. Subsequently, the U.S. Food and Drug Administration (FDA), based on the analysis of the medical records of 1.4 million patients, suggested that Vioxx may have contributed to an additional 27,785 heart attacks or sudden cardiac deaths from 1999 to 2003. Because of these findings and data from additional studies, Vioxx was (voluntarily) withdrawn from the market by the manufacturer in 2004 [4]. It is worth noting that this withdrawal occurred despite the fact that many patients derived great benefit from this drug. Hopefully, in the future emerging technologies will help to target the use of drugs such as Vioxx to individual patients who have a maximal benefit/risk profile and in this way avoid the loss of valuable drugs to patients.

Traditionally, nonclinical–toxicological assessment has been based largely on data derived from animal studies; this has all the well-known advantages and inconveniences associated with the use of animals. There is increasing pressure to reduce, if not eliminate, the use of animals for scientific experiments and to reduce the cost and time taken to develop new drugs. Ideally, therefore, animal toxicity studies should be replaced by a series of robust, highly predictive, low-cost, and simple to conduct *in vitro* and *in silico* (computational) studies. Much progress has been made in recent years toward this goal; however, we are still a long way from achieving this ideal. A range of *in vitro* studies, some of which are accepted by regulatory authorities, are now available to toxicologists; for example, the use of the 3T3 cell assay to test for phototoxicity potential [5]. In recent years, there have been great advances in decoding genes and DNA sequences from a number of organisms, a task that has been facilitated by the development of techniques such as microarrays [6, 7] and array-based comparative genomic hybridization [8, 9]. At present, one million sites in any individual's genomic DNA can be simultaneously interrogated, which facilitates study of the link between disease and genetic variation. As a result, genomic data for humans is increasingly available and important in drug development. Increased understanding of the human genome provides insight into the underlying mechanism/s of disease, which in turn supports the development of new approaches to treating and/or preventing diseases [10–12]. To illustrate this link, it is necessary for us to briefly discuss the role of genes in human disease and the effects of xenobiotics on genes. Human diseases are monogenic, chromosomal, or multifactorial in origin: *monogenic diseases* are caused by changes to a single gene [13, 14], *chromosomal diseases* are produced by changes in chromosomes [15], and *multifactorial diseases* are the most common and are caused by variation in many genes, and may be influenced by the environment. Genes are either *constitutive* or *inducible*. Constitutive genes are expressed continuously and control the ability of DNA to replicate, express, and repair itself, plus they control protein synthesis and are central to regulating metabolism. In contrast, inducible genes are only expressed intermittently [16]. During the process of gene expression, DNA is transcribed to mRNA, which in turn is translated to protein. Central to the regulation of gene expression is chromatin, a histone-DNA complex. For any given gene, the histone-DNA complex is the inactive state of the gene. One mechanism by which genes are silenced is linked to the presence of positively charged amino acids in histones, which produce zones in the histone–DNA complex that are susceptible to DNA methylation which then regulates gene expression [17, 18]. Small noncoding RNAs, for example, RNAi, may also be involved in the gene regulatory processes. This complex process requires the coordination of modifications to histones, transcription factor binding, and chromatin remodeling and results in the unwinding of the DNA in the transcription zone. As a result, the DNA is accessible to activating and repressor transcription factors (TFs), which bind to a specific DNA-binding domain and an effector domain. On binding an activating TF, the effector domain then recruits RNA polymerase II, allowing transcription of the corresponding gene/s to occur [19–21]. TFs can also activate genes by binding to the enhancer regions, which are located upstream, downstream, or in the introns of a gene. Small noncoding RNAs are also involved in controlling gene expression. Because the regulation of genes involves the interaction of a number of different regulatory cascades, by interfering with these cascades xenobiotics

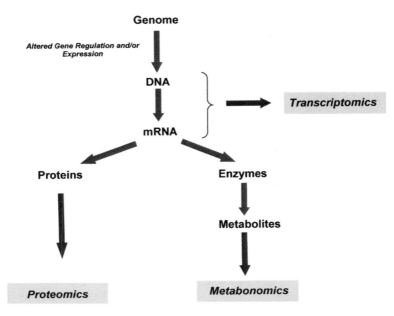

Figure 1.1. The "omics" technologies
The genome is comprised of all the genes, regulatory sequences and noncoding regions of an organism's DNA. The regulation of gene expression involves the interaction of a number of different regulatory cascades. By interfering with these cascades xenobiotics may alter gene expression, protein/enzyme production and in consequence cellular metabolism. These effects can be monitored by analysis of tissue DNA/RNA profile (Transcriptomics), protein/enzyme profiles (Proteomics) and metabolite production (Metaboniomics).

can alter gene expression and protein/enzyme production and, consequently, cellular metabolism. These effects can be monitored by analyzing tissue DNA/RNA profiles (transcriptomics), protein/enzyme production (proteomics), and metabolite production (metaboniomics) (see Fig. 1.1). Analysis of the "-omic" changes in different tissues, resulting from treating animals with a test compound may provide an early, specific indicator of toxicity [22, 23] and help to identify biomarkers of toxicity [24, 25]. This approach has great promise for developing new, specific, sensitive techniques to better characterize, and understand, the nonclinical toxicity of drug development candidates and their risk–benefit ratio. Nevertheless, despite the great strides that have been made in developing and applying these new technologies, the backbone of nonclinical safety assessment remains animal toxicity studies for the time being.

OBJECTIVES OF THIS BOOK

There is a wide range of excellent textbooks available, which review in detail individual and specialist aspects of pharmaceutical toxicology. Our focus is a more broad-based and general description of the subject. We describe, with references to key source materials, the background to, and conduct of, the principal nonclinical studies that are central to nonclinical drug development. Although the discussion is primarily based on a description of the development of the low-molecular-weight organic molecules, which have been traditionally developed as pharmaceuticals, the general process we describe is also applicable to newer drug technologies (proteins, nucleic acids, nanoparticles, and the like) linked to recent advances in biotechnology. As we emphasize in individual chapters, regardless of the source and type of test compound or route of administration, the basic toxicological questions to be asked are the same. What changes is the range of studies deployed to answer these questions. What are the relevant questions? They are questions that help:

- the drug development scientist to understand the toxicological profile of the test compound,
- the drug discovery scientist to refine the chemical motif of the test compound to optimize efficacy and reduce side effects and
- the drug development team to advance the test compound to the clinic and then to the marketplace and the patient.

In many instances, the understanding of a complex process, such as drug development, is helped by reviewing real-life cases. This presents a problem, as drug development is done case by case, but, as we show, a baseline approach is provided by regulatory guidelines. We encourage the reader to review the advice we give in this book in the light of the type of compound that they are developing and the drug development strategies deployed for drugs that are currently on the market. While our reference point is the role and conduct of nonclinical studies in the support of drug development, for the most part the subject matter we cover applies more broadly to the toxicological evaluation of chemicals. To illustrate this, we can consider the role of toxicology in the REACH (Regulation for Registration, Evaluation, Authorisation and Restriction of Chemicals) process, which was implemented in the European Union (EU) in 2007. The REACH legislation was enacted as a way of managing the risks that chemicals may pose to health and the environment. This legislation applies to chemicals used in industrial processes, cleaning products, paints, clothes, furniture, and electrical appliances. In short, the use of all chemicals in the EU is covered by REACH [26]. In order to meet their legal obligations under REACH, manufacturers and importers of chemicals *must* identify and manage risks linked to the substances they manufacture and market. To do this, they submit a Registration Dossier to the European Chemicals Agency [27]. One element of this dossier is a Chemical Safety Report (CSR), which describes the chemical safety assessment for the chemical under consideration. In the CSR, registrants must present and discuss a range of data [28]:

- substance identity
- *physicochemical properties*

- *exposure/uses*/occurrence and applications
- *mammalian toxicity*
- *toxicokinetics*
- *chemical categories*
- ecotoxicity
- environmental fate, including chemical and biotic degradation

As this list shows, some data (items highlighted in italics) are similar to the nonclinical data required in drug development. Indeed, if it is available, nonclinical toxicity data can be used. Thus, Chapters 4–10 in this book, which deal with study conduct, types of study, and reporting, also apply to generating toxicity data for the CSR. However, remember that the underlying philosophy differs and thus will alter the risk assessment process relative to pharmaceuticals. In Chapter 11, we discuss the risk management of potential drug toxicities in humans. Again, the general principles that we discuss apply to the REACH risk management process, with the added complication that REACH also requires the preparation of an environmental risk management plan, which falls outside the scope of this book. Our attention is mostly on the "scientific" aspects of nonclinical toxicology. However, Chapters 3 and 4, and, to some extent, Chapter 10, deal with administrative/organizational aspects of nonclinical studies. These activities are sometimes overlooked, or relegated to a secondary importance; this is a mistake. Time spent optimizing these aspects of nonclinical activities can produce significant savings in terms of time and resources and reduces the possibility of errors in study conduct, data interpretation, data reporting, and risk management.

REFERENCES

1. Merriam-Webster's On-Line Dictionary, 2009. http://www.merriam-webster.com/
2. *Cambridge Advanced Learner's Dictionary*, 2009. http://dictionary.cambridge.org/
3. Gilbert SG and Hayes A, 2005. *Milestones of Toxicology*. http://toxipedia.org/display/toxipedia/Milestones+of+Toxicology
4. Anon, 2009. Vioxx News at http://www.vioxxnews.com/
5. Europe, the Middle East, and Africa, EMEA, 2002. Note for guidance on phototoxicity testing. http://www.emea.europa.eu/pdfs/human/swp/039801en.pdf
6. Hon GC, and Hawkins RD, Ren B, 2009. Predictive chromatin signatures in the mammalian genome. *Hum Mol Genet 18*:R195–R201
7. Morozova O, Hirst M and Marra MA, 2009. Applications of new sequencing technologies for transcriptome analysis. *Annu Rev Genomics Hum Genet 10*:135–151
8. Wu X and Xiao H, 2009. Progress in the detection of human genome structural variations. *Sci China C Life Sci 52*:560–567
9. Waddell N, 2008. Microarray-based DNA profiling to study genomic aberrations. *IUBMB Life 60*:437–440

10. Chen X, Jorgenson E, and Cheung ST, 2009. New tools for functional genomic analysis. *Drug Discov Today 14*:754–60

11. Ioerger TR and Sacchettini JC, 2009. Structural genomics approach to drug discovery for Mycobacterium tuberculosis. *Curr Opin Microbiol 12*:318–25

12. Plump AS and Lum PY, 2009. Genomics and cardiovascular drug development. *J Am Coll Cardiol 53*:1089–1100

13. de Vries B, Frants RR, Ferrari MD and van den Maagdenberg AM, 2009. Molecular genetics of migraine. *Hum Genet 126*:115–32

14. Gasser T, 2009. Molecular pathogenesis of Parkinson disease: Insights from genetic studies. *Expert Rev Mol Med 11*:e22

15. Kalman B and Vitale E, 2009. Structural chromosomal variations in neurological diseases. *Neurologist 15*:245–53

16. Latchman DS, 2007. *Gene Regulation*. New York: Taylor & Francis

17. Spannhoff A, Hauser AT, Heinke R et al., 2009. The emerging therapeutic potential of histone methyltransferase and demethylase inhibitors. *ChemMedChem 4*:1568–1582

18. Shukla A, Chaurasia P, Bhaumik SR, 2009. Histone methylation and ubiquitination with their cross-talk and roles in gene expression and stability. *Cell Mol Life Sci 66*:1419–1433.

19. Roeder RG, 1996. The role of general initiation factors in transcription by RNA polymerase II *Trends Biochem Sci 21*:327–335

20. Nikolov DB and Burley SK, 1997. RNA polymerase II transcription initiation: A structural view. *Proc Natl Acad Sci USA 94*:15–22

21. Lee TI and Young RA, 2000. Transcription of eukaryotic protein-coding genes. *Annu Rev Genet 34*:77–137

22. Xu EY, Schaefer WH, and Xu Q, 2009. Metabolomics in pharmaceutical research and development: Metabolites, mechanisms and pathways. *Curr Opin Drug Discov Devel 12*:40–52

23. Schiess R, Wollscheid B, and Aebersold R, 2009. Targeted proteomic strategy for clinical biomarker discovery. *Mol Oncol 3*:33–44

24. Lord PG, Nie A, and McMillian M, 2006. Application of genomics in preclinical drug safety evaluation. *Basic Clin Pharmacol Toxicol 98*:537–546

25. Waring JF and Halbert DN, 2002. The promise of toxicogenomics. *Curr Opin Mol Ther 4*:229–235

26. European Chemicals Agency, 2009. REACH and CLP guidance at http://guidance.echa.europa.eu/guidance_en.htm

27. European Chemicals Agency, 2009. at http://guidance.echa.europa.eu/index_en.htm

28. European Chemicals Agency, 2008. Guidance on information requirements and chemical safety assessment. Part B: Hazard assessment at http://guidance.echa.europa.eu/docs/guidance_document/information_requirements_part_b_en.pdf?vers=20_10_08

2

THE REGULATORY ENVIRONMENT

Claudio Bernardi and Marco Brughera

INTRODUCTION

More than 400 years ago, Paracelsus (1493–1541), one of the "fathers" of the biomedical sciences, toxicology in particular, pointed out that "*all substances are poisons, and it is the right dose that differentiates a poison from a remedy.*" This assumption generally applies to natural compounds such as animal venoms and poisonous plants and to chemically or biologically derived pharmaceuticals. Subsequently, in the eighteenth and nineteenthcenturies, the "art of toxicology" was further developed by a number of scientists (M.J. Bonaventura Orfila, Claude Bernard, Louis Lewin), who are now considered the founders of modern toxicology, resulting in 1893 in the publication by Rudolf Kobert (1854–1918) of one of the first textbooks on modern toxicology [1]. However, during this time scientists investigating the mechanisms of toxicity and attempting to define rational criteria for the detection of the toxic effects of xenobiotics, used different investigative approaches, which sometimes produced conflicting and misleading results. In more recent times, when this largely academic interest in toxicology was coupled with the more pragmatic interests of the nascent pharmaceutical industry, toxicology was "standardized" and given a legal dimension. This resulted in the appearance of regulatory authorities, which have oversight of the regulatory framework for drug development and the granting of marketing approval. In short, "regulatory toxicology" was born. As a result, regulatory authorities started to define the range of experimental data

Pharmaceutical Toxicology in Practice: A Guide for Non-Clinical Development, Edited by Alberto Lodola and Jeanne Stadler
© 2011 John Wiley & Sons, Inc.

that pharmaceutical companies needed to support the conduct of clinical trials in humans with drugs in development and to obtain the authorization / permit to market new drugs.

The evaluation of experimental data for novel drugs, by an independent regulatory authority, was implemented at different times in different regions. One of the first regulatory authorities to be established was the US Food and Drug Administration (FDA), and was a result of the the Elixir Sulfanilamide disaster [2]. In 1932, it was shown that a chemical derivative of the red dye, Prontosil, had antibacterial properties and when treated with this modified dye, patients who were severely ill from a streptococcal infection made a complete recovery. Subsequently, other researchers developed modified Prontosil compounds, which eventually lead to the discovery of the so called "sulfonamide drugs." Sulfanilamide, used safely in tablet and powder form since 1936, was the first member of the sulfonamide family of drugs that are used today. In 1937, a liquid form of the drug (Elixir Sulfanilamide), using diethylene glycol to dissolve the sulfanilamide, was commercialized in the United States. In the absence of any legal requirement to do so, no additional nonclinical testing of this novel formulation was conducted, and in spite of the known toxic properties of diethylene glycol, Elixir Sulfanilamide was used to treat patients. From September to October 1937, more than 100 people died as a direct consequence of treatment with Elixir Sulfanilamide. This tragedy could have been avoided if a few, relatively simple, toxicity studies had been conducted with the reformulated drug. Japanese regulatory authorities were formed in the 1950s and in many European countries in the 1960s, following the thalidomide tragedy [3]. Thalidomide first entered the German market in 1957 as an over-the-counter remedy; the product was regarded as "completely safe" "even during pregnancy." From 1957 to 1961, thalidomide was marketed in about 50 countries and was used to treat pregnant women against morning sickness and stress, and to help them sleep. Thalidomide does not have any acute toxicity; a fatal overdose is virtually impossible, and peripheral neuropathy is probably its dose-limiting factor. However, although some studies have shown a dose dependence of peripheral neuropathy, typically after a dose of 40–50 g, in other studies neuropathy only occurred at a dose of just 3–6 g. In 1956, the wife of an employee of the drug's manufacturer (Chemie Grunenthal) assumed samples of the drug, and she gave birth to a baby born with malformations. Soon thereafter, there were additional reports of malformed children born to mothers treated with thalidomide, and a common pattern of limb deformities (principally phocomelia) emerged. In all, from 1956 to 1962, about 10,000 children were born with severe malformations to mothers who had been treated with thalidomide. Dr. W.G. McBride, at Crown Street Women's Hospital, Sydney, Australia, first raised suspicions of the link between thalidomide use in pregnant women and malformations. The drug was withdrawn from the market in 1961. Consequently, there was a rapid increase in the laws, regulations, and guidelines for reporting and evaluating the safety, quality, and efficacy data of new drugs. Against this background of national and/or regional regulatory authorities having responsibility for developing the requirements for drug registration, differences in regulatory requirements emerged; this came at a time when the pharmaceutical industry was becoming internationally orientated and was developing global marketing strategies. Indeed, the requirements for quality, safety, and efficacy data were so divergent between (national) regulatory authorities that the pharmaceutical industry sometimes had to repeat time-consuming and expensive studies to market the same drug in different countries. Given government concerns over rising health care costs, the pharmaceutical industry's concern over the escalating cost of research and development and the public's expectation of rapid access to safe, efficacious new medicines, it became apparent that there was a need to rationalize and harmonize these regulations.

THE INTERNATIONAL CONFERENCE ON HARMONIZATION

To address issues of national divergence in regulatory requirements for pharmaceutical development, the International Conference on Harmonization of Technical Requirements for Registration of Pharmaceuticals for Human Use (ICH) was established in 1990. In brief, the purpose of ICH [4] is to:

- provide a forum for regulatory authorities and the pharmaceutical industry to discuss the requirements for drug development,
- update harmonized technical requirements in the light of advances in science and technology,
- ensure that there is a harmonized approach to the development of new guide-lines/requirements,
- facilitate the adoption of new or improved research and development approaches, and
- facilitate the dissemination of harmonized guidelines and encourage common standards.

The ICH process was launched by representatives of regulatory agencies and industry associations of Europe, Japan, and the United States. The ICH Steering Committee (SC) was established to oversee the process in which expert working groups (EWGs) would engage the scientific and technical aspects of each harmonization topic. The first SC meeting decided that safety, quality, and efficacy would have been the focus for the initial harmonization activity.

Key Players in the ICH Process

Key players in the ICH process are the six parties drawn from regulatory bodies and pharmaceutical companies in Europe, Japan, and the United States:

- European Commission (EC),
- European Federation of Pharmaceutical Industries and Associations (EFPIA),
- Japanese Ministry of Health, Labour and Welfare (MHLW),
- Japan Pharmaceutical Manufacturers Association (JPMA),
- United States Food and Drug Administration (FDA) and
- Pharmaceutical Research and Manufacturers of America (PhRMA).

The EC, which represents 27 members of the nations of the European Union (EU), established the European Medicines Agency (EMEA) as the centralized regulatory authority for the EU. The EMEA is responsible for drug marketing applications and approvals using the so-called "centralized procedure" [5]. Technical and scientific support for ICH activities is provided to the EMEA by the Committee for Medicinal Products for Human Use (CHMP). The EFPIA includes members from 29 national pharmaceutical industry associations and 45 leading international pharmaceutical companies [6]. Much of the federation's work is concerned with the activities of the EC and the EMEA; a network of experts and country coordinators had been established to ensure that harmonized EFPIA views are heard within the ICH process.

Although the Japanese MHLW has responsibility for approving drugs, medical devices, and cosmetics [7], technical and scientific support for ICH activities are provided by the Pharmaceuticals and Medical Devices Agency (PMDA), the National Institute of Health Sciences (NIHS), and experts from academia. JPMA represents all the major research-based pharmaceutical manufacturers in Japan.

The FDA has a wide range of responsibilities for drugs, biologicals, medical devices, cosmetics, and radiological products [8]. The FDA consists of administrative, scientific, and regulatory staff organized under the Office of the Commissioner and has several centers with responsibility for the various products that are regulated. Technical advice and experts for ICH work are drawn from the Centre for Drug Evaluation and Research (CDER) and the Centre for Biologics Evaluation and Research (CBER). PhRMA represents US pharmaceutical companies and companies that conduct biological research related to the development of drugs and vaccines [9] and coordinates its technical input to ICH through dedicated committees of experts drawn from PhRMA member companies. In addition to the key players, there are a number of participants who have observer nonvoting status and provide a link between the ICH and non–ICH countries and regions:

- the World Health Organization (WHO),
- the European Free Trade Association (EFTA), and
- Canada (represented by Health Canada).

Additionally the International Federation of Pharmaceutical Manufacturers & Associations (IFPMA), a nongovernmental organization representing national industry associations and companies from both developed and developing countries, is closely associated with ICH and ensures contact with the pharmaceutical industry from outside ICH Regions.

The ICH Process

The ICH process is described in detailed elsewhere [4]. Following is a summary based on this detailed description. New harmonization initiatives arise from:

- ICH regional guideline workshops,

- regional and international conferences, workshops, and symposia, and
- Associations, federations, and societies linked to pharmaceutical development.

Once a proposal for harmonization has been made by one of the six parties (see above) to ICH or one of the ICH observers, the SC formally initiates the harmonization process. A concept paper (CP) summarizing the proposal is then prepared and includes at least the following information:

- proposed harmonization action,
- description of the problem,
- summary of the technical/scientific issues, which require harmonization,
- origin of the proposal, and
- type of working group that will take the proposal forward.

If the proposal is taken forward, a business plan must also be agreed on. An EWG or an IWG (Implementation Working Group) is then formed, on which the six ICH parties each have a representatives, and a topic leader and deputy topic leader are nominated. In addition, ICH Observers and interested parties may nominate representatives to the working group. A rapporteur is appointed who is responsible for keeping an up-to-date action plan and timetable with clear deliverables and deadlines. In moving from topic proposal to adoption, there are a number of steps involved:

Step 1. The rapporteur prepares an initial draft guideline based on the original CP. These drafts (and revisions) are reviewed by the EWG, and when a consensus is reached, the process moves to the next stage.

Step 2. If there is consensus within the SC, the Step 1 guideline is released as the Step 2 final document. If consensus is not reached within an agreed period, the SC either extends the timetable for discussion or suspends/abandons the project.

Step 3 . The Step 2 final document enters Step 3, at which time there is a wide-ranging regulatory consultation in the three regions. In the EU Step 3 is published as a draft CHMP Guideline; in Japan it is (translated) issued by the MHLW for internal and external consultation; and in the United States it is published as draft guidance in the Federal Register. Industry associations and regulatory authorities in non–ICH regions also comment at this time. The outcome of this consultation procedure is the Step 4 expert Document. If consensus is not achieved in previous steps, the SC may extend the period for discussion, abandon the current draft and move the project back to Step 1, or suspend/abandon the project.

Step 4. The proposed guideline is then recommended for adoption. If, however, there are major objections from one or more parties representing industry, the regulatory parties may agree to prepare a revised document.

Step 5. This is the regulatory implementation step, is in accordance with national/regional procedures, and results in the adoption of the guideline within the (legal) regulatory framework of the EU, Japan, and the United States.

This procedure adopting new or revised guidelines can lead to uncertainty as to when published drafts and/or revisions should be adopted into drug development strategies.

When existing guidelines undergo revision, it is important for users to engage with regulatory authorities (e.g., in pre-Investigational New Drug (IND) or end-of phase 2 meeting) to discuss development strategies. In general, however, waiting until Step 4 before adopting draft guidelines or revisions is commonly considered a prudent approach. It is unlikely, however, that major changes are implemented after Step 3, and generally only fine tuning occurs at these stages. Moreover, for new guidelines, the potential advantages of following preliminary recommendations may outweigh the risks of delays in the development program once the guideline enters Step 5.

THE FUTURE OF ICH

Since ICH was formed, there have been six conferences (1991, 1993, 1995, 1997, 2000, and 2003) and three public meetings (2007, 2008, and 2009) to ensure that the harmonization process is carried out in a transparent manner and that there is an open forum in which to present and discuss ICH recommendations. In general, the most significant topics addressed and followed-up outcomes from these meetings were identifying new harmonization initiatives and needs for further international harmonization, implementing the Common Technical Document (CTD), selecting new topics in a systematic manner with a focus on new technologies and innovative medicines, and considering the need for increased regulatory cooperation postmarketing. As a result, the following projects were adopted:

- to revise the M3 Guideline to reduce the use of experimental animals, in the light of alternative methods for safety evaluation, the possibility of combining juvenile toxicity studies with chronic toxicity studies, and the revision of animal studies required in support to early clinical studies (i.e., microdosing),
- to revise the S6 Guideline to address species selection, study design, reproductive/developmental toxicity, carcinogenicity, and immunogenicity,
- to define the scope of the S9 Guideline for patient selection in studies with anticancer compounds and to review the requirements for obtaining a marketing authorization, and
- to revise the S2 guideline in the light of recent advances in understanding of the genotoxicity and potential carcinogenicity of xenobiotics.

Currently, several guidelines are under revision, having recently reached Steps 2–4. Taking into account the average time required to reach *Step 5*, we can assume that it will take at least one or two years before all the guidelines under revision are adopted worldwide. In addition, discussion has started within the ICH program to identify potential new issues that need to be addressed in the near future. Several topics have already been identified (i.e., photosafety, identification and use of safety biomarkers in the preclinical studies, new cell-based therapies, and the like); additional topics will certainly be identified in the future. Sometimes, unexpectedly or following the review of a controversial dossier, regulatory authorities focus their attention on specific findings or topics. Often this focus is limited to a particular region or national authority, and the issue raised does not assume international relevance. Recent examples of this are:

- the potential risk for arrhythmias due to drug-induced QT prolongation generated much scientific debate and resulted in the release of nonclinical and clinical guidelines. Despite numerous retrospective evaluations, the development of new predictive tools and methodologies and the reliability of nonclinical QT data as a predictor of arrhythmias in humans is still superseded by a robust clinical assessment and has recently been rediscussed at the ICH [10],
- in Europe, the risk related to the detection of potentially genotoxic impurities triggered several regulatory requests for supplemental information and even delayed the marketing authorization of some drugs: this resulted in the release of new quality and safety guidelines and their adoption in United States, and
- the potential risk for phototoxicity was highlighted in some EU regions and is now subject to regulatory adoption in each region and within ICH guidelines.
- The potential carcinogenic risk of some biopharmaceuticals (e.g., growth factors) in the United States, in particular, has been highlighted and will be addressed in the S6 ICH guideline revision.

    In these instances, the issue must be discussed and resolved with the region/country involved on a case-by-case basis.

OVERVIEW OF ICH GUIDELINES

ICH guidelines are grouped into four major categories based on ICH Topic codes:

- Q: "quality topics," guidelines relating to chemical and pharmaceutical quality assurance (e.g., stability and impurity testing),
- S: "safety topics," relating to *in vitro* and *in vivo* nonclinical studies (e.g., carcinogenicity testing, genotoxicity testing),
- E: "efficacy topics," relate to the design and endpoint of clinical studies in humans (e.g., dose–response studies, good clinical practices), and
- M: "multidisciplinary topics," group together topics that do not fit into one of the above categories and that may have the other topics (e.g., the CTD)

Key nonclinical regulatory guidelines for assessing the safety of new drugs are in the "S" and "M" topics [4] and is highlighted in Table 2.1. We focus on ICH guidelines, as these reflect the consensus view on nonclinical safety requirements for novel medicines of the principal pharmaceutical-producing regions. The current set of guidelines is

TABLE 2.1. Key regulatory guidelines for the assessment of drug safety.

ICH number	Guideline
M3 (R2)	Non-Clinical Safety Studies for the Conduct of human Clinical Trials and Marketing Authorization for Pharmaceuticals
S4A	Duration of Chronic Toxicity Testing in Animals (Rodent and Nonrodent Toxicity Testing
S3B	Pharmacokinetics: Guidance for Repeated Dose Tissue Distribution Studies
S3A	Toxicokinetics: The Assessment of Systemic Exposure in Toxicity Studies
S1B	Testing for Carcinogenicity of Pharmaceuticals
SIC(R2)	Dose Selection for Carcinogenicity Studies of Pharmaceuticals
S5(R2)	Detection of Toxicity to Reproduction for Medicinal Products & Toxicity to Male Fertility
S6	Preclinical Safety Evaluation of Biotechnology-Derived Pharmaceuticals
S7A	Safety Pharmacology Studies for Human Pharmaceuticals
S7B	Safety Pharmacology Studies for Human Pharmaceuticals
S2(R1)	Genotoxicity Testing and Data Interpretation for Pharmaceuticals Intended for Human Use
S8	Immunotoxicity Studies for Human Pharmaceuticals
S9	Nonclinical Evaluation for Anticancer Pharmaceuticals

considered appropriate for preparing development strategies for the majority of new drugs and appropriate to safeguard healthy volunteers or patients enrolled in clinical studies (see Chapters 5–9). Nevertheless, a critical assessment of development issues and needs should be undertaken before deciding on the nonclinical study package to ensure that innovative technologies, scientific advances, and all available data are taken into account. However, the reader is cautioned that there are still instances of country specific guidelines (e.g., see Table 1 in Chapter 7) such that the toxicological scientist should not simply rely on ICH as the sole source of information. In our view, the current guidelines are generally well balanced. Decisions with respect to controversial and/or complex topics are made based on a sound analysis of the most up-to-date scientific data/techniques and the consensus view within the scientific community of the significance of these data/techniques.

DIFFERENCES BETWEEN GUIDELINES FOR NBEs AND NCEs

For many years, pharmaceuticals were almost exclusively represented by small chemical molecules; however, over the years the importance of biological entities (e.g., antibodies, peptides, proteins, polynucleic acids) in medicines has progressed rapidly. Although the general framework and the main objectives of the current nonclinical guidelines was originally developed and implemented to advance new chemical entities (NCEs), they are still relevant to the development of biotechnology-derived drugs (NBEs). In 1997, the ICH S6 guideline, which deals specifically with the nonclinical evaluation of biotechnology-derived pharmaceuticals, was finalized and adopted. In addition to the standard criteria and endpoints described by the existing guidelines for the development of NCEs, issues specific to NBEs were highlighted in this guideline, and specific issues arose that need to be addressed during the development of NBEs:

- cross reactivity and selection of the relevant animal species/model,
- production of antidrug antibodies and their impact on pharmacokinetic behavior,
- interference with the host immune system (i.e., immunogenicity), and
- batch-to-batch consistency of the test compound, the impact of changes in production, and impurities.

ONGOING REVISIONS TO ICH GUIDELINES

Revision of ICH guidelines is a continuous process (see above). Analysis of the proposed changes to current guidelines is of interest because given the relatively long delay between the entry into development of a test compound and delivery of the final commercial drug it can affect current development strategies. Of most interest in current revision processes (as of December 2009) are the proposed changes to the following guidelines:

1. The S6 guideline, for which a final concept paper for revision was accepted in June 2008, and for which Step 4 is expected for June 2010. Principal issues to be addressed in this review are:
   - criteria for species selection and study design,
   - reproductive/developmental toxicity,
   - carcinogenicity, and
   - immunogenicity

A detailed description of the work that will be undertaken can be found elsewhere [11].

2. The S9 guideline, currently at Step 4 for which the principal issues under discussion were:
   - an approach to setting a safe start dose for clinical trials,
   - a study design to support initial clinical development,
   - duration of repeated dose toxicity testing limited to 3 months,
   - reproduction toxicity requirements only to embryo–fetal toxicology assessment,
   - a flexible approach to evaluating the safety of metabolites and impurities, and
   - defining the scope and patient population/indication

A detailed description of the work that will be undertaken can be found elsewhere [12].

CONCLUSION

Based on current drug development regulatory guidelines and ongoing revision process that involve some of the most critical guidelines, we can conclude that great efforts have been made during the last decades to align and harmonize nonclinical drug requirements worldwide. Common and well-defined regulatory guidance facilitates drug development, avoids a needless repetition of studies, thus shortening the whole research and development process, and making new drugs available to patients in the shortest time possible and at the lowest cost possible. An additional benefit is to reduce the use of animals, consistent with the 3Rs (replace, reduce, and refine) paradigm. Nonetheless, biomedical sciences and knowledge are continuously evolving along with perceived regulatory needs and guidelines. The ICH process is central to this evolution and provides a forum for openly discussing what is ideally needed, what is possible, and what should be done. An ad hoc evolution of regulatory guidance is avoided, and each constituent (national regulatory agencies, industry, and patients) take part in the debate. Given this constant evolution in requirements, the toxicological scientist has to maintain up-to-date knowledge of national and internationally harmonized drug development guidelines.

REFERENCES

1. Doull J and Bruce MC., 1986. Origin and scope of toxicology. In: CD Klaassen, MO Andur, and J Doull, editors. *Casarrett and Doull's Toxicology: The Basic Science of Poisons*, 3rd ed. New York: Macmillan. pp 3–10

2. Ballentine C., 1981. Taste of Raspberries, Taste of Death The 1937 Elixir Sulfanil-amide Incident. *FDA Consumer* magazine June 1981 issue at http://magazine-directory.com/FDA-Consumer.htm

3. Lenz W, 1963. Das Thalidomid-syndrom. *Fortschr Med 81*:148–153

4. ICH, 2009 at http://www.ich.org/

5. EMEA, 2009 at http://www.emea.europa.eu/

6. EFPIA, 2009 at http://www.efpia.org/

7. MHLW, 2009 at http://www.mhlw.go.jp/english/

8. FDA, 2009 at http://www.fda.gov/

9. Pharma, 2009 at http://www.phrma.org/ ICH, 2009c. S9: Nonclinical Evaluation for Anticancer Pharmaceuticals

10. ICH, 2008. E14 Implementation Working Group Questions & Answers at http://www.ich.org/LOB/media/MEDIA4719.pdf

11. ICH, 2009b. Final Concept Paper S6(R1): Preclinical Safety Evaluation of Biotechnology-Derived Pharmaceuticals (Revision of the ICH S6 Guideline) at http://www.ich.org/LOB/media/MEDIA4733.pdf

12. ICH, 2009c. S9 Guideline: Anticancer pharmaceuticals at http://www.ich.org/LOB/media/MEDIA5785.pdf

3

TOXICOLOGICAL DEVELOPMENT: ROLES AND RESPONSIBILITIES

Franck Chuzel and Bernard Ruty

INTRODUCTION

Clinical studies are designed to determine with a high degree of confidence whether a developmental drug is safe for administration to humans. However, clinical trials cannot begin until the nonclinical safety of the drug candidate has been demonstrated. This involves a range of *in vivo* toxicology studies, usually in a rodent and a nonrodent, and a range of *in vitro* assays (see Chapters 5–9). Given their complexity, these studies require the concerted effort of a multidisciplinary "study team" composed of experts from a range of disciplines (Fig. 3.1) and are subject to stringent (global) regulatory requirements (see Chapter 2 for an overview). An additional complexity is that studies can be "single-site studies" (all activities and procedures related to the study are conducted in one facility) or "multiple-site studies" (one or more study related activities are done at a laboratory/facility that is geographically separated from the site at which the *in vivo* phase is conducted). Given this background, the efficient organization of study teams, and in particular a clear definition of roles and responsibilities for each contributing team member, is critical to the successful conduct of studies. Good organization and management of study teams will go a long way to avoid and, if necessary, address and overcome technical/scientific problems and interpersonal problems. Many of the problems encountered with in-house studies overlap with those occurring with contract research organizations (CRO) that specialize in toxicology studies (see Chapter 4).

Pharmaceutical Toxicology in Practice: A Guide for Non-Clinical Development, Edited by Alberto Lodola and Jeanne Stadler
© 2011 John Wiley & Sons, Inc.

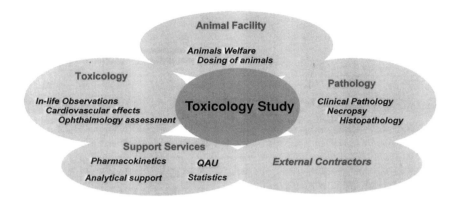

Figure 3.1. Experts from a range of disciplines form the multidisciplinary study team responsible for nonclinical study conduct and report preparation

For some issues, resolution is simpler for in-house studies, where there is control of all aspects of the study, for others it is simpler for CRO-based studies, where team dynamics may be simpler. In this chapter we review the organization needed to support in-house studies and potential issues and how they may be resolved.

INSOURCING *VERSUS* OUTSOURCING

On occasion, the expertise and/or resources necessary to support toxicity studies is not available in an organization. In this instance, this skill gap can be addressed by hiring specialist scientists or, more economically, CROs. In these cases, a well-defined outsourcing strategy allows a clear definition of activities that must be performed internally and activities that can be subcontracted to an external provider. A good starting point to support this decision is to prepare a comprehensive list of the nonclinical activities and skill profiles needed for the project in question. A matrix decision scheme can then be used (see Fig. 3.2) to help decide which activities should be conducted in house and which activities should be outsourced. Using this approach, activities are divided into four domains:

1. activities to be outsourced,
2. activities to be kept internally only if resources are available,
3. activities to be kept internally *unless* a CRO has specific expertise in this area, and
4. activities that must absolutely be kept in house.

The allocation of individual study activity to one of these four areas is then made according to two decision criteria: one is the importance of performing the said activity

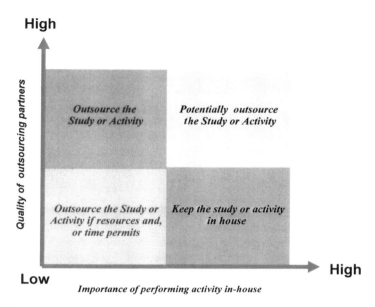

Figure 3.2. A matrix decision scheme to help decide which activities should be conducted in-house and which activities should be outsourced

internally and the second is based on the quality and expertise of potential outsourcing partners in the target activity. This type of approach ensures that all toxicology skills/activities needed for a project are made available.

THE STUDY TEAM

The conduct of a toxicology study requires a complex series of activities, tasks, and subtasks to be performed. This presents a considerable organizational complexity that can most efficiently be addressed by dedicated nonclinical toxicology study teams. We recommend that a toxicology study team be created for each study; the role of the team is to manage all aspects of the study and to anticipate and to resolve problems during the life of the study. The procedure for establishing a study team will be company specific, however, in general a "core team" should be established, composed of the scientist and technicians who will be charged with the conduct of the study, data capture, data evaluation, and data interpretation. Therefore, in addition to the study director (SD), there should also be technical team leaders (in life, clinical pathology, and postmortem activities), key members of the technical staff (who are key to the day-to-day organization of operational/technical activities). Ideally, the study pathologist should also be a member of this team (see Fig. 3.3). This core team is supported by the broader technical team/s and administrative staff. How the study team functions will vary from company to company; however, at minimum it should start by critically reviewing the study protocol. This

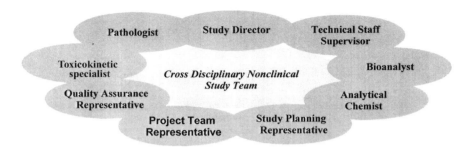

Figure 3.3. Composition of a typical nonclinical study team

review can be conducted by circulating the draft protocol to the study team, who then pass feedback to the SD and/or in one (or more) prestudy meeting. Specific study needs, potential and/or unresolved issues (scientific, resource, good laboratory practice [GLP]), questions about study-specific procedures should be reviewed and resolved. At this stage, problems can arise due to operational and/or resource constraints; for example, toxicokinetic or clinical pathology investigations may require a blood sampling schedule that cannot be supported by the number of technicians available. These exchanges are also key to a reducing/preventing errors during the study and ensuring that appropriate resources are made available to the study. Early identification, and correction, of issues with the study design will help reduce problems once the study has started. In addition to the study team, which is focused on nonclinical development, there may also be a project team, whose role is to manage the drug development project as a whole. These two teams must work in close collaboration and make sure that, at minimum, there is a free flow of information between these teams; how this "flow of information" is achieved will differ between organizations. One widely used approach is appointing a team member (a "project team representative") with specific responsibility for building and maintaining the link between the two teams and ensuring that cross-consultation occurs on key issues.

Given that the study team is composed of a number of subject matter experts, working in close collaboration under pressure of time, conditions are ideal for conflicts to arise between team members. These differences of opinion can occur at any time. In our experience, problems arise most often with respect to interpreting data, deciding on the scientific strategy to be pursued, and resolving study issues. For example, there may be disagreement on setting the No Observed Effect Level (NOAEL), findings that are used to define the NOAEL or the toxicological significance/relevance of findings. To resolve these differences, teamwork and good communication, supported by a comprehensive and meticulous analysis of data and use of the scientific literature, is needed. One of the first steps to take to resolve these conflicts to ask obvious questions:

- Is this a well-recognized and understood finding?
- Is this finding linked to the pharmacological activity of the compound?
- Is this finding relevant to humans and/or the clinical use of the compound?

- Did similar findings occur with other compounds of the same structural and/or pharmacological class?
- Does any other treatment related effect support one or other of the proposed interpretations?

Experienced members of the team may have dealt with these questions previously and know well-rehearsed strategies for dealing with it. Of course, care is needed to ensure that this does not become an excuse for lack of analysis and innovation. However, if team members cannot agree, then, as a final step, it may be necessary for management to step in and make the final decision.

Another source of conflict can be disagreements between study scientists and technicians. For many study tasks, it is the study technicians who are primarily responsible for handling animals, sampling blood, dosing animals, collecting data, and (at least) conducting a preliminary analysis. For example, recording clinical signs, recording ECGs, and analyzing friction can occur between technical staff and more senior team members when highly experienced technicians have greater practical/technical expertise than more senior (scientist) team members. As discussed earlier, prestudy discussions/meetings will help avert some of these problems, which emphasize the importance of including technical staff in these discussions whenever possible. In general, many, study/project decisions can, and should, be taken in the light of individual expertise, not seniority; however, if all else fails, supervisors or management may need to be involved. Once a decision has been made, usually a compromise in accordance with resource availability and the strategic objectives, the study team must support the decision. This may seem to contradict the GLP requirement that the SD is the "central point of accountability" for studies. However, operationally this is simply an acceptance of the fact that expertise in technical, administrative, and wider strategic constraints does not reside uniquely with the SD.

The Study Director

According to GLP guidelines [1], the SD is the pivot around which toxicity studies are organized and has overall responsibility for the conduct of a study, as well as (at least in theory) for interpreting, analyzing, documenting, and reporting the results. The principal functions of a SD fall into four main categories: technical, scientific, administrative, and GLP compliance. Therefore, any scientist with appropriate education, training, and at least a basic understanding of all the disciplines involved in nonclinical studies can be appointed an SD. An SD who has significant study experience is at a premium because formal training, even to PhD level, usually does not equip the SD with knowledge of the operational aspects of a toxicity study. For most SDs, in-house training is needed to bridge knowledge gaps, and in this respect experienced technical staff can play a key role in familiarizing the SD with the practical elements of study design and feasibility. In addition, the American Board of Toxicology has, for many years, offered a certification for toxicologists [2] and EUROTOX accord European Registered Toxicologists status [3]. Although these certifications/registrations schemes do not guarantee "quality," they are good indicators of experience in toxicology. The SD should have formal training in life sciences, a degree (ideally a PhD) in their chosen discipline. If possible, the SD group should consist of people of different backgrounds, seniority, and scientific expertise. This increases creativity, innovation, cross-fertilization of knowledge, and flexibility to support most, if not all, toxicity studies that need to be performed. If possible, the SD group should be composed of experts in general toxicity (which usually account for about 60% of the global study activity), genetic toxicology, reproductive toxicology, safety pharmacology, and toxicokinetics/metabolism studies; in practice, this range of expertise is usually only found in house in large companies. Some companies also use experienced technical staff in the role of SD. The advantage of this is that such people have a good knowledge of the technical, operational, and organizational aspects of toxicity studies. However, they may not have sufficient scientific expertise to undertake complex studies (e.g., long-term repeat-dose studies, carcinogenesis studies). This can be addressed by individualized training, focused on the theoretical aspects of toxicology. In any event, however, it is advisable that initially these SDs should be assigned to the less complex toxicity studies (e.g., single-dose or range-finding studies). Overall, this approach provides a good opportunity for high potential technical staff to be developed, and, in addition to the motivation this brings, it also increases flexibility and allows better use of specialists and more experienced SDs.

A study is assigned to the SD by management. The skills needed by the SD vary according to the criticality of the study (pivotal *versus* nonpivotal) and the type of study (e.g., general toxicity study, reproductive toxicity, immunotoxicity, and mechanistic toxicity). An experienced senior SD may have the expertise to undertake all studies for a given project, a less experienced junior SD will not. The advantage of one SD conducting all toxicity studies for a test compound is that he/she will have up-to-date knowledge of the outcome of previous studies for a given test compound and, consequently, a good understanding of the evolving toxicity profile and potential nonclinical issues. However, this approach may not be possible if the number of projects and studies to be managed by the SD results in an excessive workload. In this case, different SDs have to be used, where good communication and information transfer between SDs involved is essential. The SD must be proactive in identifying and resolving problems. If the SD does not have sufficient expertise to evaluate problems and issues affecting all aspects of the study then the integrity of the study may be compromised. Given the breadth of specialist techniques that support a nonclinical study, in general, the SD must rely on subject matter specialists; in some cases, the problem may be so specialized that the nonspecialist may not be able to fully understand the problem. Thus, the experienced SD is able to recognize what can and cannot be delegated *effectively* and *safely*. Although the SD remains the central point of accountability for the study, in reality, the SD must delegate responsibility for decision making about specific issues to subject matter experts. The SD must maintain regular contact with other members of the study team to ensure that they are aware of all major events occurring in the study. This is particularly important from a GLP perspective because, all deviations, planned and unplanned, from the study protocol must be recorded [4]. It is essential that everyone involved in the conduct of the study have sufficient trust in the SD (and management) to report errors without fear of reprisals. Any deviation to the study plan must be part of the final study report and include a statement on the impact of the deviation/s on the quality of the data and the outcome of the study. In addition to scientific and technical skills, an SD must also be able to manage the study team: strong interpersonal skills are essential. In many instances, because the SD is also the central point of toxicological expertise for the development project (particularly in a small size company where resources may be limited), the SD who is a skilled communicator (verbal and written) brings a benefit to the role.

The Study Pathologist

The study pathologist has responsibility for the characterization of the structural and functional changes in cells, tissues, and organs that are induced by the test compound; usually they also have responsibility for interpretation of clinical pathology data [5]. The pathologist must ensure the quality and integrity of the histopathology and clinical pathology data and its interpretation. Certification by the American College of Pathology (ACVP) [6] or by the European Board of Pathology is highly desirable. Even if this certification does not guarantee of experience and/or quality, it usually indicates expertise in toxicologic pathology. However, as recently pointed out by the Society of Toxicologic Pathology [7] many competent study pathologists are not board certified [8]. Although a uniform accreditation standard for toxicologic pathologists does not currently exist, and the basic requirements to qualify as a toxicologist-pathologist vary by country, there is a general consensus that practicing toxicologic pathologist must have formal training in a biomedical science (usually veterinary medicine) and postgraduate training in toxicologic pathology.

A pathologist must be nominated to a study. Although the study protocol can be issued without the nomination of a pathologist, however, we do not recommend this practice. During study protocol discussions, the study pathologist brings a unique perspective and experience and has a real role to play in finalizing the list of organs to be examined. If there is only one staff pathologist, the choice of study pathologists is obvious and has an additional advantage that the pathologist will most probably have been involved in all previous studies. We have found that it is important that the pathologist who has read previous studies or has at least participated in the peer reviewing previous studies should be nominated. The more complex the study, for example, carcinogenicity studies, the more important this is.

The significant challenge facing pathologists is maintaining diagnostic consistency within studies, between studies, and with other pathologists [9]. Histopathological diagnoses typically include some degree of subjectivity; therefore, although diagnostic terms used by different pathologists for the same lesion should be comparable, their precise use may not always be identical by pathologists. It should be noted that for carcinogenicity studies, the Registry of Industrial Toxicology Animal-data (RITA) initiative has been established to "optimize the comparability and interpretation of tumor data within and across rodent carcinogenicity studies by exploiting shared expertise and resources" [10]. If a company employs a number of pathologists, then an in-house procedure for reviewing histopathology data and nomenclature should be developed. Small companies may only employ one pathologist; in such a case, harmonization is problematic due to the comparative "isolation" of the pathologist. In this instance, it is necessary that an expert consultant pathologist performs a peer review with the (internal) study pathologist. In addition, the study pathologist must communicate clearly what are often complex and highly technical data to the SD and other members of the study team. Histopathology findings (first phase of the risk identification/evaluation) are usually accompanied by a discussion of the significance of the findings and their potential relevance to humans (the start of the risk management phase). Although differences in the risk evaluation phase are usually dealt with and/or within the pathology group, disagreement about risk management occurs at the level of the study team and can lead to conflict on occasion (see below).

The Technical Staff

It is essential to have a skilled staff of technicians with a broad range of expertise in support of a range of *in vitro*, *in vivo*, and *ex vivo* procedures. When all technical needs cannot be met internally, a clinical research organization must be used (see Chapter 4). One of the most critical skills needed by technicians who have responsibility for the *in vivo* part of studies is the ability to evaluate clinical signs. Training in the recognition of clinical signs is essential, with oversight by an experienced veterinarian or a highly experienced toxicologist to ensure proper interpretation is advisable. Ideally, experienced animal care technicians and toxicology technicians should be hired; however, when this is not possible, a combination of experienced staff working with motivated but less experienced staff is also acceptable. Technical staff should be familiar with the GLP regulations, understand good animal welfare and care procedures, and be able to handle animals to minimize stress. The humane application of euthanasia techniques is essential to avoid unnecessary suffering to animals; this is good animal welfare practice and good science. Additional benefits of well-trained staff are high motivation, resulting in a high morale, producing pride in "their studies," and good quality studies.

Management

Management plays a key role in all aspects of nonclinical study conduct and interpretation, but it is important to consider whom "management" is. First, there is direct operational management (supervisors) who are in charge of the day-to-day organization (by field of activity); here, there is a direct and hierarchical link with staff. A typical structure is that shown in Fig. 3.4a. Secondly, there is functional management (see Fig. 3.4b), which is not hierarchical, and involves cross-department/cross-line cooperation. The SD usually acts as a functional manager for the study being conducted. Most members of the study team participate in a project primarily at the operational (experimental) level while also providing (at times significant) input to the development strategy for (their) individual projects. For management, the situation is reversed; practical input is usually limited, and their focus is primarily on the strategic issues affecting individual projects within the context of the full development portfolio. The key functions of line management include but are not limited to the following:

- appointing key members of the study team,

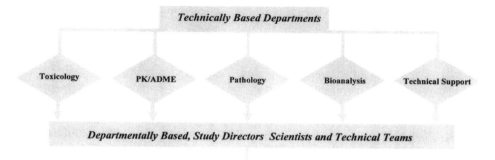

Toxicology Study

Figure 3.4a. Organizational Structures. a. Example of a *Functional Structure*

- ensuring that regional/international quality standards and guidelines are respected,
- making sure that there is sufficient (qualified) personnel available at any given time to ensure that the scheduled study workload can be met,
- implementing training program/s for all study personnel adapted to their role and their level of responsibility to ensure that they remain at the cutting edge of their discipline, and
- supporting the study team by providing advice and support on all of nonclinical strategy development, study conduct, and resolution of issues (scientific, technical, and functional). In many organizations, it is line management that usually makes key decisions in these areas.

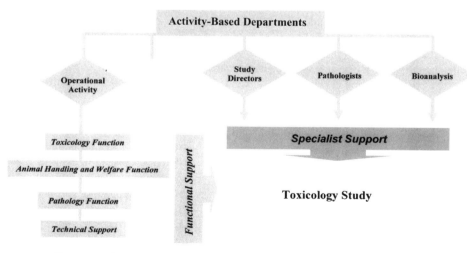

Figure 3.4b. Organizational Structures. b. Example of a *Matrix Structure*

Oversight of resources is always critical. Based on standard study designs, standard resource needs can be determined. However, although they provide good baseline data for integrated resource planning, these standardized resource needs must be reviewed and adapted to the specific study design. As part of this process, the SD and the study team must ensure that management has a clear understanding of the resources needed to support the study, and, if the need arises for additional equipment, add personnel or novel toxicology models to support his/her study. Because there are always competing demands for finite resources, management must review these needs in the light of business imperatives and the strategic needs of the drug development portfolio. Thus, a request for additional resources may be turned down, in which instance it is essential that the study team, and the SD in particular, understand the underlying rationale.

ORGANIZATIONAL STRUCTURES

There is no "best" way to organize nonclinical study activity (see Fig. 3.4). Each organization will develop the structure that suits it best and that makes maximum use of the resources available to it. However, there are several types of baseline organizational structures that can be used as a guide to commonly used approaches:

- *Functional structures:* Specific disciplines (toxicology, pathology, animal care etc) are organized in necessary functional units, which are then subdivided into subspecialties as needed.
- *Product-oriented structures:* This occurs essentially at the divisional level. Separate and dedicated nonclinical organizations are responsible for different development areas, including pharmaceutical, diagnostic reagents, and medical devices. Each area would have a full complement of dedicated nonclinical facilities/expertise. The principal drawback of this approach is that there would be a duplication of effort and a loss of economies of scale. There are also problems of scientific/technology transfer from one toxicology unit to another one and reduces the cross-fertilization of ideas to a minimum. On a positive side, toxicology activity in each area can be focused on area specific technologies and studies. In a cost-constrained environment (always the case in drug development), this is not a sustainable model.
- *Geographical focus structures*: Pharmaceutical companies are increasingly consolidating, resulting in a global market presence and dispersed research facilities. In this situation, nonclinical resources can be organized based on geographical location. Each major geographic region would have a full complement of nonclinical facilities/expertise. This approach suffers from the same problems as a product-oriented structure does. However, given its regional focus, interaction with regional regulatory bodies may be facilitated. This type of organization usually requires an overarching management structure to oversee and integrate activity globally, which creates several problems. As for product-oriented structures, scientific/technology transfers from one toxicology unit to another, reduced

cross-fertilization of ideas to a minimum, duplication of effort, and a loss of economies of scale are all problems associated with this type of structure.

Overall, a "hybrid" structure, which combines the best features from each of these basic approaches, appears to be those most commonly adopted.

CONCLUSION

Pharmaceutical companies are constantly looking for new ways to address the high attrition rate in drug development; over 90% of all drug candidates never reach the market [11]. This high rate of attrition has resulted in a lack of productivity and a dearth of new drugs reaching the patient. The recent high-profile withdrawals of marketed drugs, for example, the painkiller Vioxx and the diabetes drug Avandia, further focused attention on the importance of assessing drug safety [12]. An additional problem for pharmaceutical companies is that with many marketed drugs losing their patents in the next few years (including some so-called "blockbuster" drugs), significantly decreased revenues will result. Drug discovery and development has historically been a trial-and-error process whereby companies screen thousands to millions of compounds. There is a growing demand across the pharmaceutical industry for more rational, predictive, science-based approaches to reduce the chance of failure. There is also a demand for more cost effective and predictive toxicology studies and strategies. Regulatory authorities are supporting industry by building on existing knowledge to allow new, more cost-effective approaches to clinical development (e.g., exploratory investigational new drug, IND) [13]. These are discussed elsewhere in this book (see Chapters 5–10). To meet the benefits these new approaches bring, the organizational challenges they engender, particularly for nonclinical studies, also has to be addressed. Understanding these organizational needs is less "glamorous" to the experimental toxicologist than novel technologies and scientific discussion; however, increased productivity must involve greater (organizational/functional) efficiency and possibly reengineering of the research and development process [14]. Considerable (nonclinical) resources are often wasted in developing and validating assays and unnecessary model systems, some of which may be nonpivotal, duplicative, ineffective, and not cost effective in time or resources. Judicious, systematic planning of all nonclinical activities and optimized organization and good management of all study personnel is critical in achieving in meeting the challenges of these changes. Good organization, management of the nonclinical study team, and effective consultation/communication with other partners in drug development can reduce or even eliminate logistical *and* scientific problems. Moreover, when such problems occur, a robust organization will optimize resolution of these problems. Mistakes will still occur, but, as Winston Churchill said, "Success is the ability to go from one failure to another with no loss of enthusiasm." Therefore, although not glamorous to the toxicological scientist, the organizational and management issues we have raised should be undertaken with as much enthusiasm as the scientific challenges in developing drugs.

REFERENCES

1. Organisation for Economic Cooperation and Development, 2002. OECD series on principles of good laboratory practice and compliancemonitoring Number 13. Consensus Document of the Working Group on Good Laboratory Practice. The Application of the OECD Principles of GLP to the Organisation and Management of Multi-Site Studies. ENV/JM/MONO(99)24. http://www.iris-pharma.com/download/Multi-site-studies-OECD.pdf

2. American Board of Toxicology, 2010. Candidates. http://www.abtox.org/ABOT_candidates.shtml

3. Federation of European Toxicologists & European Societies of Toxicology, 2010. Applying to Register. http://www.eurotox.com/pag.asp?ID_pagina=81

4. Organisation for Economic Cooperation and Development, 1998. OECD series on principles of good laboratory practice and compliance monitoring. Number 1. OECD Principles on Good Laboratory Practice (as revised in 1997) ENV/JM/MONO(98)17. http://www.iris-pharma.com/download/Principles-on-GLP.pdf

5. Morton D, Kemp RK, 2 Francke-Carroll S et al., 2006. Best practices for reporting pathology interpretations within GLP toxicology studies. *Toxicol Pathol* **34**: 806–809,

6. The American Board of Pathology, 2010. http://abpath.org/

7. Society of Toxicologic Pathology, 2010. http://toxpath.org/

8. Crissman JW, Goodman DG, Hildebrandt PK et al., 2004. Best Practice guideline: Toxicologic histopathology. *Toxicol Pathol* **32**, 126–131

9. Ward JM, Hardisty JF, Hailey JR and Streett CS, 1995. Peer review in toxicologic pathology. *Toxicol Pathol* **23**:226–234

10. RITA, 2010 Registry of Industrial Toxicology Animal-data. Continuous advancement of rodent tumor data acquisition and interpretation. The road to success since 1988. http://reni.item.fraunhofer.de/reni/public/rita/#objective

11. Selick HE, Beresford AP, and Tarbit MH, 2002. The emerging importance of predictive ADME simulation in drug discovery. *Drug Discov Today* **7**:109–116

12. U.S. Food and Drug Administration, 2005. Report to the nation. Improving public health through human drugs. http://www.fda.gov/downloads/AboutFDA/CentersOffices/CDER/WhatWeDo/UCM078935.pdf

13. U.S. Food and Drug Administration, 2006. Guidance for industry, investigators, and reviewers. Exploratory IND studies. http://www.fda.gov/downloads/Drugs/GuidanceComplianceRegulatoryInformation/Guidances/ucm078933.pdf

14. Stevens JL and Beker TK, 2009. The future of drug safety testing: Expanding the view and narrowing the focus. *Drug Discov Today* **14**:162–167

4

CONTRACT RESEARCH ORGANIZATIONS

Maurice Cary

INTRODUCTION

When new drugs are developed, it is almost inevitable that a biotech or pharmaceutical company, large or small, will need the services of scientists and professionals external to their organization. In large companies, this occurs when the companies have full drug development pipelines, since as many compounds as possible are developed simultaneously, whereas small companies typically do not have sufficient laboratory capacity to develop their own compounds. The nonclinical development program may present a significant challenge for any company in terms of internal capacity, that is, animal rooms, technical staff, or both, to run every single study required to meet their needs. Even if there is sufficient capacity, it may not be the most cost-effective option. Considering the potential scarcity of (internal) resources, as well as the uncertainties inherent in drug development programs, the intelligent use of contract research organizations (CROs) increases flexibility and is good management practice even for large companies. Furthermore, despite efforts by pharmaceutical companies to recruit the best-qualified scientists and develop a wide range of special techniques internally, it is often not cost effective to develop all the specialized techniques that may be required. In fact, it may not be wise for a company to attempt to develop all such techniques internally. There is the distinct possibility that after a company directs staff, equipment, and finances to address a special need, the requirement may change, and that regulators have moved

Pharmaceutical Toxicology in Practice: A Guide for Non-Clinical Development, Edited by Alberto Lodola and Jeanne Stadler
© 2011 John Wiley & Sons, Inc.

on to require use of another technique/animal model considered to delineate more precisely the potential for a compound to be of concern in the clinic. For example, in the mid-1990s, regulatory authorities recommended the Purkinje fiber assay for assessing a compound's potential for QT prolongation. Many companies established the internal capacity to run this assay only to find that the authorities required the hERG channel assay instead. A more prudent course is to use CROs to run such specialized assays, as there is no significant long-term commitment on the part of the sponsor to invest in additional laboratory space and/or personnel that might become a surplus to need. If regulatory requirements change, they can simply hire another CRO to address the new requirement. In today's rapidly changing world of drug development, using CROs to expand internal capacity and access the technical expertise needed to address shifting development needs and regulatory requirements is a wise strategy. In any company, when suitably qualified people are not available internally, we recommend that an external consultant be hired to manage the outsourced development program.

Poor management of outsourced studies is a common reason for failure and usually occurs because the sponsor has not mastered the skills necessary to manage the outsourcing program effectively. Inefficient management of an outsourcing program leads to unnecessary delays in regulatory submissions. In addition, the real cost is not the cost of the study itself but potentially the lost revenue due to delayed market entry and lost patent time. Good CRO selection makes study monitoring easier and good monitoring makes report preparation easier. Good reports result in high quality regulatory documents and timely submissions and, most importantly, reduces delays in getting new drugs to market. Select the wrong CRO and the problems snowball. In any case, placing blame never helps in attaining a development objective. It is imperative that the sponsor be proactive and capable of being involved in the report production process to ensure that its objectives are met.

SELECTING A CONTRACT RESEARCH ORGANIZATION

The first questions to ask when selecting a CRO should be: Who is doing the selecting and are they qualified to make a proper selection? Poor selection of the CRO cannot be overcome by study monitoring, even when it is of the highest quality. A substandard study report will be the likely product. The report itself, after scientific review, may appear to be in line with international standards; however, it may be a ticking time bomb waiting for regulatory review to find significant good laboratory practice (GLP) violations. Worse, the regulatory review may find inconsistencies in the data or its interpretation that the sponsor did not find, typically because the sponsor's reviewer did not have a broad enough background to find the clues that such inconsistencies might exist. If a sponsor does not have an experienced monitor with broad experience in applying GLP principles, animal health, and husbandry practices, we recommend they delegate this activity to an external consultant.

General steps involved in initiating a study at a CRO a are summarized as follows:

- Define criteria for selection of a CRO (e.g., scientific qualifications, special technique)

- Prepare CRO candidates list
- Review curriculum vitae and training records of key personnel at each CRO
- Conduct a "qualifying visit" to ensure GLP compliance
- Include an inspection by a laboratory animal veterinarian to ensure high quality animal husbandry
- If GLP compliance and animal husbandry standards are acceptable, obtain a study cost estimate based on a draft study design
- Decide if multisite study approach will be taken
  - Select subcontractors and identify principal investigators
  - Qualify subcontractors facilities
- Finalize study details and obtain a final cost estimate
  - Include details needed by CRO and subcontractors
- Obtain a draft study protocol, including final study details
- Get approval of cost estimate by the sponsor
- Sponsor reviews draft study protocol
- Finalize protocol with CRO, obtain final quotation, and sign a contract

Most critically, in applying the initial steps for selecting a CRO selection, it is important to avoid a number of simple mistakes, which we have summarized in Table 4.1. Using cost considerations only, may be the worst criterion on which to select a CRO. For small companies, on tight budgets, lower-cost suppliers have an obvious attraction; however, this flawed approach to CRO selection can also occur in larger companies. Although larger, more financially stable companies generally understand the link between cost and quality and are able to employ experienced, knowledgeable personnel who avoid shortsighted decisions, the temptations of false economies are always present. Companies whose development decisions are only driven by costs typically place themselves in a "perfect storm," that is, low-cost low-quality CROs plus poorly paid, underskilled professionals resulting in a poor study outcome. It is equally important to realize, however, that selecting the most expensive CRO does not guarantee high quality. A sponsor should conduct a genuine, not general, inspection of the CRO prior to placing any work there. This means conducting a detailed evaluation of the three basic areas of concern when placing work at a CRO:

- GLP compliance: a sponsor should ensure there is full compliance prior to study placement and monitoring regularly thereafter,
- Animal health and husbandry practices of the highest quality: a veterinarian with industry experience should inspect and monitor these aspects of a study,
- High-quality specialist scientific disciplines: for example, formulation, toxicokinetics, and histopathology.
- Use specialist scientists to evaluate and oversee specialist techniques.

Never follow the leader. "Well known" does not necessarily translate into good or even adequate performance relative to a sponsor's specific needs. Just because other

TABLE 4.1. Mistakes to avoid when selecting a contract research organization [1].

Mistake	Comment
Financial myopia	• Cost-based selections most often expose sponsors to problems, such as study personnel of limited or insufficient experience and GLP compliance problems.
General, not genuine analysis	• There is no substitute for actual inspection of the CRO by an experienced, knowledgeable representative of the sponsor who can verify the physical plant and technical capabilities of the candidate CRO.
	• A sponsor should never rely solely on information provided by the CRO or even a trusted third party.
Following the leader	• A CRO that is perfect for one sponsor may be inadequate for another
	• A sponsor should avoid passively following others and select the CRO that will meet their needs.
Scattered approach	• Pick a few CROs to work with, but not too many
	• A sponsor will almost certainly need to work with more than one CRO
	• No CRO will likely serve all potential study/techniques needs
	• Scattering outsourcing efforts can also be counterproductive because of the inability to effectively monitor multiple scattered CROs
Relying on local CROs	• Why limit yourself to local CROs?
	• A company with global monitoring capabilities should not limit their outsourcing needs on the basis of geography
	• If the local CRO can perform the exact type of study that you need then they should be used
	• Go wherever you must to get the best study

companies are using a particular CRO does not mean that the CRO is good for you. Conduct your own inspection and make your own decision based on your assessment of the CRO and your specific needs. Using more than one CRO is good policy; however, using an excessive number of different CROs is not. This is simply a matter of logistics. Using a large number of CROs is likely to be counterproductive because more monitoring personnel will have to spend more time traveling, more often, to ensure an adequate monitoring program. With this scenario, logistical and financial challenges will be such that adequate monitoring of studies and facilities will most probably not be possible. Another potential trap is relying on local CROs. Why limit yourself to the capabilities of CROs that just happen to be in your company's vicinity? With today's communication technology, no company should be limiting their outsourcing programs based on geography alone. Naturally, if the local CRO can perform the exact type of study that you need, when you need it, and to a high standard, then they should be used. However, if a geographically distant CRO has a strong track record after years of specialization in a particular species, study type and/or technique and a reputation for producing high-quality reports it may be the best choice even if the CRO is on another continent. In the end, high quality is the objective. Go wherever you must to get it. If you are looking for a specific technique or a certain type of study (e.g., reproductive toxicology studies in primates), you may have only one real choice regardless of geographical proximity. However, before going halfway around the world to evaluate a CRO fully, assure yourself it is worth the trouble by conducting a preliminary evaluation of the CRO in question, especially that they can indeed perform the specific technique or study to the highest standard. In the case of reproductive studies in primates, one might inquire about the spontaneous abortion rate. If the CRO reports a large number of pregnancies per annum and suspiciously low spontaneous abortion rates, it looks too good to be true, and it probably is.

The selected CRO should have an extensive historical database of study parameters (e.g., the number of gavage accidents relative to number of gavage studies performed; ophthalmology, electrocardiography, clinical pathology, and histopathology data) that appear realistic. If your company lacks the personnel able to make such assessments, do not hesitate to find a consultant who can. Beware of the CRO that claims to be able to perform all techniques and all types of studies in most major laboratory animal species. A reality check is needed. If you approach a CRO about performing a technique, and you know that the technique is a recent requirement by the authorities, ask how many times the CRO has performed this technique. If the CRO has not validated the technique, they may intend to do so in your study. This is a legitimate approach to establishing new techniques: the CRO has to start somewhere. However, you should decide on a case-by-case basis if this is acceptable from a scientific and/or strategic perspective. If development and validation of a new technique is necessary, and it will be marketed to others in the future, that development cost should not be borne alone by the sponsor who went first; negotiate the cost of your study with this in mind.

ROLES AND RESPONSIBILITY

In general, focus attention principally on the technical and professional staff, that is technicians, study directors and pathologists and not on management. This is a simple, practical consideration. Management does not dose animals, they are usually not involved in the day-to-day conduct of studies, they do not necropsy animals, and they do not read slides. However, management has a vital role in setting the framework for the three core principals of a high-quality CRO: scientific excellence, GLP compliance, and good animal health standards—all this while establishing an organizational structure that ensures that these principles will be implemented. A good technical staff will ensure the implementation and application of all three principles at the bench level. In our experience, the ability of a CRO to link the vital roles of management and technical staff successfully is directly related to the critical mass of the CRO (i.e., enough resources to produce a particular result). As is often the case with any large business, when a CRO becomes too large, there can be a disconnection between these two groups because of the miscommunication between management and technical staff. The result, generally speaking, is poor to mediocre implementation of the core principles at bench level. Conversely, despite the best intentions of management, when a CRO is too small (i.e., below critical mass), there may simply not be enough technical staff to ensure implementation. Obviously, the ideal critical mass lies somewhere in between. The focus of management should, at minimum, be to:

- develop and maintain a plan for the "quality" of the physical plant
- establish and maintain high scientific standards,
- ensure a GLP compliance culture,
- maintain good animal health standards/animal husbandry practices,
- installing/validating state-of -the art data capture systems,
- create a senior staff–based report writing structure that supports junior staff,
- ensure there is an efficient approach for dealing with issues raised by sponsors and their resolutions.

The contribution of a good technical staff, is to ensure the implementation and application of the core principles, maintain the physical plant, ensure day-to-day compliance, and see that good animal health/husbandry standards are applied. Most importantly, the technical staff ensures the conduct of a high-quality study and the collection of reliable data, so that a high-quality report can be prepared on the sponsor's behalf. The first step in evaluating study personnel is to review the curriculum vitae and training records of the study directors, pathologists, senior technical staff, and any junior technical staff that may be involved in your study. In addition to education and breadth of experience, look for length of service at the CRO in question, as well as the time each individual has been in his or her present position. Assessing personnel in this manner will not only give you an idea of their technical and professional capabilities but it will also give you some idea of the stability of the staff, and thus the stability of the CRO itself. For example, you may learn that a necropsy technician has 15 years experience simply by glancing at the years of employment. Closer review may reveal that the technician actually only has 1 year experience in necropsy and 14 years as an in-life technician. Therefore, total length of experience may not be an accurate reflection of their experience and capability as a necropsy technician. The best technical teams are usually led by individuals with many years of experience. The best study teams are usually those that have been working together for many years. In the laboratory where timing and cooperation are often critical, a team that is used to working together for many years is extremely valuable.

Study Director

Ideally, the study director (SD) and the CRO should be selected at the same time. It should be borne in mind that although the CRO usually assigns an SD to a study, the sponsor could ask for a specific SD. According to GLP and OECD (Organisation for Economic Cooperation and Development) guidelines, the SD is the central point of accountability for the study (e.g., see [1]), and it is the SD's signature that makes every document official. Key qualities for a SD at a CRO are logistical and organizational ability. A large part of the SD's role is logistical, particularly when one considers the need to organize the protocol and amendments, coordinate the principle investigators (PIs) in multisite studies [2], and track shipments of study materials. If these logistical/organizational challenges are not met, the result is often a missed report deadline and possibly a missed submission deadline.

Study Monitor

A study monitor (SM) is appointed by the sponsor and should be the sole point of contact between the sponsor, the SD, and CRO management. All activities have to be communicated and coordinated through the SD and SM, otherwise chaos results. An experienced SD and a single dependable point of contact will make a sponsor's life easy, whereas an inattentive study director and multiple contacts can make life very difficult. The SM should have sufficient information to determine if the objectives of the study, and the development program itself, have been met. This is the responsibility of the sponsor and not the CRO. For example, does the planned study conform to regulatory guidelines? Has dose selection been optimized? For a carcinogenicity study, has the maximum tolerated dose been determined? If not, would the use of a maximum feasible dose be applicable in selecting the high dose for this specific test article? Such points are best addressed by the SM, and although valuable input can come from the CRO, ultimate evaluation should not be left solely in the hands of the CRO. The SM/sponsor has all the necessary background information to make such decisions. The sponsor should appoint an SM with the skills and experience to handle or understand every aspect of monitoring, from study initiation to reporting. The monitor does not have to handle every aspect personally but must have enough understanding of each study aspect to know when it has been implemented correctly. Additionally, the monitor needs to be able to identify and use any additional assistance or expertise to ensure proper conduct of the study. Although the SD is the central point of accountability of the study, in practical terms, it is the monitor, via the study director, who must lead the day-to-day running of a study. However, because the SD, for obvious reasons, does not have the background knowledge, or awareness, of the inside workings at the sponsor that the monitor has, the monitor must lead the study team. If a sponsor uses an SM who can only evaluate a study superficially, and does not have the knowledge base to be able to assess the potential for error or judge when something has gone wrong independently when evaluating the critical stages of a study, then a problem is waiting to happen. The only questions then are these: When will the problem be discovered? What impact will it have on the integrity of the study? For example, can a study monitor without specific practical experience critically assess the collection of blood samples or the quality of a necropsy? The answer is no.

The best monitors have enough business sense to understand the details of the contractual arrangements between the sponsor and the CRO and to determine where and what to negotiate with the CRO. Good interpersonal skills are necessary for a good monitor. Such a monitor can typically position him/herself as the leader of the team, including the SD and other key individuals from the CRO in the collaborative effort to complete a high-quality study successfully. This is especially necessary when one considers that the monitor is the scientific and managerial interface between the sponsor and the CRO. This leadership role is only granted to the SM by the SD and other CRO staff, based on the monitor's knowledge, experience, and technical and interpersonal skills. If any of these characteristics are lacking, collaboration between the monitor, SD and CRO staff may break down with a negative impact on the final product—the study report. Not to be underestimated is the SM's role in communicating changes in study design, development strategy (that result in new deadlines), and any other information from the sponsor deemed critical to the successful, timely preparation of a high-quality report that meets the sponsor's development needs. It is appropriate here to re-emphasize the "sole point of contact" concept mentioned earlier in this chapter. Critical changes or information should only come from one source at the sponsor, and it should be received by only one contact at the CRO. It is easy to imagine the potential for chaos when information comes from multiple sources at the sponsor and is received by multiple sources at the CRO. The CRO's ability to meet the sponsor's needs is directly related to the accuracy and timeliness of the information received from the sponsor. This is the SM's responsibility.

Management

Management by the CRO plays a vital role in the overall coordination of studies. We have found that the ability to interact easily with management at a CRO seems to be inversely related to the size of the organization. Obviously, there is a critical mass required in order for a CRO to function effectively, thus very small laboratories present their own challenges. A medium-sized laboratory whose senior management has direct knowledge and experience of the day-to-day tasks of running a study is ideal. This is especially true when something goes wrong and requires rapid attention. And things do go wrong. When they do, one does not want to weed through successive layers of management before corrective action can be initiated. Moreover, experienced managers at a CRO are often extremely valuable discussion partners with whom to address regulatory issues, study design questions, and approaches to reporting, just to name a few items.

The Pathologist

Pathologists are in short supply. Knowledgeable, experienced drug development pathologists are even scarcer. Although there are a number of collaborative activities between industry, academia, and professional organizations of pathologists to increase the availability of pathologists, as Cockerel [3] pointed out, "A 2002 employer and training program survey confirmed a critical shortage of existing veterinary anatomic and clinical pathologists, and predicted the situation would worsen in the future due to continuing deficit in supply, increases in demand, and retirements in the current workforce." We estimate that this void will not be filled in the next 10–15 years. Additionally, differences in training pathologists exist, and although some efforts have proven successful in harmonizing approaches, this is still a problem. To overcome this shortfall, a number of CROs use trainee pathologists to perform the initial histopathology examination of tissue sections in detail, essentially diagnosing not only findings that are potentially compound related but also a full spectrum of background (incidental) alterations that fall within the range of normal physiological deviation. Using this method, the pathologist reports "everything he/she sees." The data are then reviewed by an experienced pathologist, who separates treatment-related findings from incidental findings. The idea is that with increasing experience, the trainee pathologist is eventually better able to provide an accurate histopathology evaluation that discriminates treatment-related from incidental findings. Unfortunately, this is not always the case, and irrelevant details can sometimes cloud important findings.

A pathologist who monitors studies at a CRO is extremely rare. However, the best solution is to have a pathologist do the monitoring when possible, or even put one in charge of the outsourcing program. Smaller companies generally do not have this option because they typically do not employ pathologists directly and often use a consultant pathologist. Even then, it is not easy, simply because most consulting pathologists are not involved, or interested in becoming involved, in the generalities of outsourcing activities. Any company outsourcing drug development work, which does not have a pathologist intimately involved in the process, is increasing the risk in an already risky-business unnecessarily. The lesson: involve pathologists early and keep them involved. In an attempt to ensure high-quality histopathology evaluations at CROs, larger companies have adopted one of two approaches. Sponsors either have the histopathology examination done by one of their staff pathologists or have histopathology work performed at the CRO and then peer reviewed by a staff pathologist or a consulting pathologist who may or may not be included in the protocol as a PI (depending on the policies of the quality assurance (QA) group involved). The latter approach is not ideal because peer review by nature is a spot check (usually a minimum of only slides from 10% of all animals, plus slides of all target organs are reviewed), thus if the primary evaluation was substandard, the peer review will not totally correct it. Either approach depends on the experience and knowledge of the sponsor's staff pathologist. Alternatively, a company might use a multisite approach to conduct a study. In this approach, an experienced consulting pathologist will perform the primary slide evaluation and, as a PI, will submit a histopathology report to the SD for inclusion in the final study report.

LABORATORY FACILITIES

Focus on the quality of the staff should not exclude focus on the quality of a CRO's physical plant. Observe the obvious. Is the facility clean and orderly? If the place smells, has cracked paint on the walls, and appears chaotic and slovenly, then do not expect things to improve dramatically if you conduct a study there. It is better to use a CRO with well-maintained facilities. In this respect, it is important to use the services of a laboratory animal veterinarian who has experience inspecting CROs on hand for an initial inspection of the animal housing facilities and husbandry practices. A number of CROs are obtaining AAALAC (Association for Assessment and Accreditation of Laboratory Animal Care) accreditation to certify a high standard of animal husbandry (see Chapter 7). This is commendable, but it can never substitute for a prestudy inspection by an experienced toxicologist, preferably a veterinarian. It is essential that a sponsor verify the internal standards of a CRO for themselves and not become dependent on certificates. When it comes to hygiene, work practices, and routines, rigorous standards must be applied, regardless of location. Perhaps, a technician with the best intentions decides to bring in "treats" in the form of freshly cut grass or fruit for the animals inside the colony. This is not done with malicious intentions, but it can ruin a study. Such habits may take years to eliminate, if ever, because it may be recognized locally as something "good" to do. Companies exploring outsourcing opportunities in the developing world (e.g., China and India) would be prudent to apply extra vigilance in evaluating these CROs, given their relative lack of experience.

QUALITY STANDARDS AND GLP COMPLIANCE

A critical step in selecting a CRO is a so called "prequalification visit" by a representative of the sponsor, ideally by an in-house QA professional, an external QA consultant, or someone familiar with the details of GLP to determine GLP compliance. The most scientifically sound cutting-edge studies may be challenged by regulatory authorities if they do not comply with GLPs. A key question to ask at the prequalification visit is: Does the CRO perform process-based inspections, study-based inspections, or both?

Processed-based inspections focus on the workflow in a particular laboratory or area and checks that the steps in accomplishing tasks specific to that laboratory or work area (e.g., formulation analysis) are followed according to standard operation procedures. While study-based inspections focus on activities (e.g., in recording raw data that established times for clinical observations are respected or that TK samples are frozen within the time period specified in the protocol) that are specific to a study. Process-based inspections are less resource demanding than study-based inspections. There is a reduced labor cost which can subsequently be passed on to the sponsor in the form of lower priced studies. However, this potentially jeopardizes quality and may ultimately not be a savings at all if the scientific integrity and/or the GLP compliance of the study are brought into question. Essentially, process-based inspections do not focus on the details specific to a particular study, potentially missing data entry errors or dubious entries in the raw data. An example is when a technician signs *into* the study room to make the clinical observations later than the time they signed *out*, or when sample deliveries are made outside of the time specified in the protocol. In our view, CROs that promote GLP compliance based solely on process-based inspections should be avoided. GLP certification does not guarantee uniform quality per se but does depend on the experience of the government agency granting the certification. Because interpreting GLP guidelines is involved, GLP certification can result in a CRO being technically within its country-specific GLP regulations, but accepted international standards may not be met. For example, we once visited a laboratory (certified by its country's GLP authority) where it was considered acceptable that the head of QA was also an SD and reported to the head of toxicology. This is an obvious conflict of interest, as QA must be independent of other lines and report only to management and contradicts international GLP compliance standards. It is critical to determine how data are captured. Ideally, all critical data (e.g., weighing, clinical signs, necropsy, organ weights, and histopathology) should be captured using computer-automated GLP-validated systems. Doing this is needed to reduce the chance of human error. Ask to see the validation records, which verify that the software used is able to consistently, and accurately, capture and tabulate data in the desired manner and format.

Finally, if your company plans to use the CRO's archive for the long-term storage of your data, then check the archive for GLP compliance. Determine what the CRO's policy is regarding entry to the archive e.g., there be limited access that requires justification to enter and approval by management). Check the sign-in and sign-out sheets. Also, check the archive's fire protection system. It should be some form of harmless, inert gas capable of extinguishing fires. It should not be water. A fire extinguisher outside the archive is useless.

MONITORING STUDIES

Emphasis has been placed on selection of CROs because often this step is where the uninitiated and inexperienced make their biggest mistakes. If the aponsor gets the selection right, monitoring studies is significantly easier. Make the wrong selection and monitoring becomes an uphill battle. Successful monitoring is a team effort (not an adversarial one) between the CRO and the sponsor and success depends on cooperation. A team approach facilitates the communication required for successfully completing a study and, equally important, for dealing with study issues as they occur. The first step (and an absolute must) is the signing of a confidentiality agreement between the Sponsor and the CRO, enabling an open exchange of information necessary for preparing a tailored, comprehensive study protocol necessary for conducting a quality study. Such information might include clinical signs observed in earlier studies, expected toxicokinetic results, or expected histopathology findings (see Chapter 7 for - details). Even with a confidentiality agreement in place, some sponsors choose to withhold this information and give the SD at the CRO just enough information to prepare the study plan. Often, some key information is not shared with the CRO until the time the report is prepared. In our view, this is not ideal but is often the case. As a guide, Table 4.2 describes key elements involved in study monitoring and, consequently, skill sets required to monitor the various stages of a study. If the required skilled set is not available internally, then use an experienced external consultant. Good monitoring involves being able to foresee errors before they happen. Preventing problems is always preferable to correcting preventable errors. Ideally, a sponsor should deploy a monitoring team consisting of specialists in the subject matter, which, at minimum, should comprise the following:

- a veterinary pathologist with experience of monitoring in-life and postmortem aspects of studies,
- a QA specialist to ensure the overall GLP compliance of the study,
- an analytical chemist to review the preparation and handling of the test compound formulation and toxicokinetic analyses,
- other specialists deemed necessary.

TABLE 4.2. Key activities for a sponsor for monitoring and reporting toxicology studies.

Activity	Action
Prestudy Phase	
	• Dose formulation (DF) analysis set up and validation prior to first dosing of animals
	• DF analysis prior to dosing of animals
In-Life Phase	
	• Monitor first day of dosing (study monitor and GLP inspector)
	• Monitor blood sampling for toxicokinetics (TK)
	• Verify shipping and delivery of DF and TK samples
	• Regular (but not annoying) contacts with Study Director
	• Regular visits to CRO during the study
	• Frequency a function of the length of study
	• Mandatory in the event of unusual findings regardless of length of study
	• Interim data review (if applicable)
	• Ensure submission of regular updates by CRO to sponsor
	• Review and approve all scheduled protocol amendments
	• Monitor interim and final necropsies
	• Monitor histopathology process
	• Primarily applicable to chronic studies
Report Preparation	
	• Review draft study report
	• For multiple site studies:
	• Ensure the timely delivery of data and reports by Principal Investigators (PI) to the CRO
	• Review PI's report(s) in parallel with preparation of draft study report by study director
	• PI reports must be finalized prior to the target finalization date for the study report
	• Check peer review of histopathology results for irregularities
	• Circulate draft study report within the sponsor's organization for comment and consensus
	• Finalize study report and prepare the expert report summary (including tables)

The steps outlined in Table 4.2 can guide sound study monitoring. There are various options regarding the precise approach to take for each step. A detailed discussion of those options and the merits of each are beyond the scope of this chapter. Suffice it to say, if a company wants to have a successful outsourcing/monitoring program, having appropriate personnel to conduct the monitoring is key. Of course, a company will also have to have managers who are themselves capable of judging the personnel needed. In our experience, this is not the case all too often and is why some companies have ineffective, underfunctioning outsourcing programs, producing studies that are less than ideal for regulatory submission.

Obtaining references, reviewing inspection histories, and asking about CROs' communication policies are valuable and advisable, but the sponsor will not actually know how the study will proceed until it is running. Then, of course, the sponsor is already committed. An experienced SM with a skill set broad enough to pinpoint the technical details can assist the study director and the CRO staff in obtaining reliable data and producing a quality report. This is easier if the monitor also has a working knowledge of the practices and character of that specific CRO, not by name but by history. Over the years, mergers and acquisitions have created global CRO organizations from CROs that were previously separate. Although these CROs are now unified under the same organizational name, a number of CROs have maintained their premerger character, so that beyond the name, the disparity in terms of quality and performance between CROs still remains. Table 4.3 summarizes areas on which the study monitor should focus when inspecting a study. The points raised in Table 4.3 should be regarded as the main elements of a "core inspection" to which additional study specific elements may be added. Because of the range of studies that require monitoring, it is impractical to list all the steps required to monitor a study appropriately. If this is not done, differences in procedures between CROs and possibilities for something to go wrong will occur. Nonetheless, this guide is useful for the SM to help organize an approach for a specific inspection. Bear in mind that priorities may shift during successive inspections that may occur during a long study. A sponsor needs an SM capable of rapidly providing the correct input and reacting appropriately to whatever situation arises in the study on the spot at the CRO. Sometimes the SM has no choice but to react quickly with no chance for discussion with their management. An SM that does not possess the skills to do this may jeopardize the integrity and usefulness of the study. It is appropriate to emphasize that much of this chapter describes the ideal situation where a sponsor has identified one or two individuals with the broad skill set necessary to handle the placement of studies from CRO selection to necropsy. In reality, most sponsors will find it difficult to recruit such individuals either internally or externally. An alternative is to hire an individual that can cover as much of the skill base needed as possible (i.e., a junior monitor) and have the skills of the junior monitor supplemented with that of an experienced consultant or consultants. Another alternative could be breaking down the outsourcing process into individual tasks and identifying an individual monitor per task to address the need. This approach involves additional expense and the greater logistical burden of organizing the team for monitoring visits. However, this team concept, although costly and less efficient, is often the only available alternative for some sponsors.

PREPARING STUDY REPORTS AND REGULATORY DOCUMENTS

The final product of any study is to produce a scientifically robust GLP-compliant report on time. The most rigorous CRO selection program will not guarantee this. The most detailed monitoring plan possible will not guarantee this, but it will help. On the other hand, if CRO selection was poor and monitoring was ineffective, it is unlikely to result in a high-quality report that is suitable and robust enough for regulatory submission.

TABLE 4.3. Areas to review during a monitoring visit to a contract research organization.

Area to Review	Activity/Questions

General impressions	• Check:
	  • Cleanliness and housing condition of animals
	  • Treatment of animals
	• What was your impression of the fabric of the CROs?
	  • Does it look orderly?

Animal records	• Check country of origin, health screening documentation, and inoculation records • This is particularly important for primates

Animal identification	• What method is used?
	  • Chip implant, tattoo, ear clipping?
	  • If a chip implant is used, can the chips be read
	  • How was this validated?
	  • Can tattoo be read?
	  • Can the ear clips be deciphered easily?

Animal cage information	• Check the information on the cage cards for completeness and accuracy
Formulation analysis (FA) documentation	• Check the date of the FA and make sure the formulation was checked before the first dose was administered to animals • Were protocol-driven analysis intervals maintained?
Toxicokinetic sample documentation	• Were blood samples collected at the correct time and in accordance with the protocol? • Was whole blood, serum, or plasma collected? • Were the samples processed and stored as specified in the protocol?
Dose administration	• At minimum, always check this on the first day of the study • Were the body weights collected and used for calculation of the dosing volume? • Was the dose administered correctly? • Site and volume of administration, dose, and frequency?

Study room documentation	• Check the study day book
	  • If used for manually recording clinical signs, review data and check for signatures
	• Who entered the room?
	  • What time did they enter and what time did they leave?
	  • How often did the study director visit the study room?

Quality control	• What system is in place to identify errors? • Is there a designated person who does this? • How are errors recorded and handled? • Were GLP compliant measures taken?
Quality assurance	• Review all QA reports • Check in the study day book how often QA performed a study-specific inspection • What were the responses to any QA comments/citations? • If a major error/s was found, did management get involved in resolving the error/s?

TABLE 4.3 (Continued).

Area to Review	Activity/Questions
Postmortem	<ul><li>What is the condition of the necropsy room and how is it organized?</li><li>Did they tare the balance daily for collection of organ weights?</li><li>Was the euthanasia of animals humane and properly conducted?<ul><li>What method was used?</li></ul></li><li>Is the necropsy team competent and well organized<ul><li>Do they work together as a team?</li><li>How are they organized?</li></ul></li><li>How are data collected?<ul><li>Check labeling of jars and storage</li><li>What is the system for quality control of necropsy and organ weight data?</li></ul></li><li>How are mistakes, out-of-range weights or unexpected findings handled?</li></ul>

Nevertheless, preparing the study report is the last chance to try to salvage a study if CRO selection and monitoring were poor. The SM who prepares the report should guide the process with the input of information that the SD may not be aware of (e.g., expected toxicities, pharmacokinetics, pathology, drug class information). Confidentiality agreements protect the sponsor, so why leave the study director in an information vacuum while the report is being prepared? Again, it is imperative to have an SM with a knowledge base to handle most of the report review. The SM can certainly review the toxicokinetics, formulation analyses, and histopathology reports and should be able to understand the results. However, experts in the subject matter should be involved to evaluate the robustness of specialist data and to ensure that the data produced can be trusted. It is the responsibility of the SM to ensure that study objectives are clearly communicated to the SD at the CRO (see above) so that all objectives are clearly reflected in the study report. If the authorities determine that the study has not met the stated objectives, it will be the sponsor's fault and not the CRO's. In any case, placing blame never helps in attaining a development objective. It is imperative that the sponsor be proactive and actively involved in the report production process to ensure that the objectives are met. Drafts of the study report need to be produced on time. Some CROs put the draft report delivery dates in the protocol as a means of ensuring that the deadline will be met. If this is not the practice at a CRO, the SM should insist on it. For multisite studies, it is advisable to include the due dates for the reports from each PI. The protocol is the one document that all study participants will have, and this allows the participants to know when their report is due and what the due date is for the study report itself. Therefore, put the dates in the protocol; such transparency will assist in ensuring that the deadlines are met by all. If the deadline is not met, this will be highlighted in the form of an amendment or deviation to the protocol. The SM's role and impact in meeting the report deadline cannot be overemphasized. When necessary, the SM should take the initiative and organize teleconferences to discuss issues that do not lend themselves to e-mail communication. There is often no substitute for face-to-face discussion and if that is deemed necessary (and the budget permits it), these meetings should be organized when there is a need to discuss a particularly contentious, difficult report or issue. In multisite study studies, timely delivery of the reports from the PIs is an absolute must. The sooner the PI's reports are submitted and integrated into the main body of the study report, the sooner a serious review of the draft report can start. In our experience, final reports from PIs should be delivered at least a week in advance of the finalization deadline for the study report. This time is required to allow integration of the PI's report into the study report and ample time for the CRO's QA unit to inspect the fully integrated report. Typically, in a multisite study, the QA unit of the CRO delegates responsibility for the GLP inspection and certification of the PI's report to the PI's QA unit to avoid duplicate inspections.

A young SD should be matched up with an experienced knowledgeable one. It is imperative that someone in the report preparation process has the knowledge and experience to ensure the preparation of a high-quality report that accurately reflects the raw data, reasonably interprets its significance, and succinctly integrates the data into a readable narrative. It is sometimes difficult for a CRO to retain senior/experienced SDs; thus, the responsibility for the input of expert knowledge and experience in the report preparation process must be shared by the sponsor. A monitor with limited knowledge and experience can hamper preparation of the report, often unbeknown to management at the sponsor. In extreme cases, after rounds of frustrating reviews that fail to resolve critical issues, the SD gives in and reports to management that they have an unmanageable client on their hands. Then typically, the CRO's management contacts the sponsor's management. Sometimes this situation can be resolved, sometimes not. This can result in the CRO finalizing the draft report as best as possible, with little input from the sponsor. To prevent this, the sponsor must guide the process by ensuring the availability of all the necessary information needed to produce a high-quality report. If the SD is not performing to the level of your expectations, or if after repeated report reviews you do not have the quality of report you want, contact senior management at the CRO and request that someone more senior become involved. A signal that indicates things are going badly is when the SD's response is that a proposed comment/interpretation is "speculation," when in fact such speculation has been practiced for many years and is considered accepted dogma. It is clear that such a SD does not have the required knowledge base. If it has not been done already, this might be the time to use a consultant or expert to substantiate or dispute the comment /interpretation in question. Such issues need to be resolved while the study report is still at draft stage. Another signal that the reporting capabilities of the SD (or report writer, as is the case with some CROs) are suboptimal is simply the size of the document. If the SD submits a 70-page "Results and Discussion" section for an uneventful 2-week study, there is probably a problem. Typically, a very large report is the result of a regurgitation of the raw data without much integration or interpretation. Such a report serves no one well. The sponsor has paid for a certain level of quality in a first draft, and in this case has not received it. Send it back, and demand that the CRO revise it at their cost. Upon submission of the first draft of the report, internal circulation at the sponsor's organization should be done as rapidly as possible. The larger the number of people involved in the sponsor's review, the earlier this internal review should start. Obviously, the quality of the input will be dependent on the level of competence at the sponsor itself. In small companies if the SM is an external consultant and the company essentially has no internal expertise in nonclinical safety, the SM should nevertheless still be involved in the review process. If not, there is always the possibility that a critical detail relevant to the entire development program can be missed. Such an omission from the final report may precipitate the need for a final report amendment. To promote timely production of the final report, verify that the CRO has alerted its QA unit to include the report in its planning schedule well in advance of the deadline for release of the final audited report. Otherwise, there may be an unexpected delay. During the in-life phase of the study, determine the expected turnaround time for QA to complete their review of the report. Also determine how long the SD will need to finalize the report once it comes back from QA. All too often, a sponsor agrees to finalize the report and expects the report to be released by the CRO within 2–3 days. Such expectations may be out of touch with the reality of the finalization process at the CRO. Make sure you understand the report preparation/finalization process at the CRO (the process is CRO specific) in order to make sure that the reports will be delivered on time. Amendments to final reports, almost without exception, give the impression of uncertainty regarding the results and/or lack of organization on the part of the sponsor and should be avoided as these, amendments can raise questions about the reliability of the information in the report and even have a negative impact on the sponsor's reputation if it occurs consistently. Regulatory authorities are aware of sponsors' reputations. It cannot be emphasized enough that an amendment to the final report is a worst-case scenario. Of course, it depends on what is being amended. If it happens to be a minor typing error on the title page that required correction this will have no or minimal impact and will not likely arouse suspicions. However, if it turns out that the main interpretations of the study needs rewording, or even if a central point must be dropped from the discussion, accomplishing this with an amendment to the final report will definitely arouse the interest/suspicion of reviewers and may detract from the study's credibility.

Although CROs offer regulatory document preparation (e.g., common technical document, investigational new drugs, and investigators' brochures) in their list of services, it may not be the best place to produce the final (and most critical) product submitted to the regulatory authorities. Typically, individuals with the experience and skill to prepare such regulatory documents are in management at the CRO. Due to time constraints and scattered focus because of multiple responsibilities, it may not be possible to involve such individuals. If the sponsor does not have the dedicated, experienced staff to prepare such regulatory documents, then we recommend the use of consultants. There are consultants that specialize in the preparation of regulatory document, but again care should be taken in evaluating them prior to employing their services. The sponsor should review the curriculum vitae of the individuals that will be involved in their project. It is critical to assess the years of experience and the skill base and experience of the individuals concerned as discussed.

CONCLUSION

Any large company with a substantial number of compounds in the pipeline will have to use CROs at some time. Consecutive development of compounds in the pipeline simply does not lend itself to efficiently and quickly determine the most suitable compound for success in clinical trials and eventual entry into the market. We are all familiar with the concept that it takes testing of thousands of candidates to come up with one likely success [4]. This obviously requires significant resources. For large companies when internal cost of an employee (i.e., salary, benefits, pension, and insurance) is taken into account, using a CRO may be more economical. For smaller companies with limited resources (technical and financial), using a CRO may be the only option. Use of a CRO may also be the best option when special techniques are required in developing a drug, especially if there is a risk that the requirement for the study may be dropped by regulatory authorities. Why spend the time and money to equip a laboratory, including hiring personnel, just to learn in the next year that the authorities have decided that the previously requested technique was no longer required? Cost should not be the primary decision driver when selecting a CRO. Ironically, a cost-driven decision can be the most costly in the selection of CROs and could possibly ruin an entire program. Even worse are cost-driven study designs, which typically result in holes in the data that necessitate an additional study to fill the gaps. Sponsors should use CROs and the experience of their senior management to develop cost-effective study designs and development programs, but the cheapest CRO or study design may turn out to be the most expensive in the long run. Too often, management of pharmaceutical and biotech companies force cost-driven decisions, often at the expense of quality, necessitating repetition of an entire study or a new study designed to fill gaps created by the first "cheaper" design. Occasionally, this scenario is at the expense of patients, when low-quality work produces unreliable results that endanger patients because something was missed in a poorly designed, low-quality, preclinical study. The other scenario is not so obvious: life-saving medicines do not reach the market due to shoddy study performance, reporting, or both, causing unnecessary delays or even wrongly terminating the development of the candidate drug. This can occur in the smallest and largest companies and reflects a strong economic incentive, but cost cutting often proves to be shortsighted, and occasionally dangerous.

Naturally, when a company is faced with the task of developing several compounds simultaneously while facing budget constraints, economics is an issue. However, companies should not expect to develop drugs in any CRO hoping to achieve huge savings globally, especially by going to Asian CROs. The true cost savings do not come from an ultra-cheap study (typically in the thousands). The true cost savings (typically in the millions) come from developing the portfolio faster, more efficiently, with high quality, preventing the need to repeat entire studies, or parts thereof, and getting your compound to market as soon as possible. Any delays in the development program result in costs much higher than the savings achieved by running the program on the cheap.

Monitoring studies must be undertaken by experienced individuals with a broad skill set to ensure delivery of a high-quality study; at risk is not just the loss of money and time but also the loss of animals used unnecessarily when studies have to be repeated. Using inexperienced SMs can lead to underperforming, inefficient outsourcing programs. Good interpersonal skills are also necessary. If a person can criticize, be sure that the person is equally as good at praising. Let people know when they do a good job. Make sure that their management knows that they did a good job. Praise them in front of their management so that a good performance has been confirmed before all. No leader can only criticize. Become the monitor (sponsor) that the study directors like to work with, not because you are easy, but because you are competent and they can learn from you. The success of the outsourcing program depends on the knowledge, experience and skills of the monitor(s) running the sponsor's program.

REFERENCES

1. OECD, 1999. OECD Series on Principles of GLP and Compliance Monitoring Number 8 (Revised). Consensus Document The role and responsibilities of the study director in GLP studies at http://www.olis.oecd.org/olis/1999doc.nsf/LinkTo/NT00000D56/$FILE/09E98860.PDF

2. OECD, 2002. OECD Series on principles of good laboratory practice and compliance monitoring Number 13. Consensus Document of the Working Group on Good Laboratory Practice. The Application of the OECD Principles of GLP to the Organisation and Management of Multisite Studies at http://www.olis.oecd.org/olis/2002doc.nsf/LinkTo/NT00000B8A/$FILE/JT00128856.PDF

3. Cockerel, GL 2009. The ACVP/STP Coalition for Veterinary Pathology Fellows at http://www.acvp.org/training/coalition.php

4. Anon, 2003. Points to Consider in Preclinical Development at http://www.pacificbiolabs.com/tech_downloads.asp

5

SAFETY PHARMACOLOGY

Claudio Arrigoni and Valeria Perego

INTRODUCTION

Safety pharmacology has been defined as a separate and distinct safety evaluation discipline only recently [1]. It is situated between toxicology and primary (discovery) pharmacology and examines changes in organ/system functions with emphasis on acute and functional pharmacodynamic effects. It also differentiates itself from primary pharmacology, which defines the effect of a drug on the intended target in that safety pharmacology focuses on off-target pharmacological interactions, and was originally referred to as "general pharmacology." This differentiation places safety pharmacology between the disciplines of both toxicology and discovery pharmacology. With toxicology, it shares the common goal of determining the safety and tolerability of potential new drugs and protecting clinical trials participants and patients from the potential adverse effects of pharmaceuticals. In common with discovery pharmacology are the endpoints, which are pharmacodynamic rather than toxicological. The range of doses tested differentiates safety pharmacology from both primary pharmacology and toxicology. On one hand, doses must include and exceed pharmacodynamic active doses so that possible overdosing or extremely high plasma levels in patients and clinical trial participants (such as those attainable in low metabolizers or by inhibition of metabolic pathways by concurrently administered drugs) are taken into account. On the other hand, extremely high doses, which would induce toxicity, must be avoided, as organ toxicity could prevent a correct interpretation of pharmacodynamic effects.

Pharmaceutical Toxicology in Practice: A Guide for Non-Clinical Development, Edited by Alberto Lodola and Jeanne Stadler
© 2011 John Wiley & Sons, Inc.

Safety pharmacology studies are regulated by international guidelines [2, 3]. Several safety pharmacology tests are performed at different stages of the discovery process to help identify the best development candidate and provide an early insight into potential toxicities of putative development candidates (particularly toxicities linked to an exaggerated/off-target pharmacological activity of the compound). When tests have had a sufficiently high throughput, they can also be used in a structure–activity relationship (SAR) study, which can help chemists refine a molecule's chemical motifs and eliminate, or significantly reduce, unwanted effects. In this chapter, we first address regulatory requirements governing safety pharmacology studies, and then we discuss different study types in detail, drawing a distinction between studies used for developmental purposes and studies applied in a screening mode to the discovery process.

REGULATORY ENVIRONMENT

Due to its relatively recent definition as a distinct discipline, regulations covering safety pharmacology studies are also relatively recent. The first attempt at rationalizing and giving a precise structure to this testing was made by the Japanese Ministry of Health in 1995 with the *Japanese Guidelines for Nonclinical Studies of Drugs Manual 1995* [4]. This guideline classified safety pharmacology studies in two categories:

> studies that should normally be conducted for all test substances
> studies to be conducted, as necessary, in light of the results of category A studies.

A comprehensive list of the required category A studies was provided, which included assessing the effects of test compounds on general behavior, the central nervous system (spontaneous locomotor activity, general anesthetic effect, effect on convulsions, analgesic activity, effect on body temperature), autonomic nervous system and smooth muscle (isolated ileum), respiratory and cardiovascular system, digestive system, and water and electrolyte metabolism. The conduct of these studies was mandatory prior to the conduct of clinical trials and registering new drugs in Japan. At about the same time reports of a particular type of arrhythmia (torsade de pointes, TdP) and sudden death related to the use of terfenadine, a nonsedating H1-antihistamine, and of other noncardiovascular drugs, began to appear in the literature [5–8]. This arrhythmia was usually associated with prolongation of the QT interval of the ECG, ascribed to the prolongation of cardiac repolarization following inhibition of potassium channels, namely the delayed rectifier potassium channel I_{Kr} encoded by the *hERG* gene (human Ether-à-go-go Related Gene) [9]. Because of such an unwanted effect, several drugs were removed from the market or had their label revised to reflect this risk. These agents come from a wide variety of chemical and pharmacological classes, some examples are given in Table 5.1. No regulatory guideline existed at that time for studying the potential effect of drugs on cardiac repolarization. Because these arrhythmias were often elicited by drugs taken for the treatment of non–life-threatening, noncardiovascular indications, regulatory authorities became interested in how to predict which drugs might cause

TABLE 5.1. Examples of marketed drugs that cause QT-interval prolongation.

Pharmacological class	Drug	References
Antibiotics	Erythromycin, grepafloxacin	83, 84
H1 antihistamines	Terfenadine, diphenhydramine, astemizole	85, 86
Psychotropic agents	Phenothiazine derivatives, haloperidol, sertindole, risperidone	87, 88
Antifungals	Fluconazole, ketoconazole	89
Gastroprokinetics	Cisapride	90, 91

alterations in ventricular repolarization. The European Agency for the Evaluation of Medicinal Products (EMEA) was the first regulatory agency to produce testing recommendation through an ad hoc panel of experts convened in 1996 by the Committee for Proprietary Medicinal Products (CPMP). The resulting Points to Consider document [10] recommended the conduct of nonclinical and clinical studies in order to assess the potential for QT prolongation by noncardiovascular drugs. The nonclinical part of the document strongly supported the integration between the results of *in vitro* and *in vivo* models. Therefore, results from action potential duration (APD) studies in isolated cardiac tissues, such as Purkinje fibers or papillary muscle, were considered complementary to the evaluation of QT duration and T-wave morphology in animal models. A direct link between QT prolongation and arrhythmogenesis was not (and still is not) established. This fueled a debate between the pharmaceutical industry and regulatory authorities as to the scientific basis, and relevance, of the testing recommendations that had been developed. This debate resulted in an adoption of this topic by the International Conference on Harmonization (ICH) and resulted in the creation of two ICH guidelines: ICHS7A, published in 2000, and ICHS7B, published in 2005 [2, 3]. The guidelines were adopted by the United States, the European Union, and Japan (in Japan, the ICH guidelines superseded the 1995 national guideline). It is an interesting historical note that the ICH S7A guideline is the first to officially define "safety pharmacology":

> Pharmacology studies can be divided into three categories: primary pharmacodynamics, secondary pharmacodynamics and safety pharmacology studies. . . . safety pharmacology studies are defined as those studies that investigate the potential undesirable pharmacodynamic effects of a substance on physiological functions in relation to exposure in the therapeutic range and above.

The ICH S7A guideline covers the requirements for safety pharmacology testing and, as did the 1995 Japanese national guideline, it differentiates between "safety pharmacology core battery" studies to be conducted on all test substances, and "follow-up and supplemental studies" to be conducted if concerns are raised by results of the core battery studies or findings in clinical studies that cannot be explained by the existing information. Safety pharmacology core battery studies investigate the effects of a test compound on vital body functions: cardiovascular, respiratory, and central nervous systems are considered vital organ systems that should be studied. The guideline also covers test systems (species, *in vitro* systems, sample size, use of controls, and route of administration); dose levels or test compound concentrations for *in vivo* and *in vitro* studies and their duration; and addresses the evaluation of metabolites, isomers, and finished products. The ICH S7B guideline specifically deals with nonclinical testing on QT-interval prolongation liabilities; it describes a core cardiovascular study battery that, as in the Points to Consider document, includes an *in vitro* test and an *in vivo* experimental model. In almost all reported cases, drugs that prolong the QT interval do so by inhibiting the I_{Kr} potassium channel. For this reason, the *in vitro* model recommended by the S7B guideline is the patch clamp model, in which the I_{Kr} potassium channel is expressed in HEK293 or CHO cell lines that have been stably transfected with the encoding gene, for the channel, or in native cardiac cells. The recommended *in vivo* model is a telemetric cardiovascular study in conscious, freely moving nonrodents. As in the CPMP "Points to Consider" document (see above), emphasis is given to the collection of ECG interval data and to the morphological analysis of the T-wave. Rats and mice are not indicated as useful species because their cardiomyocytes lack the I_{Kr} channel (in these species the primary ionic current controlling repolarization is I_{to}). Conscious, freely moving animals are preferred over anesthetized, tethered, or restrained animals for several reasons. Anesthetic agents can prolong QT and thus mask a drug's effect [11]. Anesthetized animals normally have higher heart rates than conscious animals do, resulting in a shorter QT interval, therefore QT-interval prolongation by a drug could be balanced and hidden by the shortening caused by the anesthetic and by the change in sympathetic balance. Similarly, restraint or tethering can increase animals' stress, thereby increasing their heart rates, although training the animals before performing the experiment can reduce greatly the change in cardiac frequency in such cases. Finally, last but not least, adopting telemetry allows animals to be used again, reducing the total number of animals used.

The S7B guideline goes beyond the CPMP Points to Consider by introducing the "integrated risk assessment" concept (Fig. 5.1). For this assessment, data from the two core studies (*in vitro* I_{Kr} and *in vivo* QT study) are interpreted together with other relevant data, for example:

- primary and secondary pharmacology,
- chemical/pharmacological class (whether or not at risk of delayed ventricular repolarization), results from supplemental and/or follow-up studies,
- potency of the test substance relative to reference compounds,
- relationship between exposures associated with repolarization effects (both *in vitro* and *in vivo*) and exposures eliciting the primary pharmacological effect in nonclinical species (or the projected human therapeutic exposure), and
- impact of metabolites and metabolic differences between test species and humans.

The overall conclusion from the risk assessment constitutes "evidence of risk" for the test substance to delay ventricular repolarization and prolong the QT interval in humans. The conduct of these studies prior to a First-in-Human study (FIH) (suggested by the guideline) and the resulting integrated risk assessment supports the planning and

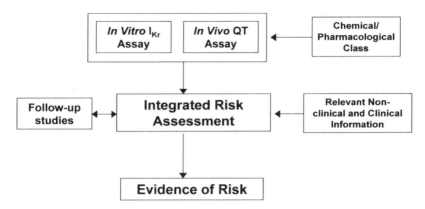

Figure 5.1. Integrated risk assessment strategy from the ICH S7B guideline [3]

interpretation of subsequent clinical studies. Supplementary and follow-up studies are also described in the S7B guideline. These studies, both *in vitro* and *in vivo*, should be conducted when inconsistent results are obtained from the core studies or between these and clinical findings. *In vitro* studies, such as APD in Purkinje fibers or papillary muscle, ventricular wedge preparations, and the Langendorff isolated heart model [12], can give information on the effects of compounds on ion channels other than I_{Kr}. When inhibiting the I_{Kr} current does not result in prolonging QT in animal models, an inhibition of the cardiac L-type Ca^{++} channel can very often be demonstrated (e.g., verapamil). In such a case, prolongation due to inhibition of the repolarizing potassium current is balanced by the concurrent inhibition of the calcium current sustaining the plateau phase of the action potential. Anesthetized *in vivo* preparations can be useful when side effects in conscious animals (such as emesis or tremors) do not allow testing at sufficiently high doses (and therefore plasma levels). In such models, an increase in heart rate can be overcome by cardiac pacing. Sustained plasma levels of the test compound can be achieved by intravenous infusion. Electrophysiology parameters (monophasic action potential (MAP) from ventricular myocytes) can be obtained in the same animals, thus allowing the effects on action potentials and surface ECG to be compared.

Compliance with good laboratory practices (GLP) is required for core battery tests by both guidelines, whereas supplementary or follow-up studies, due to their investigative nature, do not need to comply (although compliance to the greatest extent feasible is expected). It is expected that core battery studies will be conducted before FIH studies, whereas supplemental and follow-up studies (which can be triggered by clinical findings) need to be conducted in a timely fashion when needed.

EXPERIMENTAL MODELS

Following the adoption of the ICH S7A and S7B guidelines by regulatory authorities worldwide, safety pharmacology testing is routinely applied in the pharmaceutical industry. Not all companies conduct the same tests, however. Some companies, especially small and biotech companies, which have limited resources, tend to conduct only core battery tests (i.e., *in vitro* and *in vivo* cardiovascular, respiratory, and behavioral testing) and limit follow-up and supplemental studies on a case-by-case basis. Major pharmaceutical companies, on the other hand, tend to perform more testing that cover other systems (renal, gastrointestinal). In addition, the major companies can conduct some studies classified as follow-up studies (e.g., action potential duration in Purkinje fibers for *in vitro* cardiovascular, spontaneous motility for CNS) [13]. In the following sections, we describe in detail experimental models used in safety pharmacology studies. We have followed the division used in the ICH S7A guideline for "core battery studies" and "follow-up and supplemental studies."

General Considerations

Before discussing individual studies, some general points can be made that are valid for all studies:

Choice of Species, Number of Animals, and Sex.
Usually, rodent and nonrodent species used in toxicology studies are used for safety pharmacology evaluations. This allows for a better selection of the doses to be tested (see below) and an integrated safety assessment based on data from both toxicology and safety pharmacology investigations. The number of animals used in the studies must be large enough to allow small effects of the test compound on the test system to be detected. This should be defined by a power analysis that will identify the minimum number of animals required to achieve statistical significance. Following, we report the number of animals we use in studies and those that give the required power for acceptable levels of statistical significance. Although these numbers are widely regarded as sufficient to allow studies of appropriate statistical power, it is good practice to conduct a power analysis to confirm this when preparing the draft protocol for the study. If no difference in systemic exposure to test compound and toxicological effects between males and females is known or expected, only one sex can be used in safety pharmacology studies. If there is a difference, one can choose to use the most sensitive sex or to use both sexes in studies. If the latter alternative is chosen, considerations about the number of animals to be used must be applied to each sex separately, given that data analysis are conducted for each sex separately.

Choice of Test Doses/Concentrations.
Doses and test compound concentrations should be chosen such that a dose– or concentration–response relationship can be established. For *in vivo* studies, doses tested should include, and exceed (in terms of systemic exposure), pharmacologically active doses in animal models or, when available, a dose giving the expected therapeutic effect in humans. In the absence of any adverse effect on the safety pharmacology endpoints evaluated, the highest dose tested should be one that produces moderate adverse effects; depending on the study strategy adopted, this can be derived from toxicology study data. In particular, effects such as tremors or fasciculation, which may confound interpretation of ECGs, can be dose limiting. In our experience, doses similar to the ones used in repeated dose toxicology studies of up to

4 weeks long are usually enough to define the pharmacological profile of a test compound. For *in vitro* studies, the range of test compound concentrations tested should include and exceed the expected human therapeutic exposure range. In the absence of effects, the ICH S7B guideline requires that the highest concentration tested be defined by the physicochemical characteristics (i.e., maximum solubility) of the test compound. This requirement has raised some concern among pharmaceutical companies, which refute that any compound will show an apparent effect if tested at high concentrations, resulting in a number of false positives that would require further testing and discussion. Redfern et al. [14] has compared published data on I_{Kr} activity, APD, and QT prolongation in animals and QT effects and reports of TdP in humans for 100 drugs. They found that drugs with no QT liabilities show a >30-fold separation between I_{Kr} activity and unbound therapeutic plasma concentrations. Therefore, a 30-fold multiple of the expected human therapeutic level could represent the upper limit of concentrations appropriately to be tested in case of negative results.

Route of Administration. Usually, the route of administration envisaged for human use is used in studies. Anesthetized animal models, however, require a different approach, as anesthesia inhibits gastric motility, thus potentially affecting absorption of the test compound. In this case, two alternative routes are normally employed: intravenous or intraduodenal. The advantage of intravenous is to ensure the complete bioavailability of the test compound and allows testing of incremental doses in the same animal thus reducing the number of animals required for the study. Intraduodenal administration (using a cannula, surgically inserted into the duodenum) more closely mimics oral administration and takes possible first-pass metabolism into account . The choice between these two alternatives must take the pharmacokinetics (PKs) of the test compound into account.

Evaluation of Systemic Exposure. It is important to relate pharmacological side effects to systemic exposure rather than to the administered dose of test compound. This way, differences in PK between different species are taken into account and projection to the expected human therapeutic dose is possible. However, blood sampling of PK could interfere with the recording of physiological parameters that could confound their interpretation. Cardiovascular, respiratory, and central nervous systems can all be heavily affected by the stress caused by animal handling. Subjecting control animals to the same procedures does not guarantee that the parameters recorded will be interpreted correctly. For this reason, we found that it is better not to take blood samples from animals in a safety pharmacology study but to relate effects to the exposures obtained in toxicology studies in the same species, where a complete PK profile is usually generated. In rodent studies, this is practically equivalent to having satellite groups of animals for PK sampling (as is common in toxicology studies). If PK data are deemed necessary (e.g., due to high interanimal variability) in nonrodent cardiovascular studies, we suggest either obtaining a single blood sample after *t*max (to not interfere with pharmacological effects, which are usually maximal at *C*max), or redosing the same animals in a separate session solely for sampling blood. In the latter case, the amount of the compound required will be doubled, and study completion will require more time.

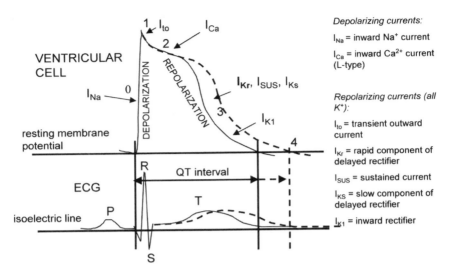

Figure 5.2. Ventricular cell action potential and surface ECG
This schematic, which is not to scale, shows how the increase of inward currents (I_{Na}, I_{Ca}) or reduction of outward currents (such as through I_{Kr} channel block) can prolong the action potential and the QT interval (dotted line).

CORE BATTERY STUDIES

In Vivo Cardiovascular Study in Nonrodents

Before describing the experimental model for cardiovascular studies in conscious nonrodents, let us review the mechanism of drug-induced alterations in the cardiac depolarization–repolarization cycle that might cause life-threatening arrhythmias such as TdP. The QT interval of the surface ECG represents action potential changes of cardiac cells during depolarization and repolarization (Fig. 5.2). Changes in the polarization state of the cell membrane are mediated by movements of ions (sodium, calcium, and potassium) across the cell membrane through a many ion channels. Rapid inward movements of sodium ions (the so-called I_{Na} current) are responsible for the depolarization that causes the phase 0 upstroke of the action potential, corresponding to the QRS complex on the surface ECG. Following the rapid inactivation of sodium channels, a transient-outward repolarizing potassium current (I_{to}) causes the phase 1 notch of the action potential and signals the beginning of cellular repolarization. The plateau characterizing phase 2 is due to the balance between inward depolarizing calcium currents (I_{Ca}) and the delayed rectifier outward (repolarizing) potassium current (I_{Kr}). This balance between inward and outward currents results in the flat S-T segment on the surface ECG. Progressive inactivation of the calcium currents and activation of other repolarizing currents (among which is the slow rectifier potassium current, I_{Ks}) lead to phase 3 of the action potential, which completes the repolarization of the cardiac cells and corresponds to the T wave on the surface ECG, and to phase 4, where the cell membrane is at its

TABLE 5.2. Gene mutations that have been shown to cause Long QT syndrome [18].

Type	Gene	Channel affected
LQT1	KCNQ1 (KvLQT1)	IKs
LQT2	KCNH2 (hERG)	IKr
LQT3	SCN5A (hH1)	Na
LQT4	ANK2 (ankyrin B)	—
LQT5	KCNE1 (minK)	IKs accessory subunit
LQT6	KCNE2 (MiRP1)	IKr accessory subunit
LQT7	KCNJ2 (Kir2.1)	IK1

resting potential. As Fig. 5.2 depicts, a prolongation of phase 3 of the action potential results in QT prolongation on the surface ECG (dotted lines). Congenital long-QT syndromes (LQTS) have been recognized for decades and are characterized by prolongation of the QT interval caused by genetic mutations. People affected by this syndrome are subject to cardiac events such as arrhythmia and syncope, leading to sudden death in some cases. At present, mutations at seven distinct genes have been identified as responsible for LQTS [15] (Table 5.2). Of these genes, three encode potassium channels, one encodes the sodium channel, and two encode potassium channel accessory subunits (the last, most recently described gene, encodes a scaffolding protein)[16–19]. LQTS2 is due to a mutation in the gene that encodes the potassium channel known as $hERG$ ($KCNH2$). The combination of the product of this gene with the product of another gene ($KCNE2$, $MiRP-1$) produces the I_{Kr} potassium channel (the fast component of the delayed rectifier current) [20]. Antiarrhythmic drugs with class III action (sotalol, amiodarone, dofetilide) selectively block the I_{Kr} channel. The same effect has been demonstrated for several noncardiovascular drugs shown to prolong the QT interval and, in some cases, to cause TdP [14]. The recognized gold standard for cardiovascular evaluation is the telemetry model in conscious, freely moving nonrodents, as shown in Fig. 5.3. Animals are implanted subcutaneously or intraperitoneally with sensors that collect blood pressure, ECG, body temperature, and activity data and transmit them to a receiver placed within the cage/kennel in which the animal is housed. Surgery for transmitter implantation should take place at least 2–3 weeks before the animals are assigned to a study to allow complete recovery from the surgical procedure. The receiver is connected to a remote computer, on which an acquisition program collects and analyzes the physiological signals and reports the results of the experiment. Animals are free to move within their cage/kennel without any tethering or restraint. In a standard study design, four animals of the same sex usually receive four treatments: vehicle and three different doses of the test compound on different study days. Treatments are performed following a Latin square crossover or an ascending-doses design (Table 5.3). In the former, all treatments are given to different animals each day, whereas in the latter all animals receive the same treatment each day. Of the two, the Latin square design gives more statistical power to the study, as it takes into account the difference between days. The ascending-doses design is favored when little information is available on the half-life of the test compound; with each animal receiving the same treatment on the same day, possible carryover effects

TABLE 5.3. Latin square crossover and ascending-dose study designs.

| | \multicolumn{4}{c}{Latin square crossover} | \multicolumn{4}{c}{Ascending dose} |
	Animal 1	Animal 2	Animal 3	Animal 4	Animal 1	Animal 2	Animal 3	Animal 4
Day 1	Vehicle	Dose 1	Dose 2	Dose 3	Vehicle	Vehicle	Vehicle	Vehicle
Day 2	Dose 1	Dose 2	Dose 3	Vehicle	Dose 1	Dose 1	Dose 1	Dose 1
Day 3	Dose 2	Dose 3	Vehicle	Dose 1	Dose 2	Dose 2	Dose 2	Dose 2
Day 4	Dose 3	Vehicle	Dose 1	Dose 2	Dose 3	Dose 3	Dose 3	Dose 3

In the Latin square crossover design, all treatments are given to different animals in the same day. In the ascending dose design, all animals receive the same treatment in the same day; vehicle is given in the first experimental day, then the drug from lowest to highest dose are given on subsequent days.

due to a long half-life of the compound will be similar in all animals. With both designs, a washout period is observed between treatments in order to avoid carryover effects from the previous treatment. Five half-lives are usually considered sufficient, but when information on the PK of the compound are scarce, it is advisable to observe at least a 1-week washout between doses. Telemetry allows physiological signals to be recorded continuously for long periods of time, the only limitation being space available on the computer for data storage. Because each animal serves as its own control, adequate basal recordings (before each treatment) are essential. In our experience, a 1-hour recording before treating the animals is sufficient. Continuous recording should be carried out for at least 24 hours after treatment; this will allow data to be collected during periods of

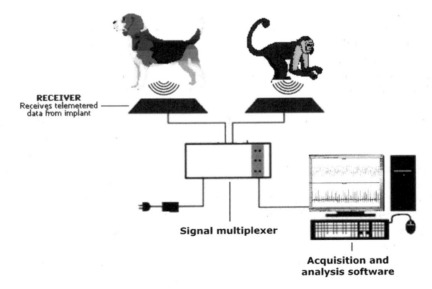

Figure 5.3. Configuration of used in the cardiovascular telemetry model
A radio signal from an implanted transmitter is received by an antenna and sent to the acquisition and analysis software through a signal multiplexer

high and low heart rate (day and night, respectively), an important aspect of QT/RR relationship analysis (see following). The data will then require careful review/analysis and reduction in order to isolate experimentally relevant portions of the complete data set. All commercially available acquisition and analysis programs (see following) allow the user to choose which data to extract and at which frequency. The approach we use consists of extracting data for at least 10 seconds (or at least 15 cardiac cycles) every 15 minutes before treatment, then 10 seconds every 30 minutes (oral administration) or every 15 minutes (intravenous administration) up to 1–2 hours post-Cmax. The remaining data, up to 24 hours after treatment, is analyzed only if recovery from any treatment-related effect is not achieved.

QT Correction and QT/RR Analysis

Due to the inverse relationship between QT and heart rate, the need to normalize QT duration for the effects of cardiac frequency is widely acknowledged. The resulting parameter, calculated with mathematical formulas, is called QTc (QT corrected). However, there is no consensus on the best correction formula. Bazett's formula [21] and Fredericia's formula [22] are widely used, notwithstanding the recognition of their inadequacy at high and low heart rates (they both overestimate corrected QT at high heart rates and underestimate it at low heart rates):

$$\text{Bazett's formula: } QTc = QT^*RR^{1/2}$$

$$\text{Fredericia's formula: } Qtc = QT^*RR^{1/3}$$

A canine toxicity study data [23] demonstrated that pretest data for large studies can be used to derive a correction model based on the analysis of covariance (ANCOVA) method, which provides a near-zero slope for the QTc–HR (heart rate) relationship. The limitations of this approach are that the study sample size is usually insufficient to describe the QT–HR relationship accurately, especially at high and low heart rates, and the correction formula varies from study to study, hindering comparisons between studies and test compounds. An alternative is to use the ANCOVA method after compiling a (large) historical database of QT–HR data for animals from previously conducted studies to describe fully the normal QT and HR relationship within a species [24]. Using this approach, and providing that QT data are collected for the widest possible HR range (thus the importance of collecting ECG data at high hearts rates during the day and at low heart rates at night), we found that the log–log formula for correcting the QT interval for heart rate is best for describing the QT–HR relationship and the best at achieving a zero slope for the QTc–HR relationship in both beagle dogs and cynomolgus monkeys (Fig. 5.4). The log–log correction has the advantages of using the ANCOVA method as described in [23] and further, since corrections are derived from a large historical database, they allow use of this method with smaller studies such as those used commonly for safety pharmacology studies. Data drawn from an historical database can also be used to describe the population distribution of QT values within discrete HR bins (Table 5.4) so that an outlier analysis, similar to that proposed by

TABLE 5.4. QT distribution per heart rate class in beagle dogs.

HR	No. of complexes		QT (msec)	
	Males	Females	Males	Females
21–40	95	162	239 ± 17.9	246 ± 16.9
41–60	1277	1129	227 ± 16.0	228 ± 16.9
61–80	1523	1409	218 ± 18.6	219 ± 18.1
81–100	1526	1529	212 ± 19.3	212 ± 19.6
101–120	1616	1308	205 ± 19.1	207 ± 21.1
121–140	1047	771	196 ± 18.7	196 ± 18.2
141–160	340	403	189 ± 20.0	184 ± 18.4
161–180	133	189	181 ± 21.6	169 ± 14.9
181–200	56	69	168 ± 15.9	162 ± 19.7
201–220	8	20	162 ± 8.7	154 ± 11.8
221–240	2	18	165 ± 2.1	145 ± 12.2
241–260	0	4	—	137 ± 16.7

Distribution of QT duration (mean ± S.D. from the number of complexes indicated) in discrete (10 beats/min) classes of heart rate (Accelera s.r.l., Nerviano, Milan, Italy).
— = No data.

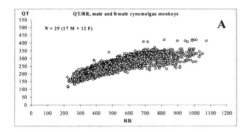
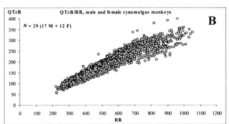
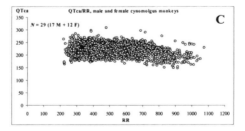

Figure 5.4. The application of correction formulas to QT-interval data from cynomolgus monkeys
The data is taken from the Accelera srl (Nerviano, Milan, Italy) in-house historical database, for cynomolgus monkey, cardiovascular parameters of. The same correction can be applied to data from beagle dogs
A: QT/RR plots show inverse relationship between QT and RR
B: Correction with Bazett's formula does not solve the inverse relationship
C: Analysis of covariance correction normalizes QT and gives a near zero slope

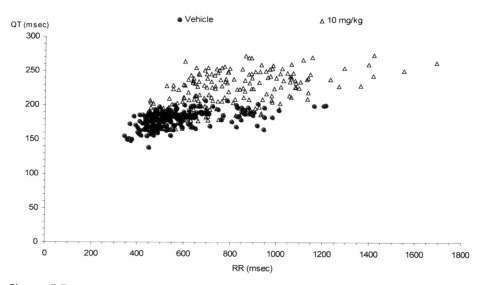

Figure 5.5. QT/RR interval relationship on a beat-to-beat basis
Oral administration of sotalol in an individual dog causes a prolongation of the QT interval, which is shown by the upward shift of QT/RR points. The data analyzed was generated in-house at Accelera srl (Nerviano, Milan, Italy)

Osborne and Leach [25], can be used in reviewing data, allowing one to interpret QT effects independent of any correction method. Correction-free interpretation of QT data can also be obtained by means of beat-to-beat QT/RR analysis [26] as illustrated in Fig. 5.5. By plotting absolute, noncorrected QT and RR values on a graph, QT prolongation results in an upward shift of the QT/RR points. The best-integrated QT analysis can, therefore, be achieved by combining the heart rate correction of QT, QT/RR analysis, and outlier analysis. Data Sciences International (DSI, www.datasci.com) and Integrated Telemetry Systems (ITS, www.itstelemetry.com and www.dissdata.com) are the major providers of telemetry equipment. Other companies include Telemetry Research (www.telemetryresearch.com), Transonic Systems (www.transonic.com), and Endosomatic Systems (www.endosomatic.com). There is a wide range of implants offered—the simplest implant includes one catheter for blood pressure (usually implanted in the femoral artery) and two electrodes for ECG recording (one lead); the temperature and activity probes are placed in the body of the transmitter. Other models offer two blood pressure channels (giving the opportunity to collect intraventricular pressure), up to six biopotential channels (which allow for multiple-lead ECG recordings), and one or two flow probes. All companies offer surgical manuals on their Web sites and organize surgery workshops. There is a wide choice of acquisition and analysis software, including Notocord (www.notocord.com), Ponemah (www.datasci.com), and CArecorder (www.itstelemetry.com). Other popular software suppliers are Buxco (www.buxco.com) and Emka (www.emka.com).

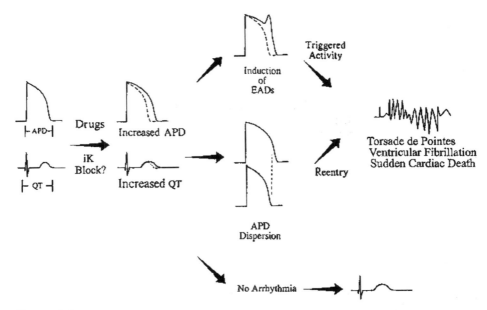

Figure 5.6. Relationship between delayed repolarization and Torsade de Point
An increase in action potential duration (APD) causes a prolongation of the QT-interval and an increase in repolarization dispersion, which can trigger arrhythmias and (Torsade de Point) TdP

In Vitro Cardiovascular Study (*hERG* Inhibition)

The QT interval measures the duration of ventricular depolarization and repolarization. When ventricular repolarization is delayed and the QT interval is prolonged, there is an increased risk of ventricular tachyarrhythmia, including torsade de pointes, particularly when combined with other risk factors (e.g., hypokalemia, acidosis, structural heart disease, bradycardia) (Fig. 5.6). Thus, much emphasis has been placed on the potential proarrhythmic effects of pharmaceuticals that are associated with prolonging the QT interval (e.g., dofetilide, terfenadine, cisapride) [27–30]. Ventricular repolarization, determined by the duration of the cardiac action potential, is a complex physiological process and is the net result of the activities of many membrane ion channels and transporters. Prolonging the action potential can result from decreased inactivation of the inward Na^+ current, increased activation of the Ca^{++} current, or inhibition of one or more of the outward K^+ currents. The most common mechanism of QT interval prolongation by pharmaceuticals is inhibition of the delayed rectifier potassium channel responsible for the I_{Kr} current. The *hERG* (*KCNH2* in the new nomenclature) gene encodes the pore-forming alpha subunit of a voltage-gated potassium channel expressed in the heart and in nervous tissue responsible for I_{Kr} [31]. An *in vitro* screening approach, using *hERG*-transfected cells, followed by *in vivo* measurement of QT intervals in laboratory animals (see above) is recommended by regulatory authorities [3].

Patch-clamp electrophysiology is the gold standard for studying interference of test compounds with the I_{Kr} channel. The patch-clamp electrophysiological assay measures the K^+ current in *hERG*-transfected cells and is considered the most accurate method for evaluating the drug inhibition of functional, voltage-gated K^+ channels. However, the methodology for such an assay has not been standardized, and some discrepancies in the literature are due to the use of different test systems [32]:

- native I_{Kr} channel expression in cardiac myocytes,
- heterologous *hERG* expression in *Xenopus* oocytes, and
- heterologous *hERG* expression in mammalian cell lines, such as HEK-293 or CHO.

When using *Xenopus* oocytes for heterologous expression of proteins, several considerations should be kept in mind. Frog oocytes express endogenous channels and transporters at low levels. These endogenous proteins can interfere with the analysis of expressed proteins in at least two ways: (1) they can be up-regulated by expression of exogenous proteins and interfere with the analysis of the protein of interest, and (2) they can form heteromultimers with the proteins translated from injected RNA. Finally, cellular environment, signaling pathways in particular, may differ from that of the cell where the ion channel of interest is normally expressed calling for extreme caution when studying channel modulation by secondary messengers in oocytes [33]. Although most cases of drug-induced TdP are associated with the *hERG* channel block, the reverse—that all drugs that block the *hERG* channel cause TdP—is not true. Indeed the major disadvantage of the patch-clamp electrophysiological assay is that tests may yield false positives; this may be due to the technique itself, for example, rundown of the current or the blockage of inward currents (I_{Ca} and I_{Na}) in the same concentration range of *hERG* current block. Notable examples are verapamil and amiodarone, which are both potent *hERG* current inhibitors (IC50 < or = 1 mM) without associated TdP [34].

Unfortunately, cloned ion channels lack the native conditions and structural architecture that make a fully functional *hERG* channel *in vivo*. Thus, screening compounds on the cloned *hERG* alone could generate misleading results (e.g., verapamil), suggesting that an *hERG*/I_{Kr} blockade alone is not sufficient to predict TdP in humans. The guinea pig ventricular myocyte, which has ion channels relevant to human cardiac myocytes, is a potential model cell for screening compounds that affect the duration of QT intervals. This assay has many advantages, such as functional measurement of all ion channels underlying the cardiac action potential in their native state and cost effectiveness compared to the use of Purkinje fibers or isolated heart preparations [35].

The Standard Patch-Clamp Protocol. Petri dishes containing cells to be used for electrophysiological study are mounted on the stage of an inverted microscope and superfused with the vehicle in which the test compound will be administered to the cells (usually Tyrode's solution). Membrane currents are recorded in the whole-cell

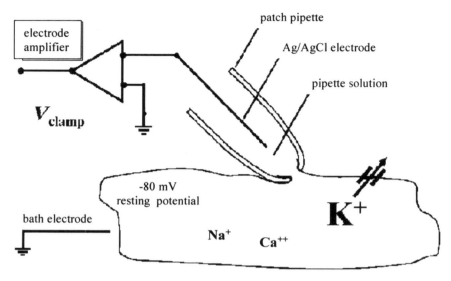

Figure 5.7. Whole cell patch clamp

configuration by using suction pipettes made from borosilicate glass capillary tubing and filled with a pipette solution that mimics the intracellular environment. Once a stable patch is achieved, recording is started in voltage–clamp mode using a commercial patch-clamp amplifier, with the cell initially clamped at –80 mV. Series resistance and capacitance are compensated (Fig. 5.7). Cells are perfused through a microperfusion system, allowing solution changes to occur within about 1 second. Experiments are performed at either room temperature (20–24°C) or near-physiological temperature (37 ± 1°C). The onset and the steady-state block of the $hERG$ channel current (I_{Kr}) due to the test compound are monitored using a pulse pattern with fixed amplitudes (first depolarization: -50 mV, second depolarization: $+20$ mV, and hyperpolarization: -50 mV). This pulse pattern is repeated every 15 seconds. Current amplitude at the onset of the second step to -50 mV ("peak tail current") is monitored until a steady state is obtained. The steady-state peak tail current is monitored and recorded in the vehicle solution, and then the test item is applied to the bath solution. At the end, a positive control substance is applied to block 100% of the current for determination of the current "leak." Current amplitude is continually monitored through the onset of the voltage step to -50 mV until a new steady-state level of current is achieved. For more details on experimental conditions, the reader is referred to the literature [36–38].

At least three ascending concentrations of the test compound should be tested until a concentration–response curve has been established or physicochemical effects become concentration limiting. Ideally, the duration of exposure should be sufficient to obtain steady-state electrophysiological effects unless precluded by the viability of the cell or tissue preparation. Positive control (e.g., E4031, cisapride) substances should be used to establish the sensitivity of the *in vitro* preparation for ion channel and action potential duration assays as well as to confirm that the ion channels of interest are present and stable. For a test compound belonging to a chemical/pharmacological class that is associated with QT interval prolongation in humans, using a concurrent reference compound (member of the same class) for *in vitro* studies should be considered to facilitate ranking the potency of the test substance in relation to its comparators.

Factors that can confound or limit the interpretation of *in vitro* electrophysiology studies include the following:

- Use of high concentrations of the test substance can be precluded by limited solubility in aqueous physiological salt solutions.
- Test substance concentrations can be limited by the cytotoxic or physicochemical properties of the test substance that disrupt cell membrane integrity so that electrophysiological endpoints cannot be obtained.
- Cardiac cells and tissues have limited capacity for drug metabolism, and therefore *in vitro* studies using the parent substance do not provide information on the effects of metabolites.

When *in vivo* nonclinical or clinical studies reveal QT interval prolongation that is not corroborated by *in vitro* studies using the parent substance, testing metabolites in *in vitro* test systems should be considered.

High-Throughput Systems. The classical patch-clamp assay is perceived as being labor and skill intensive, time consuming, and having low throughput. However, this situation is rapidly evolving through the development of a range of high-throughput electrophysiological systems [39]. High-throughput screening is necessary to identify potential *hERG* liability when potentially thousands of compounds are under consideration for lead optimization. Automated patch-clamp systems have been developed. Among these systems currently marketed are the PatchXpress (Axon Instruments/Molecular Devices) and IonWorks HT (Molecular Devices). There are also a number of non–patch-clamp methods with higher throughput; however, they do not measure functional *hERG* blocks. They do include displacement of a high-affinity radioactively labeled ligand blocker ([3H]dofetilide), atomic absorption measurement of rubidium (Rb^+) flux, and membrane potential using fluorescent voltage-sensitive dyes [40]. These approaches do not identify whether the test compound is an agonist or an antagonist of the *hERG* channel and for some, IC_{50}s are orders of magnitude higher than with classical patch clamp. For these reasons, these methods are not accepted by regulatory authorities in substituting classical patch-clamp studies; they are widely used by pharmaceutical companies in discovery to rank compounds and/or classes of compounds, however.

RESPIRATORY STUDY IN RODENTS

Plethysmography in conscious rats is the most widely used approach for the conduct of respiratory safety pharmacology studies by far [41–44]. In the "whole-body setup," the animal is placed in an airtight plethysmographic chamber in which it is free to move

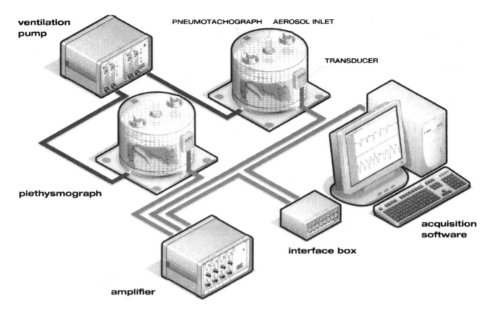

ventilation pump

PNEUMOTACHOGRAPH AEROSOL INLET

TRANSDUCER

plethysmograph

acquisition software

interface box

amplifier

Figure 5.8. Configuration used in whole body plethysmography
Schematic representation of the connections between plethysmographic chambers, ventilation pump and hardware and software

(Fig. 5.8); in the "head-out setup," the body of the animal is placed in an airtight plastic cylinder, while the head is outside the cylinder. Using this method the airflow in and out of the sealed, airtight chamber or cylinder is measured, as this flow is due to the thoracic movements occurring during respiration [45]. The head-out model has the advantage of reduced air volume in the acquisition and analysis software cylinder in comparison to the volume of the plethysmographic chamber, therefore allowing for measurements that are more precise. Because the head of the animal is outside the measuring cylinder, sniffing does not interfere with the respiratory signal. On the other hand, with the whole-body model continuous measurements for up to 6–7 hours are possible, as animals remain in the chamber continuously. The head-out model only allows short (a few minutes) recording periods, as animals are placed in the cylinder for the measurement time and are then removed. This difference in methodology also accounts for reduced stress in the whole-body chamber. With both methods, the parameters obtained include respiratory rate, respiratory volumes and flows (tidal and minute volume, peak inspiration, and peak expiration flow), respiratory times (inspiration, expiration, and relaxation time), and enhanced pause (Penh, a unitless index of airway hyperreactivity [45]). Neither method, however, allows for the determination of airways mechanics. However, this can be achieved with double-chamber plethysmography, in which the body and the head of the animal are in different chambers. Each chamber has a pneumotachograph and a flow transducer for measuring nasal and thoracic flows independently. The two chambers are separated by an elastomeric neck seal. The two flow signals can be processed separately to report common flow-derived parameters, along with specific airway resistance and its reciprocal, specific airway conductance. Combining any plethysmographic model with a pleural pressure signal acquired by telemetry will also allow the calculation of lung compliance.

In our experience, eight animals/dose group is the minimum required to achieve acceptable statistical power in these studies. Data are recorded before treatment (basal values, internal control) and up to 1–2 hours post-C_{max}. In the case of the whole-body technique, data are acquired continuously, then data reduction is applied as described for the cardiovascular telemetry study. If the head-out technique is used, data reduction is not necessary, as parameters are recorded at discrete intervals of time.

CENTRAL NERVOUS SYSTEM

There are extensive tests available for studying the effect of chemicals on the central nervous system (CNS). The majority of these tests focus on a particular aspect: for example, learning, memory, convulsive potential, electrophysiology (EEG), locomotion, pain, abuse liability, and so on. Behavioral observation tests, on the other hand, allow for the simultaneous monitoring of several parameters in the autonomic, neuromuscular, sensorimotor, and behavioral domains. Therefore, these are the preferred tests for core battery safety pharmacology CNS studies. Two experimental models are available for neurobehavioral studies: Irwin's test [46] and the Functional Observation Battery (FOB) [47, 48]. Both methods consist of behavioral observations carried out before and after treatment using a standardized observation grid containing items such as mortality, sedation, excitation, convulsions/tremors, stereotypes, aggression/passivity, reaction to stimuli (touch, noise), pain threshold, muscle tone, reflexes (corneal, pinna, righting), gait, respiration, and rectal temperature. For an in-depth description of the FOB, the reader is referred to the abundant literature [47–51]. A classical Irwin's test is conducted in steps going from the lowest to the highest invasive observation.

Step 1 includes observations made in the animals' home cage of such parameters as piloerection, bizarre behavior, exophthalmus, respiration, tremors, twitches, and convulsions,

Step 2 is performed in the open field to which the animals are moved from their home cage and includes observations on locomotor activity, alertness, body position, Straub tail, gait, palpebral opening, startle, and touch response,

Observations in step 3 are made following simple manipulation of the animals to determine passivity, visual placing, grip strength, pinna, cornea, and flexor reflex and include close observation of skin color, limb and abdomen tone, pupil size, lacrimation, salivation, and provoked biting, and finally

Step 4 observations include more invasive manipulation of the animals to establish the response to pain (tail pinch), righting reflex, ease of handling, fear, and aggressiveness. The last parameter recorded is rectal body temperature.

Throughout the observation procedure, vocalization and the number of urine pools and fecal pellets is recorded. All these behavioral signs (with the exception of body temperature) are scored according to an arbitrary scale [46]. Each laboratory has adapted an evaluation scale based on their experience, but the scale allows for scoring signs/symptoms with a value from 0 to 8. Factors present in normal animals (e.g., alertness, mobility, and the like) are scored as 4; potentiation or depression of these factors is indicated as higher or lower integers, respectively. Factors absent in normal animals are scored from 0 (normal) to 8.

In our experience, five to six animals per group are enough to detect effects due to the test compound under study. Studies involve a control group administered with the vehicle and at least three doses. Observations must be made pretreatment and at one or more time points after treatment. We recommend at least two observation sessions after treatment: one at t_{max} and one 24 hours later to demonstrate recovery from the effect. Additional observations between these two time points allow better definition of the duration of the effect. If 24 hours after treatment effects are still present, extending the observation period for up to 72 hours is useful to define the CNS liability of the test compound better.

FOLLOW-UP STUDIES

In vitro Models for Cardiovascular Findings

The APD model using Purkinje fibers or papillary muscle is by far the most popular *in vitro* model among follow-up cardiovascular studies [52]. Indeed, several companies routinely conduct this study as part of the battery of core safety-pharmacology tests before entering phase I clinical trials. This model is complementary to the I_{Kr} testing, as it provides information on possible interactions of the test compound with other ion channels (Na^+, Ca^{++}) involved in the depolarization/repolarization cycle of cardiac cells. This is particularly useful in cases when an inhibition of the I_{Kr} channel is not confirmed *in vivo* by prolonging the QT interval. In such cases, a multichannel interaction by the test compound is very likely. Inhibition of the Ca^{++} channel sustaining the plateau phase of the action potential would result in a shortened APD and QT interval, for example. This shortening could mask a prolongation effect due to inhibition of the I_{Kr} channel. Several drugs are known to behave in this way, the most studied is verapamil, which despite an IC_{50} on *hERG* in the range of 100–200 nM, is known not to prolong the QT interval in nonclinical species and in humans [53, 54]. Another feature of the APD model is that, in case of compounds that prolong action potential, the APD model can detect early afterdepolarizations, which are considered indicators of proarrhythmia *in vivo*. This is not possible with the classical I_{Kr} test, which only measures the current through the channel.

Purkinje fibers from rabbit or guinea pig papillary muscle are normally used in these experiments. Rabbits, notwithstanding their reported high sensitivity to I_{Kr} inhibitors [53], are preferred to other sources of Purkinje fibers given the extensive literature available; the use of dog or nonhuman primate tissue carries with it ethical and financial considerations that have limited their use. Papillary muscle from the guinea pig has the appropriate size to prevent ischemia in the middle of the preparation, which would compromise the experiment. The primary endpoint for detecting disturbances of

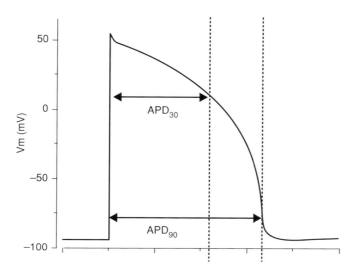

Figure 5.9. Calculation of action potential duration: APD30 and APD90
The difference between APD90 and APD30 has been proposed as a more accurate way for detecting QT prolongation

repolarization is an effect on the duration of the action potential, defined as the time from depolarization to a predefined percentage of repolarization, usually 90% (APD90) (Figs. 5.9). A more recent approach has been proposed by the PRODACT initiative [55]. Some drugs known to prolong the QT interval in humans by blocking the I_{Kr} channel were found not to prolong APD90 in Purkinje fibers or papillary muscle (e.g., astemizole, terfenadine, pimozide) [56]. It has been shown that an I_{Kr} block prolongs the action potential between 30% and 90% repolarization [57, 58]; therefore, Hondeghem and Hoffmann [58] have suggested it is better to focus on this repolarization interval by calculating the difference between APD90 and APD30 (the so-called triangulation). In this way, they were able to demonstrate APD prolongation also by astemizole and pimozide (but not terfenadine).

Another, more sophisticated *in vitro* model is the ventricular wedge preparation first described by Antzelevich et al. [59]. This model consists of a section of ventricular wall from which the transmural ECG is recorded using electrodes placed at the epicardial and endocardial surfaces of the preparation. At the same time, the duration of the action potential is recorded from epicardial, endocardial, and midmyocardial cells (M cells) using three separate intracellular electrodes. The duration of the cardiac action potential is different in the different regions of the ventricular wall, being longer in M cells compared to both endo- and epicardial cells; this is called repolarization dispersion, an increase in which, concomitance with APD prolongation, is thought to be among the determinants of arrhythmias. Measuring the transmural ECG together with the action potential across the ventricular wall and the repolarization dispersion is probably one of the most sophisticated *in vitro* approaches for determining the drug potential for QT prolongation and proarrhythmic potential. Its limited use in pharmaceutical development is due to its experimental complexity, which makes it accessible only to specialized laboratories. A simpler model that gives simultaneous determination of ECG and action potential is the isolated heart according to Oscar Langendorff. In addition, the influence of the test compound on rhythm and contractility can also be investigated in this model, making it very useful for second-tier mechanistic studies.

IN VIVO MODELS FOR CARDIOVASCULAR AND RESPIRATORY FINDINGS

Before the advent of telemetry, it was common practice to test the cardiovascular effects of drugs in anesthetized animals. This model is still valid for follow-up studies, as it provides the possibility of collecting a wide range of hemodynamic, cardiovascular, and respiratory data. Animals are instrumented to allow simultaneous monitoring of systemic, intracavitary (left ventricle) and pulmonary artery blood pressure, blood flows (arterial, femoral, renal, carotid), ECG, and respiration. Typically, a pressure transducer is inserted into the femoral artery and advanced to the descending aorta for systemic arterial pressure; a transducer is inserted into the femoral vein and advanced, through the right atrium and ventricle, to the pulmonary artery; and a third transducer is inserted into the carotid artery and advanced into the left ventricle. Blood flow probes can be placed on femoral, renal, and/or carotid arteries (as needed) to record regional blood flows and peripheral resistances. An additional flow probe can be placed on the aorta or pulmonary artery, thus allowing monitoring of cardiac output and stroke volume. Respiratory rate, volumes, flows, and times can be monitored connecting a tracheal cannula to a plethysmograph; simultaneous recording of intrapleural pressure allows calculation of pulmonary compliance and respiratory resistances. All leads (limb and precordial) of surface ECG can be collected by means of an electrocardiograph. The advantage of this model in comparison with telemetry is in the number of parameters that can be collected. Simultaneous recording of central, peripheral and intracavitary blood pressure, blood flows, and central and peripheral vascular resistances can give a full hemodynamic picture of the effects of a compound on the cardiovascular system; coupling collection of respiratory data and pulmonary arterial pressure allows for the integration of cardiovascular and respiratory effects. There are numerous disadvantages, unfortunately. First, anesthesia by itself can affect cardiovascular and respiratory parameters. Barbiturates have a profound depressing effect on respiration and on the cardiovascular system. Gaseous anesthesia is better, although some respiratory depression is associated with its use. Measurement of blood gases throughout the experiment is always advised in order to monitor the level of blood oxygenation to detect and counter the effects of anoxia if needed. Moreover, animals are stable for a limited time. Surgical preparation of the animal can take up to 1 hour and basal data collection lasts at least another hour to let the preparation stabilize. The effect of the test compound can be followed for no more than 6 hours after treatment in the best situation. Animals are sacrificed at the end of the study; therefore, there can be many animals used in each experiment. Three is the minimum number of animals per dose level; testing of vehicle and three dose levels would therefore require the use of 12 animals. A way of reducing animal use is to administer the same animal the vehicle and all dose levels of the compound under study with an appropriate time interval between successive administrations. This is simplified by intravenous administration, which also overcomes the inhibition of gastric motility caused by anesthesia, a feature that could compromise compound's absorption (see above).

The same cardiovascular and hemodynamic parameters can be obtained from chronically instrumented animals. In this model, pressure and flow sensors are implanted in animals and exteriorized through skin buttons to which wires are attached during the experiment to connect the sensors to the recording machines. In this way, the experiment can be conducted in conscious animals without the interference of anesthetics; however, the animals are tethered to the recording machines, and therefore their movements are limited. The stress associated with this model can be reduced, but not eliminated, by training the animals in advance of the study. Respiratory parameters can only be obtained by putting a mask on the animal's muzzle, a situation that again increases the stress to which the animals are subjected.

CENTRAL NERVOUS SYSTEM FINDINGS

The nervous system is involved in regulating all vital functions; therefore, practically all organs/systems are in some way controlled by it. Accordingly, the number of experimental *in vitro* and *in vivo* models available to study the effect of drugs on the central, peripheral, and autonomic nervous systems is very high, and an exhaustive description of each experimental protocol would require a book on its own. Here, we briefly cover only the most frequently used, referring to the literature for detailed descriptions.

In Vitro Models

Binding studies are the simplest and least expensive way of getting information on the possible interaction of test compounds with receptors. These studies are usually performed in screening mode during the discovery phase of drug development and are not really part of safety pharmacology. However, they can indicate to the safety pharmacologist possible interactions between test compounds and receptors. Because binding studies are not functional measurements, a positive binding result does not necessarily mean that the compound will act as an agonist/antagonist to that particular receptor. A positive result in a binding study needs to be confirmed functionally in specific agonistic/antagonistic tests. Isolated organs (trachea, uterus, aorta, ileum, and so on) challenged by the test compound in the presence and absence of specific agonists and/or antagonists will confirm or deny the results of binding studies.

In Vivo Models

Testing spontaneous locomotor activity is the most popular follow-up CNS study and is used by some investigators as part of the core battery. Locomotor activity can be quantified in rodents by a variety of methods; interruption of photoelectric beams, video image analysis, and telemetry [60], for example. Activity is measured by placing the animals in an open field for 5–10 minutes before and after test compound or vehicle administration. As for Irwin's test and the FOB, locomotor activity should be measured at least two times to detect the peak effect and time to recovery. As for all nervous system experimental models, care must be taken to ensure constant experimental conditions (time of day, noise level, degree of manipulation, environmental conditions) to obtain reproducible and reliable results. The endpoints of this experiment can be time spent in movement and time spent in each area of the open field (center, corners, walls), rearing, sniffing, grooming, stereotypes. Specific software is then used to calculate these endpoints when using beam interruption or video image analysis models. In telemetry, usually only a rough "motility" index is given (time spent moving versus time spent still). Motor coordination is often tested in follow-up CNS studies. The most commonly used model is the so-called "rotarod" [61]. Animals are placed on a rod rotating at a fixed (or sometime increasing) speed for a few minutes. The endpoint of the study is the time required for the animal to fall off the rod or the number of animals staying on the rod for the whole test. To decrease test variability, animals must be trained to stay on the rod before performing the experiment; it usually takes only one or two sessions for the animals to learn the task; animals not able to stay on the rod for the test time are usually removed from the experiment. The effect of test compounds on nociception can be studied with different experimental models: tail flick, plantar test, and hot plate detect aversion to externally applied stimuli [62]. Pain due to inflammation can be induced by the injection of chemicals (carrageenan, Freund's adjuvant, capsaicin) [1, 63, 64]; neuropathic pain can be induced surgically, usually through lesions to or ligature of the sciatic or spinal nerve [65]. In safety pharmacology, usually only the simplest models are applied, such as the hot plate, plantar test, and tail flick. These models measure the time of withdrawal of the part of the body (the plantar region of the paws or the tail) affected by a noxious stimulus: a heated metal plate on which the animal is placed, a radiant heat emitted by a focused beam, a pinch with a metal clip. Higher cognitive functions, such as learning and memory, are assessed by means of more complex and time-consuming tests, such as passive avoidance and water or radial mazes. These tests, due to their complexity, are only conducted in later phases of development if cause for concern on the impairment of these functions results from clinical or preclinical findings. The basic principle of the passive avoidance test is that the animal receives an aversive stimulation (such as a brief electric shock) in a recognizable environment (e.g., moving from the lit to the dark compartment of a two-compartment box); its response following a second challenge after treatment will show whether the test drug has affected memory and/or learning. In the water maze [66] animals are put in a circular tank containing opacified water containing an escape platform below the surface of the water that the animals has to find to leave the water; in subsequent challenges following treatment, the animal must find the same platform in a short time. The radial maze [67] consists of a central platform with arms radiating from it. Food is placed at the end of some of the arms (always the same throughout the experiment). Upon rechallenge following treatment, animals must first visit the arms in which they have found food.

Recently, regulatory authorities have focused on potentials for drug abuse and dependence, especially for certain classes of compounds (CNS stimulants, opioids, sedatives, and anxiolytics); requirements for such testing are included in the ICH M3(R2) guideline [68] and in an EMEA guideline on the nonclinical investigation of the dependence potential of drugs [69]. The tests available are very specialized (precipitated withdrawal, place preference, drug discrimination, self-administration), and their in-depth description goes beyond the scope of this book. Briefly, withdrawal tests on the potential for drug dependence look for withdrawal signs that arise after discontinuance of the drug (e.g., jumping following short repeated administration of μ opiate antagonists; weight loss, decreased food consumption, hyperthermia following long repeated administrations of benzodiazepines, cocaine or morphine), preference for an environment to which the animal has been exposed during drug administration, pressing on one of two levers to obtain drugs, or intravenous self-administration of a drug by pressing on a lever are all tests that indicate a drug's potential for abuse. For detailed descriptions, the interested reader is referred to the literature [1, 70–75].

RENAL FINDINGS

Renal function is usually investigated as part of repeated dose general toxicity studies when urine is collected to determine the parameters of urinalysis. Therefore, this test is not usually part of the safety pharmacology package of studies. In some cases, however, investigations on the renal function are required because of unexpected findings in nonclinical or clinical studies. Safety pharmacology studies, usually performed following a single administration of the test drug, allow testing of higher doses than those explored in toxicology studies, and longer collection periods (up to 24 hours) to investigate the time course of the finding better. Twenty-four hour urine can be collected in fractions, for example, 0–5 hours and 5–24 hours, allowing discrimination between early (more pharmacology driven, diuretics) and late (more toxicology driven) effects. The glomerular filtration rate (GFR) can be determined accurately from the rate of creatinine or inulin clearance. Specific markers of kidney damage, such as N-acetyl-β-d-glucosaminidase (NAG) [76, 77], can be investigated. Minimal endpoints of such studies are serum concentrations of electrolytes (Na^+, K^+, Cl^-), urea, and creatinine; urine concentrations and partial (0–5 hours and 5–24 hours) and total (0–24 hours) excretions of electrolytes (Na^+, K^+, Cl^-), urea, and creatinine; urine volume, specific gravity, and color; and creatinine clearance and GFR. Eight animals per treatment group are required. Animals are housed in metabolic cages up to 24 hours after treatment without access to water. Two water loads are given to each animal, one immediately after treatment and one after the 5-hour urine collection. To decrease variability, it is advisable to empty each animal's bladder manually with a gentle pressure over the lower abdomen before putting them into the metabolic cages. Experimental groups usually include one control and three treatment groups. It is advisable to validate the model with a range of reference compounds to cover different effects and modes of action with diuretics, antidiuretics, and nephrotoxic compounds. Once the method is validated, a reference control group should be added to a study once or twice a year to demonstrate consistency of response over time.

GASTROINTESTINAL FINDINGS

Oral drug administration can damage the gastric mucosa, which is easily detected by visually inspecting the excised stomach at necropsy or by histopathological examination. The systemic effects of drugs can affect other gastrointestinal functions, such as gastric acid secretion, gastric emptying, gastrointestinal motility, and biliary excretion. Several *in vitro* and *in vivo* methods are available for investigating these effects [78, 79]. Gastric acid secretion can be measured in rats using Shay's method [80], in which the pylorus is ligated following drug administration, then the stomach is excised and the secretion collected in the stomach is measured for volume and pH. In dogs, a gastric fistula can be surgically created with a metal cannula and gastric juice collected continuously following treatment for measurement of the same endpoints. Gastric emptying can be studied in rats by administering a nonabsorbed dye or a semisolid protein-rich meal and calculating the percentage remaining in the stomach after a fixed period of time [81, 82]. In the same way, intestinal motility can be investigated by administering a nonabsorbed colored meal (usually charcoal powder in arabic gum suspended in water) to rats or mice and measuring the percentage of small intestine that the meal traveled in a fixed time. Telemetry can be used to measure electromyograms (EMGs, which record the electrical activity of muscles during peristalsis) from the intestine. Biliary excretion is measured in anesthetized rats by collecting the bile from a cannula inserted into the animal's bile duct.

CONCLUSION

Safety pharmacology is a separate and distinct safety evaluation discipline, situated between toxicology and primary (discovery) pharmacology, which examines changes in organ/system functions with emphasis on acute and functional pharmacodynamic effects. It is regulated by international guidelines (ICH S7A and ICH S7B), which identify core battery studies, required before FIH clinical trials, and follow-up and supplemental studies, to be conducted on a case by case basis when concerns from core battery studies or clinical trials arise.

   Core battery includes studies on the cardiovascular, respiratory and central nervous systems, defined by the guidelines as vital organ systems. Cardiovascular investigations are conducted by means of an *in vitro* study on the potential for inhibition of the I_{Kr} channel and an *in vivo* study in conscious, freely moving nonrodents focused on potential effects on blood pressure, heart rate, and ECG intervals (i.e., QT interval). Experimental models widely recognized as gold standards for these studies are patch-clamp electrophysiology for *in vitro* and telemetry for *in vivo*. The respiratory function is commonly investigated in conscious rodents by means of plethysmography (either "whole body" or "head out"), which allows monitoring of respiratory rate and volumes (tidal volume, minute volume), respiratory flows (inspiratory and respiratory), respiratory times (inspiration, expiration, and relaxation time), and bronchoconstriction (through a unitless index called Penh). For CNS investigations, a neurobehavioral test (either modified Irwin's test or FOB) is conducted, monitoring items such as mortality, sedation, excitation, convulsions/tremors, stereotypies, aggression/passivity, reaction to stimuli, pain threshold, muscle tone, reflexes, gait, respiration, rectal temperature. Follow-up studies are defined as studies conducted on the same organ systems (cardiovascular, respiratory, and nervous) as in-depth investigations planned to clarify findings from core battery tests or from clinical trials. The duration of action potentials in Purkinje fibers, papillary muscles, or ventricular cardiomyocytes from guinea pig or rabbit and the isolated Langendorff heart are common *in vitro* models used in this setting. Action potentials allow determination of possible effects on cardiac ion channels other than I_{Kr} on contractility and rhythm of the heart. Cardiovascular and respiratory systems can be studied together in anesthetized nonrodents; this model allows full hemodynamic investigation, which includes such parameters as systemic, intracavitary (ventricular), and pulmonary artery pressures; central (aortic, coronary) and peripheral (femoral, renal, carotid) blood flows; ECG and parameters derived from these endpoints, such as heart contractility, cardiac output and stroke; and vascular resistances. Respiration mechanics (including respiratory resistances and lung compliance) can be monitored in the same animals in addition to the respiratory parameters obtained with plethysmography. Activity on central and peripheral nervous system receptors can be investigated *in vitro* through binding studies and functional agonist/antagonist experiments in isolated organs. *In vivo* follow-up studies can cover locomotor activity, motor coordination, nociception, learning and memory, drug dependence, and abuse potential. Supplemental studies are defined as those conducted on organ systems other than cardiovascular, respiratory, and nervous. The most commonly used are a diuresis test, which measures urine and electrolyte output in the 24 hours, together with glomerular filtration rate measured as inulin or creatinine clearance, and experimental models on the gastrointestinal tract, covering effects on the gastric and duodenal mucosa, on gastric secretion and gastrointestinal motility.

REFERENCES

1. Porsolt RD, Picard S, and Lacroix P, 2005. International safety pharmacology guidelines (ICH S7A and ICH S7B): Where do we go from here? *Drug Dev Res* **64**:83–89

2. ICH, 2000. ICH S7A guideline. Safety pharmacology studies for human pharmaceuticals (ICH step 5). http://www.ich.org

3. ICH, 2005. ICH S7Bguideline. The non-clinical evaluation of the potential for delayed ventricular repolarization (QT interval prolongation) by human pharmaceuticals (ICH step 4). http://www.ich.org

4. Anonymous, 1995. *Japanese Guidelines for Nonclinical Studies of Drugs Manual 1995*, Pharmaceutical Affairs Bureau, Japanese Ministry of Health and Welfare, 71–80, Yakuji Nippo Ltd., Tokyo

5. Fermini B and Fossa AA, 2003. The impact of drug-induced QT prolongation on drug discovery and development, *Drug Discov* **2**:439–447

6. Davies AJ, Harinda V, McEwan E, and Ghose RR, 1989. Cardiotoxic effect with convulsions in terfenadine overdose. *Br Med J* **298**:325

7. Monahan BP, Ferguson CL, Killeavy ES et al., 1990. Torsades de Pointes occurring in association with terfenadine use. *JAMA* **264**:2788–2790

8. Kemp JP, 1992. Antihistamines—Is there anything safe to prescribe? *Ann Allergy* **69**:276–280

 9. Roy ML, Dumaine R, and Brown AM, 1996. HERG, a primary human ventricular target of the non-sedating antihistamine terfenadine. *Circulation* **94**:817–823

10. Committee for Proprietary Medicinal Products, 1997. Points to Consider: The assessment of the potential for QT interval prolongation by non-cardiovascular medicinal products, CPMP/986/96. http://www.emea.eu.int/home.htm

11. Hammond TG, Carlsson L, Davis AS et al., 2001. Methods of collecting and evaluating non-clinical cardiac electrophysiology data in the pharmaceutical industry: results of an international survey. *Cardiovasc Res* **49**:741–750

12. Johna R, Mertens H, Haverkamp W et al., 1998. Clofidium in the isolated perfused rabbit heart: A new model to study proarrhythmia by class III antiarrhythmic drugs. *Basic Res Cardiol* **93**:127–135

13. Lindgren S, Bass AS, Briscoe R et al., 2008. Benchmarking safety pharmacology regulatory packages and best practices. *J Pharmacol. Toxicol Methods* **58**:99–109

14. Redfern WS, Carlsson L, Davis S et al., 2003. Relationships between preclinical cardiac electrophysiology, clinical QT interval prolongation, and torsade de pointes for a broad range of drugs: Evidence for a provisional safety margin in drug development. *Cardiovasc Res* **58**:32–45

15. Bass AS, Tomaselli G, Bullingham R, and Kinter LB, 2005. Drugs effects on ventricular repolarization: A critical evaluation of the strengths and weaknesses of current methodologies and regulatory practices. *J Pharmacol Toxicol Methods* **52**:12–21

16. Curran ME, Splawski, Timothy KW et al., 1995. A molecular basis for cardiac arrhythmia: HERG mutations cause long QT syndrome. *Cell* **180**:795–803

17. Wang Q, Shen J, Splawski I et al., 1995. SCN5A mutations associated with an inherited cardiac arrhythmia, long QT syndrome. *Cell* **80**:805–811

18. Chiang CE and Roden DM, 2000. The long QT syndromes: Genetic basis and clinical implications. *J Am Coll Cardiol* **36**:1–12

19. Mohler PJ, Gramolini AO, and Bennet V, 2002. The ankyrin-B C-terminal domain determines activity of ankyrin-B/G chimeras in rescue of abnormal inositol 1, 4, 5-triphosphate and ryanodine receptor distribution in ankyrin (–/–) neonatal cardiomyocytes. *J Biol Chem* **277**:10599–10607

20. Abbott GW, Sesti F, Splawsky I et al., 1999. MiRP1 forms IKr potassium channels with HERG and is associated with cardiac arrhythmia. *Cell* **97**:175–187

21. Bazett HC, 1918. An analysis of the time-relations of electrocardiograms. *Heart* **7**:353–370

22. Fredericia LS, 1920. Die systolendauer im elektrokardiogramm bei normalen menschen und bei herzkranken. *Acta Med Scand* **53**:469–486

23. Spence S, Soper K, Hoe CM, and Coleman J, 1998. The heart rate corrected QT interval of conscious beagle dogs: A formula based on analysis of covariance. *Toxicol Sci* **45**:247–258

24. Cooper MM, Branch C, Bastianse R et al., 2001. Mathematical correction for the inverse relationship between QT interval and heart rate in conscious beagle dogs and cynomolgus monkeys. *Toxicol Sci* **60**:A1251

25. Osborne BE and Leach GDH, 1971. The beagle electrocardiogram. *Food Cosmet Toxicol* **9**:857–864

26. Fossa AA, Depasquale MJ, Raunig DL et al., 2002. The relationship of clinical QT prolongation to outcome in the conscious dog using a beat-to-beat QT-RR interval assessment. *J Pharmacol Exp Ther* **202**:828–833

27. Cubeddu LX, 2003. QT prolongation and fatal arrhythmias: A review of clinical implications and effects of drugs. *Am J Ther* **10**:452–457

28. Sanguinetti MC and Jurkiewicz NK, 1990. Two components of cardiac delayed rectifier K+ current. Differential sensitivity to block by class III antiarrhythmic agents. *J Gen Physiol* **96**:195–215

29. Honig PK, Wortham DC, Zamani K et al., 1993. Terfenadine-ketoconazole interaction. Pharmacokinetic and electrocardiographic consequences. *JAMA* **269**:1513–1518

30. Michalets EL and Williams CR, 2000. Drug interactions with cisapride: clinical implications. *Clin Pharmacokinet* **39**:49–75

31. Trudeau MC, Warmke JW, Ganetzky B et al., 1995. HERG, A human inward rectifier in the voltage gated potassium channel family. *Science* **269**:92–95

32. Kirsch GE, Trepakova ES, Brimecombe JC et al., 2004. Variability in the measurement of hERG potassium channel inhibition: Effects of temperature and stimulus pattern. *J Pharmacol Toxicol Methods* **50**:93–101

33. Bianchi L and Driscoll M, 2006. Heterologous expression of C. elegans ion channels in Xenopus oocytes, WormBook, ed. The C. elegans Research Community, WormBook, doi/10.1895/wormbook.1.117.1 (August 1)

34. Yang T, Snyders D, and Roden DM, 2001. Drug block of IKr: Model systems and relevance to human arrhythmias. *J Cardiovasc Pharmacol* **38**:737

35. Davie C, Pierre-Valentin J, Pollard C et al., 2004. Comparative pharmacology of guinea pig cardiac myocyte and cloned hERG (IKr) channel. *J Cardiovasc Electrophysiol* **15**:1302–1309

36. Cavero I, Mestre M, Guillon JM, and Crumb W, 2000. Drugs that prolong QT interval as an unwanted effect: Assessing their likelihood of inducing hazardous cardiac dysrhythmias. *Expert Opin Pharmacother* **1**:947–973

37. Cavero I and Crumb W, 2001. Native and cloned ion channels from human heart: Laboratory models for evaluating the cardiac safety of new drugs. *Eur Heart J Suppl* **3**:K53–K63

38. Witchel HJ, Milnes JT, Mitcheson JS, and Hancox JC, 2002. Troubleshooting problems with in vitro screening of drugs for QT interval prolongation using HERG K+ channels expressed in mammalian cell lines and Xenopus oocytes. *J Pharmacol Toxicol Methods* **48**:65–80

39. Finlayson K. Witchel HJ, McCulloch J, and Sharkey J, 2004. Acquired QT interval prolongation and HERG: implications for drug discovery and development. *Eur J Pharmacol* **500**:129–142

40. Wible BA, Hawryluk P, Ficker E et al., 2005. HERG-Lite: a novel comprehensive high-throughput screen for drug-induced hERG risk. *J Pharmacol Toxicol Methods* **52**:136–145

41. Drorbaugh JE and Fenn WO, 1955. A barometric method for measuring ventilation in newborn infants. *Pediatrics* **16**:81–87

42. Pennock BE, Cox CP, Rogers RM et al., 1979. A non-invasive technique for measurement of changes in specific airway resistance. *J Appl Physiol* **94**:399–406

43. Murphy DJ, 1994. Safety pharmacology of the respiratory system: Techniques and study design. *Drug Dev Res* **32**:237–246

44. Lundblad L, Irvin C, Adler A and Bates J, 2002. A reevaluation of the validity of unrestrained plethysmography in mice. *J Appl Physiol* **93**:1198–1207

45. Lomask M, 2005. Respiration measurement in the whole body plethysmograph, 1–17. www.buxco.com/Resources.aspx?Page=WhitePapers

46. Irwin S, 1968. Comprehensive behavioral assessment: 1a A systematic quantitative procedure for assessing the behavioral and physiologic state of the mouse. *Psychopharmacologia* **13**:222–257

47. Moser VC, 1989. Screening approaches to neurotoxicity: a functional observation battery. *Int J Toxicol* **8**:85–93

48. Haggerty CG, 1989. Development of tier I neurobehavioral testing capabilities for incorporation into pivotal rodent safety assessment studies. *Int J Toxicol* **8**:53–69

49. Moser VC, McCormick JP, Creason JP et al., 1988. Comparison of chlordimefon and carbaryl using a functional observation battery. *Fundam Appl Toxicol* **11**:189–206

50. Haggerty CG, 1991. Strategy for and experience with neurotoxicity testing of new pharmaceuticals. *Int J Toxicol* **10**:677–688

51. Redfern WS, Strang I, Storey S et al., 2005. Spectrum of effects detected in the rat functional observation battery following oral administration of non-CNS targeted compounds. *J Pharmacol Toxicol Methods* **52**:77–82

52. Gintant GA, Limberis JT, McDermott JS et al., 2001. The canine Purkinje fiber: An in vitro model system for acquired long QT syndrome and drug-induced arrhythmogenesis. *J Cardiovasc Pharmacol* **37**:607–618

53. Guth BD, 2007. Preclinical cardiovascular risk assessment in modern drug development. *Toxicol Sci* **97**:4–20

54. Yuill KH, Borg JJ, Ridley JM et al., 2004. Potent inhibition of human cardiac potassium (HERG) channels by the anti-estrogen agent clomiphene without QT interval prolongation. *Biochem Biophys Res Commun* **318**:556–561

55. Kii Y, Hayashi S, Tabo M, et al., 2005. QT PRODACT: Evaluation of the potential of compounds to cause QT interval prolongation by action potential assays using guinea-pig papillary muscles. *J Pharmacol Sci* **99**:449–457

56. Hayashi S, Kii Y, Tabo M et al., 2005. QT PRODACT: A multi-site study of in vitro action potential assays on 21 compounds in isolated guinea-pig papillary muscles. *J Pharmacol Sci* **99**:423–437

57. Hondeghem LM, Carlsson L, and Duker G, 2001. Instability and triangulation of the action potential predict serious proarrhythmia, but action potential duration prolongation is antiarrhythmic. *Circulation* **103**:2004–2013

58. Hondeghem LM and Hoffmann P, 2003. Blinded test in isolated female rabbit heart reliably identifies action potential duration prolongation and proarrhythmic drugs: Importance of triangulation, reverse use dependence, and instability. *J Cardiovasc Pharmacol* **41**:14–24

59. Antzelevich C, Sun ZQ, Zhan ZQ, and Yan GX, 1996. Cellular and ionic mechanisms underlying erythromycin-induced long QT intervals and torsade de pointes. *J Am Coll Cardiol* **28**:1836–1848

60. Reiter LR and McPhail RC, 1979. Motor activity: A survey of methods with potential use in toxicity testing. *Neurobehav Toxicol* **1**:53–66

61. Dunham NW and Miya TS, 1957. A note on a simple apparatus for detecting neurological deficit in mice and rats. *J Am Pharm Assoc* **46**:208–209

62. Eddy NB and Leimbach D, 1953. Synthetic analgesics: II-Dithienylbutenyl and dithienyl-butylamines. *J Pharmacol Exp Ther* **107**:385–393

63. Gavva NR, Tamir R, Qu Y et al., 2005. AMG 9810 [(E)-3-(4-t-butylphenyl)-N-(2, 3-dihydrobenzo[b][1,4]dioxyn-6-il)acrylamide], A novel vanilloid receptor 1 (TRPV1) antagonist with antihyperalgesic properties. *J Pharmacol Exp Ther* **313**:474–484

64. Honore P, Chandran P, Hernandez G et al., 2009. Repeated dosing of ABT-102, a potent and selective TRPV1 antagonist, enhances TRPV1-mediated analgesic activity in rodents, but attenuates antagonist-induced hyperthermia. *Pain* **142**:27–35

65. Wang LX and Wang ZJ, 2003. Animal and cellular models of chronic pain. *Adv Drug Deliv Rev* **55**:949–965

66. Morris RGM, 1981. Spatial localization does not require the presence of local cues. *Learn Motiv* **12**:239–260

67. Olton DS, 1986. The radial maze as a tool in behavioral pharmacology. *Physiol Behav* **40**:793–797

68. International Conference on Harmonisation of Technical Requirements for Registration of Pharmaceuticals for Human Use, 2008. ICH M3 (R2) guideline. Nonclinical safety studies for the conduct of human clinical trials and marketing authorization for pharmaceuticals. http://www.ich.org

69. International Conference on Harmonisation of Technical Requirements for Registration of Pharmaceuticals for Human Use, 2006. Guideline on the non-clinical investigation of the dependence potential of medicinal products, EMEA/CHMP/ SWP/94227/2004. http://www.emea.europa.eu/pdfs/human/swp/ 9422704en.pdf.

70. Balster RL, 1991. Drug abuse potential evaluation in animals. *Brit J Addict* **86**:1549–1558

71. Saelens JK, Granat FR, and Sawyer WK, 1971. The mouse jumping test, A simple screening method to estimate the physical dependence capacity of analgesics. *Arch Int Pharmacodyn Ther* **190**:213–218

72. Shoaib S, Stolerman IP, and Kumar RC, 1994. Nicotine-induced place preference following prior nicotine exposure. *Psychopharmacology* **113**:445–45

73. Brady JV and Fischman MW, 1985. Assessment of drugs for dependence potential and abuse liability: An overview. In: Seiden L. S. and Balster R. L. editors. *Behavioral Pharmacology: The Current Status*. New York: Alan R. Liss. pp. 361–382

74. Balster RL and Bigelow GE, 2003. Guidelines and methodological reviews concerning drug abuse liability assessment. *Drug Alcohol Depend* **70**:S13–S40

75. Ator NA and Griffiths RR, 2003. Principles of drug abuse liability assessment in laboratory animals. *Drug Alcohol Depend* **70**:S55–S72

76. Price RG, 1992. The role of NAG (N-acetyl-β-d-glucosaminidase) in the diagnosis of kidney disease including the monitoring of nephrotoxicity. *Clin Nephrology* **38**:S14–S19

77. Price RG, 1992a. The measurement of urinary N-acetyl-β-d-glucosaminidase (NAG) and its isoenzymes; methods and clinical applications. *Eur J Clin Chem Clin Biochem* **30**:693–705

78. Harrison AP, Erlwanger KH, Elbrønd VS et al., 2004. Gastrointestinal-tract models and techniques for use in safety pharmacology. *J Pharmacol Toxicol Methods* **49**:187–199

79. Kirouac A, Rue C and Mason S, 2008. Assessment of pharmacological effects on the gastrointestinal system. *J Pharmacol Toxicol Methods* **58**:175

80. Shay H, Sun DC and Gruenstein M, 1954. A quantitative method for measuring spontaneous gastric secretion in the rat. *Gastroenterology* **26**:906–913

81. Osinski MA, Seifert TR, Cox BF, and Gintant GA, 2002. An improved method of evaluation of drug-evoked changes in gastric emptying in mice. *J Pharmacol Toxicol Methods* **47**:115–120

82. Asai T, Mapleson WW, and Power I, 1998. Effects of nalbuphine, pentazocine and U50488H on gastric emptying and gastrointestinal transit in the rat. *Brit J Anesth* **80**:814–819

83. Granberry MC, Gardner SF, 1996. Erythromycin monotherapy associated with torsade de pointes. *Ann Pharmacother* **30**:77–78

84. Katapadi K, Kostandy G, Katapadi M et al., 1997. A review of erythromycin-induced malignant tachyarrhythmia—Torsade de pointes. A case report. *Angiology 48*:821–826

85. Koh KK, Rim MS, Yoon J, and Kim SS, 1994. Torsade de pointes induced by terfenadine in a patient with long QT syndrome. *J Electrocardiol 27*:343–346

86. Sakemi H and VanNatta B, 1993. Torsade de pointes induced by astemizole in a patient with prolongation of the QT interval. *Am Heart J 125*:1436–1438

87. Wilson WH and Weiler SJ 1984. Case report of phenothiazine-induced torsade de pointes. *Am J Psychiatry 141*:1265–6

88. O'Brien JM, Rockwood RP and Suh KI, 1999. Haloperidol-induced torsade de pointes. *Ann Pharmacother 33*:1046–1050

89. Albengres E, Le Louët H, and Tillement JP, 1998. Systemic antifungal agents. Drug interactions of clinical significance. *Drug Safety 18*:83–97

90. Keller GA and Di Girolamo G, 2010. Prokinetic agents and QT prolongation: A familiar scene with new actors. *Curr Drug Saf 5*:73–78.

91. Vitola J, Vukanovic J, and Roden DM, 1998. Cisapride-induced torsades de pointes. *J Cardiovasc Electrophysiol 10*:1109–1113

6

FORMULATIONS, IMPURITIES, AND TOXICOKINETICS

Claude Charuel

INTRODUCTION

When implementing any nonclinical strategy, a very critical consideration is the degree of systemic exposure of experimental animals to the test compound or to its major, potentially active or reactive, metabolites. The composition and quality of the formulation used to dose the compound in nonclinical studies can greatly influence its oral bioavailability and its kinetic profile, depending on the physicochemical properties of the active moiety and target tissues. At the same time, when we strive for a test compound that is appropriately pure, the technical limitations of purification procedures and the degradation of the active ingredient and/or excipients make it inevitable that impurities will be present in the test formulations, and ultimately in the commercial drug substance and/or drug product. The sooner these impurities are identified and qualified, the better.

The purpose of this chapter is not to review in detail all types of formulations that can be used in nonclinical studies, or the theoretical considerations underpinning impurity guidelines or toxicokinetic models. We focus on some practical aspects that will help the reader to identify problems or discrepancies that emerge during the various stages of nonclinical testing and to fix them rapidly by making the best possible use of the information progressively assembled in nonclinical and early clinical studies. In particular, the systematic estimation of plasma drug levels allows the toxicologist to verify the degree of absorption, and the consistency/reproducibility of exposure to test

Pharmaceutical Toxicology in Practice: A Guide for Non-Clinical Development, Edited by Alberto Lodola and Jeanne Stadler
© 2011 John Wiley & Sons, Inc.

compound. These toxicokinetic measurements also give early warning of potentially active/reactive metabolites and provide key information on the linearity of the dose response, potential gender differences, and phenomena linked to autoinduction or drug accumulation. In contrast, toxicokinetic data, notably exposure multiples, are not helpful and should not be used to qualify impurities or degradation products except when the latter also appear to be significant circulating metabolites.

FORMULATIONS

Liquid formulations (solutions and suspensions) are generally used in preliminary pharmacological assays and early toxicity studies (typically up to 6 months in rodents and 1 to 3 months in dogs or monkeys), using oral, intravenous, subcutaneous, topical, intranasal, or inhalation routes of administration. Most of these formulations are prepared in a dedicated dispensary, close to the animal house if possible, either extemporaneously (if no stability data are available) or once weekly if no degradation has been demonstrated. At the early stages of development, formulations are often relatively simple, consisting primarily of pH-adjusted aqueous solutions or suspensions. Some cosolvents may be added. Although diverse mechanical mixing procedures exist for preparing suspensions, the use of a pestle and mortar is often required to break aggregates, wet the test compound, and achieve homogeneity. At this stage, short-term stability studies can be undertaken to make sure that excessive degradation does not occur during the course of the study. However, the presence of reasonable levels of impurities (see the Impurity section, following), such as synthetic by-products or degradants, may actually be desirable, as toxicity studies can qualify these impurities over the course of the development process. For longer-term and carcinogenicity studies (6–24 months), solid formulations are most often used, particularly diet mixes or pellets for rodents and capsules or tablets for dogs. As pharmaceutical development progresses, clinical formulations progressively integrate appropriate salts, the desired polymorph, and more advanced excipients designed to provide the intended formulation characteristics. Ideally, regulatory studies should be conducted with the commercial form. Although this is often feasible in nonrodents, it is not always practicable in rats or mice. Therefore, rigorous and extensive toxicokinetic data are needed at each stage of the nonclinical program to demonstrate that the bioavailability of the test compound is consistent within species and across studies. If necessary, specific toxicokinetic studies can be conducted to investigate the bioequivalence of different test formulations using small groups of animals and a crossover study design. It is also important to ensure that the formulations used in safety pharmacology and *in vivo* genotoxicity studies produce test compound concentrations that are in the same range as those expected in toxicity species.

LIQUID FORMULATIONS

Before the start of any toxicity study, we need to know the physicochemical properties of the test compound, particularly its capacity to dissolve, or form a uniform and stable suspension, in the vehicles most commonly used in nonclinical studies. In the unlikely event that such data are not available, it is worthwhile testing the solubility of the compound in water and a selection of water-miscible and nonmiscible solvents. Such tests, incidentally, may also serve to guide the selection of a mobile phase for the liquid chromatographic (LC) analysis of the test compound if no analytical method is yet available. Small proportions of dimethyl sulfoxide, ethanol, glycerol, propylene glycol, polyethylene glycols (PEG), and polysorbate (Tween) are acceptable in subacute studies, whereas lipophilic vehicles (oils, solutol, myglyol), and substituted cyclodextrins such as hydroxypropylbetacylodextrin (HPBCD) are of value for poorly soluble drugs. One should bear in mind, however, that Tween is poorly tolerated by dogs [1] and PEG concentrations above 20%–30% v/v are likely to produce diarrhea, especially in mice and dogs. Similarly, oils may affect the gastrointestinal tract and reduce or perturb food intake. High doses of cyclodextrin may lead to renal vacuolation or nephrotoxicity, depending on route of administration [2], and chemical substitution (the lower the degree of substitution, the higher the risk of renal toxicity).

For single-dose or dose-finding studies, adding hydrochloric acid or sodium hydroxide to aqueous vehicles often improves dissolution when the drug substance is a simple free base or free acid with low solubility at neutral pH. For the intravenous and, to some extent, the intramuscular route, a careful balance is needed between pH (typically in the 3–9 range) and molarity of test solutions in order to minimize local (often concentration dependent) intolerance or reprecipitation with the risk of phlebitis. Concentration is also an important factor for topical, subcutaneous, or intranasal administration. In addition, crystals should be avoided in inhalation sprays, as they may injure the respiratory mucosa. Small pH adjustments can also considerably improve the quality of suspensions. The latter are usually prepared using methylcellulose or carboxymethylcellulose (2000–4000 cps) at concentrations (about 0.5% w/v) sufficient to produce reasonable viscosity. Adding a small amount (0.1%–0.2% v/v) of surfactant such as Tween 80 improves the dispersion of the test substance. Stock solutions of methylcellulose can be stored refrigerated for at least a week, and suspensions of test compound are prepared extemporaneously or for several days if stability has been shown to be acceptable. Obtaining samples of the test suspension at different levels of the storage container (top, middle, and bottom) is critical when verifying homogeneity and physical stability. Ultimately, toxicokinetic measurements play a major role in demonstrating that bioavailability is optimal and reproducible from one animal to the other in a same dosage group, or from one study to the other. Nonlinear kinetics too often reflect improper absorption linked to inhomogeneous suspensions or poor solubility at higher doses.

For subsequent toxicity studies, a range of salts and buffers is available. Many counter ions can be used for their preparation. The most common anions (e.g., chlorides, bromides, sulfates, phosphates, tartrates, citrates, acetates, and fumarates) are present in many marketed drugs, are known to be well tolerated, and are accepted by regulatory authorities. However, there may be concern over the use of some anions due to toxicity or potential reactivity. For example, lactates may affect blood pH and ionic balance, and (di)maleates may produce nephropathy at oral doses above 10 mg/kg in dogs [3]. Similar or higher doses of bromides can cause thyroid disorders [4]. Bromides can also interfere with the measurement of plasma chloride levels by competing with chlorine on the electrode detection system used in plasma chemistry analyzers. Although not necessarily toxic per se, mesylate and tosylate salts are often problematic in drug development because carcinogenic alkyl derivatives can be formed on long-term storage or during the final steps of synthetic processes involving strong acids or alcohols. As far as cations are concerned, sodium, potassium, calcium, and magnesium are the most commonly used counter ions in the preparation of salts. For most other cations, there is a lack of regulatory precedence or key safety data, although some cations have been used in foodstuffs or occur naturally in the body (e.g., choline, glycine, arginine, and lysine [5]). Still other cations have an inherent pharmacological activity (e.g., piperazines), or attributes that render them undesirable as primary options: benzathine and diethylamine have the potential to form nitrosamines and, like ethylene diamine, are potential sensitizers. When data on long-term safety, genotoxicity, or reproductive toxicity of counter ions are missing, careful consideration must be given to their use. In these cases, a thorough evaluation of alternative uses of the moiety being considered as a food additive for example, route of administration, and structural features (absence of genotoxic alerts) is helpful in deciding whether the moiety should be developed or not.

All these observations show that changing a salt or a formulation during the development of a drug or a generic equivalent is not a trivial exercise. Such changes may not only affect the absorption and kinetics of the test compound but also affect its toxicity profile.

Solid Formulations

Capsules can be filled by hand using standard excipients (lactose, maize starch) or manufactured specifically by pharmaceutical scientists. End users should be aware of any additives (stabilizers, antioxidants) or any unusual ingredient used in the formulation. PEG-containing soft gel capsules, although not strictly solid, are useful for poorly soluble drugs. Tablets often use the same ingredients as solid capsules but offer additional options (e.g., they can be coated or fractionated). However, their production requires specialized equipment. The same applies to pellets whose manufacture involves moistening and heating steps that can accelerate degradation of the test compound. In contrast, diet mixes can be prepared easily in a dispensary, generally on a weekly basis. A preblend is made using an ad hoc mixer or a pestle and mortar to incorporate the bulk powder into a small quantity of feed or appropriate vehicle. The preblend is then transferred to a blender where the remainder of the feed is added in one or more steps. Samples of the final diet mix should be retained for concentration and homogeneity testing.

Concentration and Homogeneity Testing

Solutions and suspensions should be tested before the start of a study, at least once during the course of short-term studies (≤ 30 days) and at regular intervals for studies of longer length. The sampling frequency is adapted according to the consistency of the analytical results. Samples (1/dose for solutions, 3/dose for suspensions) should be analyzed immediately after collection for test compound content and homogeneity or stored frozen if no degradation is anticipated. It is important to ensure that the analytical samples are collected under conditions as close as possible to those used during dosing of animals and to check that suspensions are maintained under constant agitation during sampling and before analysis. It is advisable not to dilute suspensions to obtain lower dose strengths and to prepare control and active formulations either separately or by ascending concentration in order to minimize cross-contamination. In addition, careful attention should be paid to the analytical process. Data dispersion (results more than ±15% of expected) is often due to pipetting errors during the analysis—withdrawing 50-μl aliquots of a viscous suspension using a capillary pipette that can be easily obstructed by a few aggregates, for example.

For dietary administration, experimental mixes need to be prepared to verify the dispersion, homogeneity, and recovery of the test compound in the final mix over a wide range of concentrations. Usually, three samples are taken for analysis, from the top, middle, and bottom of the mix, each in triplicate. The mixing procedure thus defined is used in prechronic studies (generally 3-month dose-finding studies in rodents). For carcinogenicity studies, revalidating the mixing process should take place only if the lowest dose corresponds to a test compound concentration below the range already tested. To ensure the homogeneity of the test compound at concentrations close to or below 10 parts per million (ppm), vehicles such as lactose, microcrystalline cellulose, or maize starch are often required to prepare premixes. Given these constraints, many laboratories prefer to conduct their chronic studies using the same route of administration as that used for their subchronic program. Although this approach may accelerate the overall development process in the short term, it also presents potential drawbacks that merit consideration. In a carcinogenicity study, when the test compound is administered by gavage, the time needed to intubate 600 animals 7 days a week for 2 years is not negligible, and there is an increased risk of mortality and nonspecific pathological changes due to regurgitation, pulmonary lesions, or stress. From a toxicokinetic viewpoint, absorption of test compound from the diet is often more regular than that observed after gavage—there is a lower peak concentration and sustained exposure [5]. While there are exceptions (hormones, for example), this profile is generally more representative of the clinical situation than the quick surge and short-lived plasma levels of the test compound often seen after oral gavage in rodents. Consequently, larger doses can be used by the dietary route, minimizing drug holidays, if any, and optimizing the chance to detect and evaluate toxicity linked to sustained exposure rather than undesirable extrapharmacological effects related to peak plasma levels of the test compound.

Stability of Test Compound Formulations

A range of information is needed on the batch of the test compound used to treat animals: physical characteristics, certificate of analysis, shelf life of bulk and formulated material, formulation records, storage conditions, and stability data over a range of concentrations in appropriate vehicles. To save time and to cover future studies, it is useful to test the widest possible concentration range at the beginning of the nonclinical program. For example, solutions can be tested up to the limit of solubility and suspensions from 0.1 to 500 mg/ml. The stability of the solutions/suspensions is verified over at least 10 days to enable weekly preparation of dosing formulations. After the study has been completed, samples of all formulated materials (or when necessary bulk powders) are returned to the analytical laboratory for "exit assays" that determine a posteriori the level of degradation products present in the batches tested. This information may be used later to qualify the degradants concerned. For dietary studies where it is difficult to anticipate the choice of dose levels at the beginning of compound development, the lowest possible concentration is critical, as homogeneity is difficult to achieve and/or quantify below 10 ppm as already stated.

IMPURITIES

Acceptance criteria for impurities are based on the ICH Q3A(R2) guideline for drug substances [7] and the ICH Q3B(R2) guideline for drug products [8]. The ICH qualification process should be used to ensure that the impurity profile of a test substance or product does not present a risk at its registered limits. However, in order to retain some flexibility, higher thresholds are desirable during the early stages of compound development. At this time, analytical tools for identification of impurities are usually not fully developed, validated, or optimized. Analytical rigor increases with time, and supporting data for the qualification of impurities are progressively assembled in nonclinical and early clinical studies.

Qualification is defined as "the process of acquiring and evaluating data that establishes the biological safety of an individual impurity or a given impurity profile at the level(s) specified", whereas the qualified level is the level deemed to be safe for human consumption. Qualification is based on risk assessments supported by nonclinical and clinical studies, scientific publications, or predictive databases such as DEREK (Deductive Estimation of Risk from Existing Knowledge) [9], an adaptable system that identifies chemical functional moieties (structural alerts) that are correlated with mutagenicity (other signals being much less specific). By the time the test compound enters full development, much information with respect to identification and qualification of likely impurities and degradation products becomes available. The objective, from this point on, should be to meet the limits set out in the guidelines [7, 8].

Early Development

Impurities related to the synthetic process should be closely monitored and controlled. Particular attention should be paid to likely by-products, starting materials, or intermediates with potential genetic toxicity. It is critically important to remain vigilant in considering the impact of any changes in synthetic route or formulation on the impurity profile. Close collaboration between analytical scientists and toxicologists is needed to identify potentially problematic impurities in the test compound as early as possible in

TABLE 6.1. Qualification of impurity levels for human based on toxicity data for the rat.

Species	Body Weight (Kg)	Test Compound Dose Level (mg/kg)	Impurity in Test Compound Concentration (%w/w)	Dose (mg/kg)	Safety Factor
Rat	0,25	100	0.3	0.3	
Human	75	0.2 (15 mg toto)	0.5	0.001	300

the drug development process. Derisking strategies can then be developed to qualify, limit (purge), or eliminate those impurities. Internal target limits for impurities may also be used to provide a greater level of control. For example, when the same impurity is present in the drug substance and in the drug product, a tighter control over the level in drug substance may be required to ensure a satisfactory shelf life for the product. Degradation products generally arise because of a breakdown of the test compound due to chemical instability or the action of light, temperature, or humidity. Additionally, the test compound may react with an excipient or, more rarely, with a foreign molecule (lubricant, substance leached from storage containers). As a rule of thumb, individual impurities should not exceed 1% w/w and total impurities 5% w/w in batches of test compound used for early development. To meet these requirements, analytical methods should provide a suitable resolution of analytes (e.g., liquid chromatography with mass spectroscopic (LC-MS) or nuclear magnetic resonance (LC-NMR) detection) and be sensitive enough to attain the desired limits of quantification (typically between 0.01% and 0.05% w/w). Whenever single impurities are anticipated to exceed the 0.10% ICH threshold (0.05% for drugs expected to exceed a human dose of 2 g/day), attempts should be made to isolate and identify the compounds concerned. Other impurities will be regarded as unspecified unless there are concerns about their structures. Typical structural alerts include aryl derivatives, nitrosamines, carbamates, epoxides, lactones, hydrazines, and halides [9].

For nonclinical programs, a balance is required between the desire to qualify impurities likely to be present in future batches and the need to preserve the integrity of the studies. Whereas 1% w/w or even 5% w/w of a pharmacologically inactive, DEREK alert-free impurity does not raise credible risks in general toxicity studies, 0.1% of a (potentially) genotoxic impurity should not be disregarded, particularly for batches of test compound destined for clinical use (see the discussion on genotoxic impurities following). Because the safety of volunteers and patients is paramount, selecting test batches for use in clinical studies should be based on a range of assessments, including DEREK screens and data from genotoxicity and early animal studies (usually up to 1 month), performed either with the test compound containing the suspect impurity or with the impurity itself. As Table 6.1 shows, the qualified level is primarily derived by comparing doses used in animals and humans. This example illustrates that rats administered 100 mg/kg of a test compound containing 0.3% w/w of an impurity are exposed to a dose of this impurity that is 300-fold greater than that ingested by a 75-kg human given 15 mg of a clinical batch of test compound containing 0.5% w/w of the same impurity. If the 100-mg/kg dose corresponds to the no-observed adverse effect level in rats, the impurity is amply qualified. When the impurity is also a significant metabolite of the test compound in some, if not all, toxicity species and in genotoxicity assays, it is almost automatically qualified by existing nonclinical data (see discussion on metabolites and genotoxic impurities following). This implies that reasonable efforts have been made to measure the levels of the metabolite in the various species. This is probably the only instance where toxicokinetics are used to qualify impurities. Trying to monitor trace impurity levels in blood samples systematically obtained from animals in routine nonclinical studies does not make sense in our view because (1) the detection of such levels would necessitate extremely sensitive analytical methods and (2) there is no guarantee that the impurities concerned are absorbed.

Full Development and Commercialization

For clinical studies in support of full development, thresholds for identification, reporting, and qualification of new impurities should comply with ICH Q3A and B guidelines [7, 8]. When impurity levels exceed guideline thresholds, the options are either to reduce/eliminate the impurity through a modified synthetic process/formulation or to seek additional toxicology data to qualify the higher impurity levels. If the data does not exist, performing qualification studies should be considered according to ICH recommendations (i.e., a specific 1-month toxicity study in a single species and/or additional genotoxicity testing). However, it should be borne in mind that such studies are not without risks, as toxicology is not an exact science with fully reproducible endpoints. New findings unrelated to the test compound or impurities may emerge due to different environmental conditions such as time elapsed between pivotal and qualification experiments or genetic drift in the animal strains being used.

A variety of factors can lead to qualitative or quantitative changes in the purity profile. These changes result from modifications to chemical synthesis (scale-up or change of synthetic route, process, or starting materials), chemical instability of the test substance or product, or improvements to analytical methods leading to changes in impurity profiles or quantities. In addition, several circumstances exist where case-by-case evaluations are recommended. These include atypical dose levels (below 10 mg or above 1000 mg), unusual routes of administration (inhalation, topical), specific target populations (oncology, pediatrics), or clinical scope (life threatening, acute treatments) and novel excipients. Overall, it is necessary to be constantly aware of the changes affecting the quality/composition of the test compound under development to avoid the late discovery of a genotoxic impurity/degradant and delays and added costs to the nonclinical development program.

Genotoxic Impurities

For most impurities, where there is little or no information on genotoxicity and carcinogenicity, a pragmatic approach is needed to identify potential gene toxins as soon as possible in the development process while maintaining flexibility for selecting doses in the exploratory clinical phase. In early development, it is critical to recognize that the presence of very low levels of a genotoxic impurity might be without appreciable risks. Once the toxic potential of all starting materials, identified impurities, and synthetic intermediates has been assessed through a literature survey or search of the DEREK database, decisions are needed on how to proceed and handle the data. The options include analytical control, process control, or additional *in vitro* or *in vivo* testing [10]. This process should be initiated before the release of the first regulatory batch of test compound, which is generally used in genetic toxicity and early animal toxicity studies as well as in first-in-human studies. During the course of development and through submission of a market application, all impurities and reagents (including metals and solvents) should be assessed using the same process. Often, the toxicologist is confronted with alerting structures of unknown genotoxic or carcinogenic potential (i.e., there are no published data). If the alerting functional moiety is shared with the parent structure, the impurity can be considered qualified by the genotoxicity studies conducted with the test compound, provided the alerting substructures present similar chemical constraints/environment. In all other cases, because of the uncertain relevance of structural alerts, qualification should be based on the nature of the alert (e.g., DEREK does not differentiate enantiomers), specificity of alerting moiety (eliminating whenever possible irrelevant alerts like aromatic amines), chemical constraints/environment, or additional experiments. Regulatory authorities generally require that complementary bacterial mutation assays (Ames test) be performed using isolated impurities and testing them up to regulatory limits (5000 µg/plate). If this is not practicable, the impurity can be evaluated as part of the test substance, as long as its concentration is at least equivalent to 250 µg/plate—a level at which known mutagenic carcinogens are typically detected [11]. Whenever *in vitro* cytogenetic assays are performed, the findings should be interpreted with caution, as these assays produce a high rate of false positive responses and poor correlation to rodent carcinogenicity data [12, 13]. Further investigation of the potential for a threshold-mediated process such as oxidative damage or protein interactions (e.g., aneuploidy because of interaction with the spindle apparatus, inhibition of topoisomerases or DNA synthesis, saturation of defense mechanisms) may allow safe exposure levels to be determined. If none of these investigations demonstrates toxicity, the impurity will be treated as a standard one. Otherwise, it will follow the procedure applicable to genotoxic substances.

Impurities known to be carcinogenic and/or mutagenic should be controlled to levels appropriate for the stage of compound development if they cannot be eliminated by reprocessing. However, there is substantial disagreement in principle and variability in practice concerning the initiation of this process and control limits to be used. A staged approach has been proposed, based on data published by [14] and [15], which advocates daily intakes decreasing from about 100 µg for early short-duration clinical trials to less than 1.5 µg for registration and commercialization. In concentration terms, 100 µg/day means that the daily dose of a drug would have to exceed 1 g for the concentration of the impurity to reach 100 ppm (or 0.01%). For registration, the 1.5-µg/day value corresponds to the threshold of toxicological concern (TTC) recommended by the European Committee for Human Medicinal Products (CHMP) in their guidelines [16]. The TTC concept was originally developed by the U.S. Food and Drug Administration (FDA) for foodstuffs [17, 18] and was derived by simple linear extrapolation from the carcinogenic potencies (measured as the dose giving a 50% tumor incidence, TD50) of more than 700 carcinogens. The methods and assumptions used to obtain the TTC were very conservative, using TD50 data from the most sensitive species and sites. Originally, a TTC figure of 0.15 μg/day was associated with a 1 in 10^6 lifetime cancer risk and was termed "a virtually safe dose." A higher limit of 1.5 μg/day giving a 1 in 10^5 lifetime risk was considered acceptable for pharmaceuticals, as there is a benefit associated with their intake and the underlying estimates were very conservative. However, the CHMP guideline indicates that some structural groups of compounds would require control levels lower than the TTC due to their unusually high carcinogenic potency (aflatoxin-like, N-nitroso-, and azoxy compounds). The guideline also indicates that a level higher than 1.5 μg/day may be acceptable for short-term exposure and in circumstances such as life-threatening conditions with no safer alternatives, short life expectancy, or significant exposure to the impurity from food sources. A set of questions and answers [19] clarifies regulatory expectations and indicates European acceptance of the staged approach described by Mueller et al. [15].

REACTIVE METABOLITES

Due diligence is needed in order to identify metabolites as soon as possible to make sure they do not represent safety hazards. Reactive metabolites in particular may have genetic toxicity that could have implications for the outcome of carcinogenicity studies. Therefore, it is important to examine when human metabolites should be examined for genotoxicity based on the progress of drug metabolism studies during the drug development cycle and how the metabolites can be qualified. The degree of thoroughness and sophistication of metabolic investigations increases throughout the discovery and development process. Emerging qualitative and quantitative data determine the strategy to be used for qualifying the metabolite. Initially, metabolic information is derived from early animal studies and *in vitro* experiments using liver subcellular fractions. Such data are rarely quantitative except in cases where the metabolite is a suspect electrophile or is thought to contribute to the pharmacological activity of the test compound. Unless there is a compelling reason (species differences in metabolic profiles, low enzymatic turnover coupled with low recovery of unchanged drug in urine and bile) to expedite the preparation of the ^{14}C labeled test compound, radiolabel investigations in animals rarely start before Phase I clinical trials and human metabolism studies before Phase II. These studies, particularly in humans, provide the first comprehensive view of the fate of the test compound and quantitative assessments of metabolite exposure and test compound disposition. A complete picture of all metabolites is obtained, definitive structure assignments can be made, and routes of metabolism can be deduced from the excretory metabolite profile. At this stage, careful analysis of metabolic data across species is required. If additional genetic safety testing is needed, it should specifically focus on those human blood/excreta metabolites that are abundant, unique, and/or chemically reactive. The quantitative cutoffs (metabolites that represent at least 10% of parent compound exposure in the circulation and excreta) are aligned with current guidelines for metabolite identification [20, 21] and represent pragmatic limits that use current technologies while not compromising scientific integrity. In some cases, early signals may be obtained on potentially reactive electrophiles (e.g., Michael acceptors, epoxides, quinones, imines, and isocyanates) that are present at less than 10%. These and other structures that can be further metabolized to electrophiles (e.g., anilines, formamides, imides, alkenes, thiophenes, and furans) should also be considered in evaluating genotoxicity.

For metabolites suspected of being genotoxic, as for suspect impurities, two potential hazards, mutagenicity and clastogenicity, should be evaluated. The mutagenic potential is assessed initially using a chemical structure–driven literature search and DEREK analysis. If a metabolite presents a unique alert, incubating the test compound with an appropriate metabolic activation system can be performed under the standard conditions for *in vitro* genotoxicity assays. The objective of such a study is to measure the concentrations of metabolite that are generated and to demonstrate retrospectively that it was present in all genotoxicity assays conducted with the test compound, and is thus qualified. Suitable metabolic activation systems consist of liver S9 fractions ($9000 \times$ g supernatant from a liver homogenate) that can be obtained from rats or alternative species treated or not with a nonspecific liver enzyme inducer (e.g., aroclor). If qualification by incubation of test compounds in the Ames assay with induced rat S9 or an alternative activation system is ruled out, the metabolite can be synthesized and tested directly to limits set by ICH guidelines (see Chapter 8). Clear positive findings are likely to signal the end of development for the test compound unless an explanation can be provided relative to mechanisms and/or context [22].

To address clastogenicity, the results of the *in vivo* micronucleus test performed with the test compound are used for qualification, provided sufficient amounts of the metabolite are formed in the test species, generally the rat. If the rat is not appropriate, a mouse micronucleus assay should be conducted. It is also important to consider the results of the S9 assays carried out *in vitro*. If the metabolite is generated from the parent structure with induced rat S9, qualification may be supported by the genotoxicity package obtained with the parent compound. If necessary, safety multiples can be worked out by comparing metabolite exposures in rodents and humans. When qualification in rodents or through *in vitro* tests with induced rat S9 is ruled out, the only remaining option is to test isolated metabolites in standard *in vitro* cytogenetics assays. However, the nature and magnitude of the genotoxic response need to be very carefully examined, especially if the findings are weak, unrelated to dose, or seen in a single *in vitro* test only. This may indicate the presence of a contaminating impurity or mechanisms (cytotoxicity) irrelevant to humans. As we already mentioned, *in vitro* cytogenetic findings suffer from a high rate of false positives with poor correlation to rodent carcinogenicity. Therefore, responses that are not clear-cut or validated *in vivo* should not hinder the pursuit of the nonclinical program. Ultimately, carcinogenicity studies confirm the absence of tumorigenic potential of a test compound and its metabolites. If necessary, the process can be accelerated and risks/costs reduced by investigating the development and incidence of tumors in short-term studies (6 months) using transgenic animal models (see Chapter 7).

METAL AND SOLVENT RESIDUES IN THE TEST COMPOUND

Metals have traditionally been detected and quantified according to pharmacopoeial procedures and limits. However, metals used as reagents or catalysts have varying levels of toxicity and are generally more toxic using parenteral routes (intravenous, inhalation) than orally or topically, due to poor gastrointestinal or transdermal absorption. In addition, some metals (e.g., lead, cadmium) are cumulative toxins, whereas others, particularly the essential elements (iron, for example), are excreted or metabolized efficiently. Accordingly, it makes sense to avoid cumulative toxins, to monitor some metals more closely than others, and to set lower limits parenterally (about 1–100 ppm) than orally (about ×10 parenteral levels). This approach formed the basis of the CHMP guideline on limits for residual metal catalysts [23]. Similar to the residual solvent guideline on which it was founded, this approach uses the concept of permitted daily exposure (see following).

The 1-ppm limit just quoted corresponds to metals known to be toxic (platinum, palladium) or for which there are only limited toxicity data available (rhodium, osmium, nickel, chromium). These metals should be monitored in all steps of the synthetic process or at least during the last few steps. Synthetic intermediates that might later become starting materials should also be examined unless these materials have already been tested by the suppliers and shown to be safe. In some cases, specific limits already exist for inhalation exposure. Hexachloroplatinic acid, the most allergenic platinum salt [24], is limited to 70 ng/day based on a daily breathing volume of 20m3 and 8-hours exposure. Similarly, chromium VI and nickel have occupational limits of 10 and 100 ng/day, respectively, because they have been associated with carcinogenicity when inhaled. Chromium illustrates best the problems inherent to speciation that is the existence of multiple molecular forms linked to the oxidation state, coordinating ligands, and solvation. This property leads to some uncertainty over the likely form of metal residues present in tissues or biological fluids. In addition, toxicity may vary greatly depending on the aqueous solubility of the particular metal salt used for toxicological evaluation ([25]. More relaxed standards are applied to metals with little or no safety concerns (copper, manganese, iron, zinc) that need not be specifically monitored at any stage of development. It should be noted, however, that iron has the potential to affect the appearance and stability of parenteral products. Finally, if a nontoxic metal is used as a counter ion (sodium, calcium, potassium), it should be controlled as any other counter ion (see section on Formulations).

The control of solvents used in the manufacturing process for the drug substance and/or drug product should be conducted in the spirit of the ICH Q3C(R4) guideline [26] for residual solvents. One interesting aspect of this guideline is the concept of permitted daily exposures (PDEs), which provide safe limits for solvents with known toxicity findings. PDEs are derived by applying a safety or uncertainty factor (usually ranging from 1 to 10) to the designated lowest-observed effect level (LOEL) or no-observed effect level (NOEL). This process is described in Appendix 3 of the ICH Q3C(R4) guideline [26]. For a solvent with a NOEL of 5 mg/kg in a rat carcinogenicity study, the

PDE in a 50-kg human subject would be

$$PDE = (5 \times 50)/(F1 \times F2 \times F3 \times F4 \times F5)$$

where

F1 = 5 (an extrapolation factor for rats to humans)
F2 = 10 (used to account for variability between individuals)
F3 = 1 (applied to long-term studies)
F4 = 10 (to account for the severity of findings)
F5 = 1 (because a no-effect dose has been established)

thus

$$PDE = 250/5 \times 10 \times 1 \times 10 \times 1$$

therefore,

$$PDE = 0.5 \, mg/day$$

Although uncertainty factors are generally accepted by most regulatory authorities, they should be handled with care. Deciding on the magnitude and significance of these factors remains a judgment call in many cases.

TOXICOKINETICS

As part of the drug-discovery process and candidate selection, early metabolism and pharmacokinetic studies are undertaken to assess metabolic stability across species, to determine the potential for good oral bioavailability and length of action, and to aid in the understanding of the relationship between concentration and pharmacological effect (PK/PD relationship). Accordingly, the metabolic stability of the test compound is studied *in vitro* using tissue fractions/slices, isolated cells, or recombinant systems expressing human CYP450s. In addition, the kinetic profile is determined in various animal species, ideally using intravenous and oral dosing. This provides useful information on the absorption, half-life, clearance, and metabolism of the test compound and preliminary information on the potential routes of excretion and any gender or interspecies differences. Studies that are conducted using doses that are small multiples of the anticipated clinical dose (or known efficacious dose) must be supported by an assessment of the oral bioavailability at higher doses and with the formulation (particularly for suspensions) that will be used in subsequent toxicology studies. Nonlinear increases or low/variable increases in systemic exposure to the test compound with increasing doses can often be overcome by using a different salt or an alternative formulation. In the following sections, we focus on studies using the oral route of administration. The other routes are generally limited to short-term studies and present fewer toxicokinetic problems (e.g., the intravenous route) or have specific issues that must be examined case by case. For instance, dosing by inhalation usually mimics intravenous administration but is often associated with problems linked to the delivery system, particle sizing, or oral ingestion. Similarly, topical administration often mimics oral treatment, although the skin may constitute a more complex barrier than the intestine would.

Range-Finding Studies

Data from 7- to 15-day oral range-finding studies in rodents and nonrodents are critical in that they offer the first comprehensive view of exposure to a test compound and target organ toxicities at an early stage of the nonclinical program. An essential part of these studies is recovering blood samples to assay for the test compound. A frequent limitation at this stage of development is the quantity of active substance available. To save the compound in rat studies, the number of additional animals used to obtain toxicokinetic data can be limited to five males per dose level. Considering the very high doses being tested in such studies, and the sensitivity of current analytical methods (LC-MS), 1-ml aliquots of blood can be collected on five occasions (e.g., 1, 3, 6, 10, and 24 hours after treatment) without producing too much stress or blood volume loss in the test animals (see the discussion in Chapter 7). Considering interanimal variations, the quality of toxicokinetic data obtained from a single group of rats subject to repeat blood sampling in such conditions is often better than that observed with separate subgroups (i.e., different animals per time period). The 24-hour blood sample is critical for evaluating the half-life and estimating the plasma clearance and potential variations in clearance after repeat treatment. Data for female rats should also be generated if the test compound has been shown to exhibit sex-related differences in pharmacology or early drug metabolism studies. In dogs or monkeys, the situation is simpler, as toxicokinetic investigations are generally performed on blood samples taken from the animals of the main study groups.

Toxicokinetic data for the first dose provides key information on the extent (by referring to intravenous data) and quality (low vs high, variable vs stable, related vs unrelated to dose) of absorption. If the results are unsatisfactory, these two elements should alert the toxicologist to the need to reconsider the administered formulation. If oral bioavailability is satisfactory and approximately dose related, it is worth looking at the dose response curve more carefully in both sexes to try and quickly identify significant gender differences and sub- or superproportional increases in drug exposure vs dose (see Interpretation of Toxicokinetic Data following). The data collected after the last dose are equally important, as they either confirm/amplify first-dose observations or reveal new effects—for example, an increase in the test compound exposure relative to day 1 at one or more doses (so-called "accumulation") or a decrease in exposure linked to induction by the test compound of its own metabolism (usually referred to as "autoinduction"). Considering the inherent variability of pharmacokinetic measurements in animals, these changes should reach at least $\pm 50\%$ (relative to expected values) to be convincing. Analytically, these changes may be accompanied by the appearance of additional peaks due to the presence of new, sometimes pharmacologically active, metabolites. Changes in the clearance of the test compound secondary to extrapharmacological effects (due, for example, to changes in blood flows) or target organ toxicity (e.g., impaired liver or kidney function) are also likely to be identified at this stage.

All these elements contribute to defining the variation of test compound kinetics with respect to species, gender, time, and dose level. Robust monitoring of toxicokinetics at the beginning and end of early toxicity studies is a sound practice and critical for determining dose levels for subsequent studies.

Subchronic Studies (1–6 Months)

Toxicokinetic measurements in these studies essentially serve to confirm the data generated in previous dose-finding studies and to verify that new salts or changes in test compound formulation, if any, have not affected the kinetic profile (i.e., a demonstration of bioequivalence). Because doses used in these studies are often lower than those of shorter studies, it is important to establish consistency with existing results i.e. whether drug concentrations align with previous ones and whether steady-state levels are achieved. It may be of value to monitor plasma concentrations of a test compound on several occasions (e.g., at 2-month intervals in a 6-month study) if complex dose or time-dependent kinetics have been uncovered during early studies. When accumulation or autoinduction has occurred, it is critical to determine when the phenomena culminate or saturate to appreciate better the clinical and commercial risks associated with cumulative effects, loss of efficacy, or drug–drug interactions.

In-Diet Range-Finding Studies

The objectives of 3-month rodent studies, usually the first using a mixture of the test compound in animal feed, are comparable in many respects to those for dose-finding studies. The studies should be designed to provide a robust estimation of the area under the time–concentration curve (AUC), using supplementary animals (3/dose/time period) from which blood samples are taken every 4 or 5 hours toward the end of the study. As already mentioned, in-diet dosing usually results in lower plasma peak concentrations of the test compound and in a more prolonged exposure relative to gavage administration. Therefore, a wider range of doses than those used for 1- or 6-month (gavage) studies needs to be explored to establish relative toxicity profiles and systemic exposures (oral feed vs oral gavage) prior to 24-month studies in rodents. The FDA's Carcinogenicity Advisory Council is likely to scrutinize these data before approving the design and dose levels of carcinogenicity studies (see Chapter 7).

Carcinogenicity Studies

Carcinogenicity studies provide information on the carcinogenic potential of a test compound and on the influence of aging or long-term therapy on toxicity and toxicokinetics. There are sound reasons for testing the influence of aging [27]. Drugs acting on the cardiovascular system may modify blood flows and liver extraction more dramatically in old than in young animals due to reduced drug metabolism capacities in the former. The volume of distribution of highly lipophilic drugs may be affected by the change in the ratio between fat and lean mass that occurs with aging. In contrast, water-soluble drugs or drug-derived materials that are excreted by the kidneys may be cleared less efficiently as renal function decreases. Increasing drug exposure in aged animals does not necessarily jeopardize a study or adversely influence the interpretation of the results. However, it may affect the quality of the data by increasing mortality or undesirable effects due to an extension of the pharmacological action. It is worthwhile, therefore, to consider at the outset the need for toxicokinetics at one or several time points during chronic studies. The midpoint of the carcinogenicity study is generally a good compromise, as metabolic changes related to aging are already in place and animal survival is optimal, with little or no bias, linked to the development of spontaneous or treatment-induced tumors. Alhough they are time consuming and costly, supplementary toxicokinetic groups can be added to the study or, alternatively, single blood samples can be collected from main group animals in rat studies.

Developmental and Reproductive Toxicology

During maternal toxicity studies in rodents and nonrodents (usually rabbits), the tolerance of the dams to the widest possible range of doses is tested. These doses are often close to those used in early dose-finding toxicity studies unless specific problems (e.g., cardiovascular or gastrointestinal intolerance in rabbits) arise in a particular species. At this stage of compound development, the pharmacokinetic profile of the drug is generally well established in (nonpregnant) rodents and in nonrodents (usually the dog or monkey), whereas little or no data are available for rabbits. Therefore, it may be useful to conduct specific studies in nulliparous or pregnant rabbits in order to investigate potential interspecies differences in test compound disposition or the influence of pregnancy on absorption and clearance.

In embryofoetotoxicity studies, groups of pregnant rats and rabbits (typically four to five per dose level) are sacrificed at the end of treatment (day 16–18 postinsemination) to demonstrate drug exposure in dams and (if deemed appropriate) fetuses. Blood samples from dams can be taken 24 hours after the previous dose and up to 5 or 7 hours after the last dose, allowing a timely collection of fetuses. Fetal levels of test compound are generally measured only once, and they often correlate with maternal plasma concentrations. Experience indicates that many compounds cross the placental barrier and are present in fetal tissues at concentrations that essentially reflect their lipophilicity and/or protein binding; concentrations of test compound are generally lower in amniotic fluid than in fetal plasma or homogenates. It may also be useful to obtain toxicokinetic data in fertility (ICH Study 1/Segment 1) or pre- and postnatal (ICH Study 2/Segment 3) studies, especially when unexpected findings or adverse effects are observed. This should be decided case by case.

ANALYSIS OF BIOLOGICAL SAMPLES

A brief overview of analytical methodology and practice is provided here (there are many texts on this subject [28]). Blood or tissue samples are generally stored at $-20°C$ and analyzed for drug concentration within 2 months of collection. Most analytical methods use liquid–liquid or solid–phase extraction and liquid chromatography (LC) coupled to various modes of detection, notably UV, fluorescence, electrochemical, diode array, and, most importantly, mass spectrometry (LC-MS or LC-MS/MS). More recently, novel approaches have been developed to determine quantitatively circulating drug concentrations using dried blood spots (DBS) on paper, rather than conventional plasma samples. This assay requires small blood volumes (15 μl) and uses simple solvent extraction of a punch taken from the DBS sample, followed by LC-MS/MS [29]. Validation of the analytical techniques used is documented in a dossier that details the selection of the analytical column, mobile phase, detection mode, extraction mode, yield, linearity and recovery of calibration samples, repeatability, blind spikes, and stability at $-20°C$ for up to 2 months. Calibration samples and blind spikes (calibration samples that are given blinded to the operator) are prepared using fresh tissues (e.g., blood, organs, or amniotic fluid) from untreated animals. Experimental samples are then analyzed using the validated assay method. Each analytical run uses at least five calibration samples (plus internal standard) and two blind spikes, which ensures quality control. Drug concentrations are calculated by referring to the calibration curve. The use of one calibration curve per run allows analysts to spot changes rapidly in analytical performance. Duplicate samples are run whenever drug concentrations exceed the calibration range or if blind spikes produce unsatisfactory results ($\pm15\%$–20% of expected). Analyzing blood samples from the control group helps evaluate potential contaminations. The latter are generally limited or inexistent in intravenous and gavage studies, less so in inhalation, topical, or dietary studies where environmental conditions are more difficult to control (contaminated fur, licking of treated areas, generation of airborne powder during change of food containing hoppers). At least three blood samples per control animal are needed in order to distinguish random contaminations (isolated findings) from systematic ones or misdosing. The consistent presence of the test compound in blood samples from control groups at concentrations less than those found in the low-dose group usually signal systematic contamination. In contrast, consistent or erratic test compound concentrations in the range of those measured in treated animals are likely to reflect a mislabeling or a dosing error.

A number of mathematical models can be used to calculate pharmacokinetic characteristics. The latter are usually derived by log linear regression of the experimental data, using single or multiple compartments [28]. However, such models should be handled with care, as at least three to four data points per phase (absorption, distribution, elimination) are required to produce credible linear regressions, which is rare in small animals.

INTERPRETATION OF TOXICOKINETIC DATA

It should be borne in mind that the animals used in toxicology studies, early studies in particular, are often in a situation of 'overdose,' which can modify the absorption and the kinetics of the test compound. Bioavailability can be altered by poor dissolution of suspensions or solid formulations or by saturation of metabolism. Distribution of the test compound can be affected by binding to plasma proteins and/or tissues. Test compound metabolism may become rate limiting due to saturation of detoxification enzymes and inhibition/induction phenomena. Finally, disposition of the test compound can be compromised by extraphysiological or pathological changes in the gastrointestinal and cardiovascular systems or in the major organs of excretion. Hypothermia, anorexia, or increased water consumption are also common complications of overdose, affecting disposition.

Absorption

Even when a test compound is administered as a solution, absorption can be variable depending on the physicochemical properties of the active moiety and target tissues. In contrast to polar molecules, lipophilic substances that freely permeate the membranes are likely to be absorbed readily, blood flow at the absorption site governing the degree of absorption. If active transport occurs, the absorption may be retarded or decrease at high concentrations of the test compound. To anticipate such effects, diverse isolated-cell models (e.g., CaCo-2 cells) can be used to estimate cell permeability [30]. The influence of pH on absorption depends on the pKa of the test substance. Weak acids (pK$a > 8$) remain predominantly unionized in the gastrointestinal tract (which has a pH of 1–8) and in the urine (which has a pH of 4–9), whereas the absorption of free bases is likely to be pH sensitive if their pKa is between 5 and 11 [31]. Administration of suspensions or solid formulations, the most frequent treatment modes in toxicology studies, requires that dissolution (a prerequisite to passage across the gut wall) is complete. In rats, large doses of poorly soluble compounds and/or large volumes of administration often cause delays in absorption and time-to-peak blood concentration (C_{max}), particularly if linked to a decrease in gastric emptying and gastrointestinal motility. Consequently, clearance of the test compound is frequently slower at the high-dose levels used in toxicology studies than predicted from low-dose pharmacokinetic studies. Peak levels of circulating test compound can be delayed and distribution/elimination prolonged, resulting in much longer apparent half-lives than anticipated. One should therefore be careful not to overinterpret low-dose pharmacokinetic data and make sure that they do not lead to erroneous conclusions and decisions such as selecting the wrong species for studies or withdrawing a compound prematurely from being developed. Gastrointestinal intolerance (diarrhea, emesis), degradation in the gut lumen or by enzymes in the gut wall, and first-pass metabolism by the liver can also result in loss of the test compound.

   All these considerations emphasize the need for carefully selecting candidates based on their physicochemical properties and for defining proper pharmaceutical strategies (e.g., developing an appropriate formulation, pH adjustments, and salts.) as early as possible in the compound development process.

Distribution

The distribution rate is influenced by delivery of test compound to tissues (perfusion), membrane permeability (diffusion), and binding to blood components and tissues. Sustained exposure to high concentrations of a test compound enhances/expands delivery to tissues and increases the chances of forming irreversible cellular/molecular binding and eliciting target organ toxicity. However, polar molecules may diffuse poorly through relatively impermeable membranes (CNS, muscle, kidney, placenta). This may be critical for drugs that need to cross the blood–brain barrier to exert their activity, as well as for polar molecules or reactive metabolites that may be teratogenic or carcinogenic. Binding of test compound to plasma proteins is generally very rapid and reversible and depends on the affinity constant (K_a) and concentrations of drug and protein. Acidic drugs bind to serum albumin. Basic compounds bind to alphaglycoproteins, which are less abundant and more rapidly saturated than albumin. The concentration of systemic free drug (not bound to plasma proteins) is important because it often serves to calculate exposure multiples in humans relative to animals, especially when there are major differences in binding capacities across species. Once plasma protein binding has been determined in all species over a large range of drug concentrations (to detect variability or saturation), plasma drug concentrations measured in pivotal animal studies can be corrected for protein binding and compared to free human concentrations at the efficacious dose.

Binding to red blood cells can also be a significant factor for compounds that are known to interact with erythrocytic enzymes (e.g., carbonic anhydrase inhibitors) or that exhibit high volumes of distribution ($V_d > 5$ L/kg). In such cases, it is usually advisable to measure test compound concentrations in whole blood rather than in plasma.

Liver and Renal Elimination of a Test Compound

The Extracting of test compounds from the systemic circulation by the liver is governed by hepatic blood flows at the entry and exit of the organ and by hepatic metabolism and biliary excretion (bearing in mind that the latter is best predicted by dogs; rats do not have a gall bladder). Blood flows can be affected by suprapharmacological action, such as sustained hypotension, as well as by physiological or pathological conditions (e.g., pregnancy, age, cardiac changes, and organ damage). Reduced hepatic clearance generally results in an increase in systemic bioavailability and can be due to saturation of metabolism enzymes, inhibition of enzyme activity by the test compound or its metabolites, exhaustion of essential cofactors (e.g., glutathione), or enzyme destruction (e.g., binding of troleandomycin products to CYP450) [32]. In contrast, induction of metabolism enzymes accelerates hepatic clearance. Estimating such variations by measuring plasma concentrations of a test compound after repeat dosage and by looking at specific enzymes, primarily hepatic CYP450s, is an essential part of early toxicity assessment. This can be done *in vitro* using cellular models expressing specific CYP450s or *in vivo* by measuring total microsomal CYP450 content [33] in liver samples collected from main-group animals in dose-finding studies. The differential induction of specific CYP450 subforms can be determined by immunoblotting. Induction of hepatic CYP450 is a very frequent occurrence after treatment of rodents with xenobiotics but less so in dogs. Generally, a two- to threefold increase in total hepatic microsomal CYP450 content occurs, often accompanied by liver enlargement and sometimes by lipid deposits. Frequently, thyroid hypertrophy also occurs due to increased hepatic thyroxin clearance and feedback stimulation of the thyroid via the hypothalamus and the pituitary. These effects are generally regarded as an adaptive rather than toxic response to treatment. In chronic rodent studies, this can give rise to hepatic and/or thyroid tumors. Supported by mechanistic studies, this type of finding should not hinder the further development of a drug candidate. Because several (moderate) enzyme inducers have received regulatory approval, it appears as though the regulatory authorities are generally ready to accept such drugs, provided safe doses have be identified and reasonable mechanistic data provided. If necessary, exploratory studies can be conducted to provide supporting data. For example, thyroid function can be monitored by measuring thyroid hormone levels (e.g., T3, T4, and TSH) and inducible xenobiotic metabolism enzymes (CYP450 and UDPGT). In all situations, it is important to identify strong enzyme inhibitors or inducers, as they have the potential to produce drug–drug interactions that require specific clinical investigations with reference drug substrates.

Renal excretion is characterized by glomerular filtration, active secretion of (many) acids and bases, and reabsorption of lipophilic molecules. These processes may be sensitive to subtle changes in the ionic balance affecting urinary pH or urine composition. For example, carbonic anhydrase inhibitors (diuretics) tend to acidify the blood pH and render urine more alkaline while increasing urinary output and modifying the excretion of sodium, potassium, or phosphates. At high doses, these effects may become irreversible and lead to stone formation and nephropathy. Toxic changes can also be induced by aminoglycosides [34] or vehicles such as cyclodextrins that accumulate in the kidneys, thereby affecting their own clearance or modifying the renal function. Simplistically, one can assume that total body clearance of the test compound most often reflects liver and/or renal clearances and can be used to predict human clearance owing to allometric scaling methods. The latter are based on the fact that cardiac output, blood flows, and drug-metabolizing capacities tend to decline with increasing body weight across species. Total clearance does not scale in a proportional manner but to a power function of about 0.7, regardless of species. For example, if the mean plasma clearance in a 0.25-kg rat is 10 ml/min, then for a 70-kg human:

$$\text{Human clearance estimate} = (\text{clearance in rat} \times \text{body weight human})/$$
$$\text{body weight rat})^{0.7}$$
$$= (10 \times 70/0.25)^{0.7}$$
$$= 250 \, \text{ml/min or } 3.6 \, \text{ml/min/kg}$$

From this value, we can estimate drug exposure for a given human dose from the equation:

$$\text{AUC} = \text{dose/clearance}$$

Dose, Time, and Sex Dependencies

By examining C_{max} and AUC, it is possible to determine if there are gender differences in experimental animals and to relate exposure to length of treatment and to dose. Gender differences give indications on potential differences in metabolic pathways involved in drug clearance particularly in rats where we know that a number of xenobiotics are metabolized by sex-dependent CYP450 isozymes of the 3A and 2C families [35]. This results in higher levels of unchanged drug in females and of metabolites in males. If a metabolite is pharmacologically active, regulatory authorities may recommend using the combined AUC of the parent drug and metabolite (rather than the drug AUC alone) in order to compare genders and define safety margins better. As fewer or no sex-related

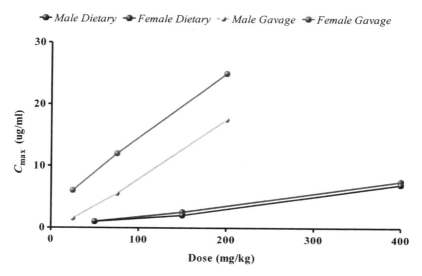

Male Dietary *Female Dietary* *Male Gavage* *Female Gavage*

Figure 6.1. Effect of route of administration on maximal plasma drug concentrations (C_{max}) of a dihydropyridine derivative in rats.

differences are seen in other species, the relevance of (male) rat data to the human situation may sometimes be questioned. However, these differences often diminish with age and increasing dose levels due to decrease/saturation of liver metabolizing enzymes. In addition, the route of administration may influence the metabolic or toxic response by increasing or decreasing peak effects. The same oral dose may produce clear gender differences after gavage treatment, whereas little or no effects are seen after dietary administration (Fig. 6.1). Such changes need to be factored in when switching from gavage to dietary administration before carcinogenicity studies.

The relation between dose and exposure is evidenced by linear or nonlinear kinetics. Linear kinetics is characterized by dose-proportional increases in AUC or C_{max}; they indicate that toxicokinetic parameters are independent of dose or test compound concentration. In practice, toxicokinetic data from consecutive toxicology studies can be superimposed when normalized for dose level. In contrast, super- or subproportionality is indicative of changes occurring in absorption, distribution, excretion, or metabolism. Quite often, however, superproportional increases in exposure indicate a reduction in hepatic clearance with increasing dose, whereas subproportional increases suggest poor absorption or autoinduction. The latter is defined as the capacity of a drug to increase the synthesis of the enzymes responsible for its own metabolism. Autoinduction can be detected a few hours after treatment is initiated or after several days, leading to clear reductions of AUCs on repeat treatment. The observation needs to be repeated, however, as autoinduction may be inconsistent and vary with species, sex, dose, or duration of treatment. In a single toxicity species, a given drug can cause autoinduction at lower doses and accumulation at higher levels (Fig. 6.2), the point of inflexion corresponding to the dose beyond which metabolism enzymes are saturated. In toxicological terms, this complex profile can lead to a rapid buildup of toxic effects beyond the point of inflexion

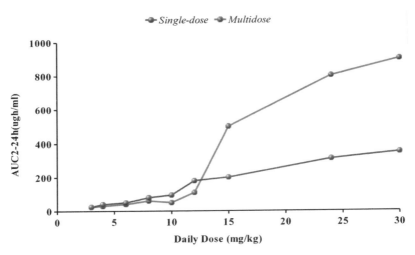

Figure 6.2. Variation of exposure (AUC) with dose level on single and multiple dosing of an azole derivative in dogs.

whereas little or no toxicity occurs at low, clinically relevant, concentrations. Accumulation of plasma concentrations with time is another frequent response to drug treatments. It may be due to pharmacokinetic reasons (long half-life) or to drastic changes in drug clearance at higher dose levels. In all situations, it is important to determine drug concentrations at steady state, which is generally achieved after four to six half-lives and depends on dosing frequency.

CONCLUSION

Toxicokinetic data generated throughout the drug development process offer the toxicologist the possibility to adjust formulations, interpret toxicity findings, and design subsequent studies.

Toxicokinetics support the choice of formulations being given to experimental animals and demonstrate bioequivalence when the route/mode of administration is modified. By measuring plasma drug concentrations regularly, preclinical scientists can verify the degree of absorption across species and the consistency/reproducibility of the drug exposure and effects across studies, thereby validating the route of administration and the choice of species. In turn, the quality of the formulations may influence drug bioavailability and kinetics, depending on the physicochemical properties of the active moiety and target tissues. It is therefore desirable to select drug candidates carefully according to their physicochemical properties and to define proper pharmaceutical strategies (pH adjustments, buffers, salts) as early as possible in the development process. However, changing a salt or a formulation during the life cycle of a drug should not be regarded as a trivial exercise; such changes are susceptible not only to affect a drug's disposition but also its toxicity profile, sometimes dramatically. In addition, new formulations introduce new impurities or degradation products that need to be carefully monitored and qualified. Qualification is based on risk assessments supported by nonclinical or clinical studies, scientific publications, or predictive databases such as DEREK. The main risk that needs to be addressed is mutagenicity, an indirect indicator of carcinogenicity. Impurities and residual solvents that present no structural alerts can be treated along ICH guidelines, recognizing that some flexibility is needed for early development. Impurities that are known to be carcinogenic and/or mutagenic should be eliminated or controlled to low ppm levels according to CHMP recommendations. Similarly, metal residues should be controlled to CHMP-recommended levels: these CHMP guidelines are being progressively accepted by most major regulatory authorities. Finally, due diligence is needed to identify and qualify reactive metabolites.

Toxicokinetic studies help to identify such potentially active/reactive metabolites. Most importantly, these studies provide key information on the linearity of the dose response, gender differences, and phenomena linked to autoinduction or drug accumulation. Inspecting AUCs and C_{max} versus dose across species is an excellent way to compare the data and establish realistic safety margins on clinical usage of the drug. We point out, however, that no single safety factor can be relied upon exclusively. Like efficacy, toxicity may not relate to plasma concentration profiles but to drug levels in the target tissues or, more simplistically, to dose when activity or toxic manifestations are due to a metabolite. As toxicology and clinical programs unfold, more information becomes available on drug disposition in animals and humans. Radiolabel and tissue distribution studies provide a framework for addressing the need to monitor metabolites. Excretion data help decide whether plasma concentrations represent a significant proportion of the administered dose or not and contribute to explain interspecies differences in drug disposition.

Overall, toxicokinetic studies provide reassurance as to the use of the no-effect dose level in the safety evaluation process. The design of these studies must be flexible with attention given to assay validation, matrix, formulation, sampling times, duration, and type of study and relevance of metabolites and dose levels.

REFERENCES

1. Marks LS and Kolmen SN, 1971. Tween 20 shock in dogs and related fibrinogen changes. *Am J Physiol* **220**:218–221

2. Perrin JH, Field FP, Hansen DA et al., 1978. β-Cyclodextrin as an aid to peritoneal dialysis. Renal toxicity of β-cyclodextrin in the rat. *Chem Pathol Pharmacol* **19**:373–376

3. Everett RM, Descotes G, Rollin M, Greener Y, Bradford JC, Benziger DP, and Ward SJ, 1993. Nephrotoxicity of pravadoline maleate (WIN 48098-6) in dogs: Evidence of maleic acid-induced acute tubular necrosis. *Fundam Appl Toxicol* **21**(1):59–65

4. Sangster B, Blom JL, Sekhuis VM et al., 1983. The influence of sodium bromide in man: A study in human volunteers, with special emphasis on the endocrine and the central nervous system. *Food Chem Toxicol* **21**:409–419

5. Harper AE, Benevenga NJ, and Wohlhueter RM, 1970. Effects of ingestion of disproportionate amounts of amino acids. *Physiol Rev* **50**:428–558

6. Charuel C, Comby P, and Monro AM, 1992. Diurnal exposure profile in rats from dietary administration of a chemical (Doxazosin) with a short half-life: interplay of age and diurnal feeding pattern. *J Appl Toxicol 12*, 7–11

7. International Conference on Harmonization, 2002. Impurities in new drug substances. http://www.emea.eu.int/pdfs/human/ich/273799en.pdf

8. International Conference on Harmonization, 2003. Impurities in new drug products. http://www.emea.eu.int/pdfs/human/ich/273899en.pdf

9. Greene N, 2002. Computer systems for the prediction of toxicity: An update. *Adv Drug Deliv Rev 54*:417–431

10. Leblanc B, Charuel C, Ku W, and Ogilvie R, 2004. Acceptability of low levels of genotoxic impurities in new drug substances. *Int J Pharm Med 18*:215–220

11. Kenyon MO, Cheung JR, Dobo KL, and Ku WW, 2007. An evaluation of the sensitivity of the Ames assay to discern low-level mutagenic impurities. *Regul Toxicol Pharmacol 48*:75–86

12. Müller L and Kasper P, 2000. Human biological relevance and the use of threshold-arguments in regulatory genotoxicity assessment: experience with pharmaceuticals. *Mutat Res 464*: 19–34

13. Snyder RD and Green JW, 2001. A review of the genotoxicity of marketed pharmaceuticals. *Mutat Res 488*:151–169

14. Bos PMJ, Baars B, Marcel TM, and van Raaij TM, 2004. Risk assessment of peak exposure to genotoxic carcinogens. *Toxicol Lett 151*:43–50

15. Mueller L, Mauthe RJ, Riley CM et al., 2006. A rationale for determining, testing, and controlling specific impurities in pharmaceuticals that possess potential for genotoxicity. *Regul Toxicol Pharmacol 44*:198–211

16. Committee for Medicinal Products for Human Use, 2006. Guideline on the limits of genotoxic impurities. http://www.emea.europa.eu/pdfs/human/swp/519902en.pdf

17. Munro IC, Kennepohl E, and Kroes RA, 1999. Procedure for safety evaluation of flavouring substances. *Food Chem Toxicol 37*:207–232

18. Kroes R, Galli C, Munro I, Schilter B et al., 2000. Threshold of toxicological concern for chemical substances present in the diet: a practical tool for assessing the need for toxicity testing. *Food Chem Toxicol 38*:255–312

19. Committee for Medicinal Products for Human Use, 2007. Questions and answers on the CHMP guideline on the limits of genotoxic impurities. http://www.emea.europa. eu/pdfs/human/swp/43199407en.pdf

20. Center for Drug Evaluation and Research, 2008. Safety testing of drug metabolites. http://www.fda.gov/downloads/Drugs/GuidanceComplianceRegulatoryInformation/ Guidances/ucm079266.pdf

21. Baillie TA, Cayen MN, Fouda H et al., 2002. Drug metabolites in safety testing. *Toxicol Appl Pharmacol 182*:188–196

22. Smith DA and Obach RS, 2009. Metabolites in safety testing (MIST): Considerations of mechanisms of toxicity with dose, abundance and duration of treatment. *Chem Res Toxicol 22*:267–279

23. Committee for Medicinal Products for Human Use, 2008. Guideline on the specification limits for residues of metal catalysts. http://www.emea.europa.eu/pdfs/human/ swp/444600.pdf

24. Malo JL, 2005. Occupational rhinitis and asthma due to metal salts. *Allergy 60*:138–139

25. Kerger BD, Finley BL, Corbett GE et al., 1997. Ingestion of chromium (VI) in drinking water by human volunteers: Absorption, distribution and excretion of single and repeated doses. *J Toxicol Environ Health* **50**:67–95

26. International Conference on Harmonisation of Technical Requirements for Registration of Pharmaceuticals for Human Use, 1997. Impurities: Residual Solvents. http://www.emea.eu.int/pdfs/human/ich/028395en.pdf

27. Schmucker DL, 1985. Ageing and drug disposition: An update. *Pharmacol Rev* **37**:133–148.

28. Kwon Y, 2001. *Handbook of Essential Pharmacokinetics, Pharmacodynamics and Drug Metabolism for Industrial Scientists*. New York: Springer-Verlag, Inc.

29. Spooner N, Lad R, and Barfield M, 2009. Dried blood spots as a sample collection technique for the determination of pharmacokinetics in clinical studies: Considerations for the validation of a quantitative bioanalytical method. *Anal Chem* **81**:1557–1563

30. Hubatsch I, Ragnarsson EG, and Artursson P, 2007. Determination of drug permeability and prediction of drug absorption in Caco-2 monolayers. *Nat Protoc* **2**: 2111–2119

31. Smith DA, Humphrey MJ, and Charuel C, 1990. Design of toxicokinetic studies. *Xenobiotica* **11**:1187–1199

32. Pessayre D, Descatoire V, Konstantinova-Mitcheva M et al., 1981. Self-induction by triacetyloleandomycin of its own transformation into a metabolite forming a stable 456 nm-absorbing complex with cytochrome P-450. *Biochem Pharmacol* **30**:553–558

33. Omura T and Sato R, 1964. The carbon monoxide binding pigment of liver microsomes. *J Biol Chem* **239**:2370–2378

34. Charuel C, Faccini J, Monro AM, and Nachbaur J, 1984. A second peak in uptake of Gentamicin by rat kidney after cessation of treatment. *Biopharm Drug Dispos* **5**:21–24

35. Smith DA, 1991. Species differences in metabolism and pharmacokinetics: Are we close to an understanding? *Drug Metab Rev* **23**:355–373

7

GENERAL TOXICOLOGY

Alberto Lodola

INTRODUCTION

A wide range of molecules are evaluated in drug development. In the past, these were usually new chemical entities (NCEs) [1]. More recently, new biological entities (NBEs), such as proteins, antibodies, oligonucleotides, and viral vectors for gene therapy, are also being developed as pharmaceuticals [2–6]. Regardless of the chemical or pharmacological class of the substance under consideration, its toxicity is related to one or more of the following factors:

- chemical structure of the molecule
- dose administered
- duration of exposure
- route of administration
- sensitivity of the test species to the molecule
- age and gender of the test species
- absorption, distribution, metabolism, and excretion of the molecule
- interaction with other chemicals

The impact of these factors on the toxicity of a test molecule is characterized in a series of animal toxicity studies of increasing complexity and duration. To facilitate

Pharmaceutical Toxicology in Practice: A Guide for Non-Clinical Development, Edited by Alberto Lodola and Jeanne Stadler
© 2011 John Wiley & Sons, Inc.

comparisons between different molecules, a number of parameters are derived from studies [7–9], including the following:

- LD50: dose at which half of all animals treated with a single dose of test compound die
- NOAEL (no-observed adverse effect level): highest dose at which treatment-related findings occur but that are not considered to be adverse
- NOEL (no-observed effect level): highest dose at which no treatment-related findings occur
- MTD (maximum tolerated dose): highest dose tolerated by test animals

Understanding the toxicity of a drug candidate is essential for safe progression into the clinic and onto the market. The NOAEL from the most sensitive toxicology species is used to set the starting dose for Phase 1 clinical studies, using a range of allometric scaling approaches [10]. Toxicity data also provide valuable support to discovery scientists in identifying safer, follow-up molecules for development if the lead candidate fails and is central in reducing compound attrition [11, 12]. Current toxicity studies rely heavily on the use of animals, while significant effort is focused on finding alternatives to animals the current situation will probably not change in the near future. Toxicity studies are conducted within a regulatory and legislative framework overseen by national agencies. In the United States, the responsible agency is the Food and Drug Administration (FDA); in the European Union, it is the European Medicines Agency (EMEA) and country-based agencies. In Japan, the Ministry of Health, Labour and Welfare (MHLW, the so called "Koseirodosho") is responsible for pharmaceutical regulatory affairs and is supported by the Pharmaceuticals and Medical Devices Evaluation Center (the so-called "Evaluation Center"), which is part of the National Institute of Health Sciences. A comprehensive discussion of the principal national regulatory authorities and country submission requirements for new drugs is provided by Chalmers [13]. For many years, drug development guidelines were developed locally by country-based agencies, leading to a lack of harmonization, reducing efficiency, increasing costs, and delaying the arrival of new drugs to market. The International Conference on Harmonization (ICH) process (see Chapter 2 for a detailed discussion) was established to address this issue. As a result, a set of internationally harmonized guidelines now covers most aspects of the drug development and registration process. These have been incorporated into the regulatory framework of ICH-participating nations. A complete review of all the regulatory guidelines is outside the scope of this discussion; however, a selected list of key nonclinical guidelines is given in Table 7.1. Because these guidelines (harmonized and national) are revised at intervals, the toxicologist must keep abreast of the changes. These guidelines do not limit the number, or range, of studies that are conducted or do they say that it is necessary to conduct all the studies in Table 7.1. The guidelines do not describe an all-encompassing toxicology study strategy for developing drugs. Not all drug development situations are covered by the guidelines; in some cases, the guidelines lag behind the evolution in the types of pharmaceuticals under development (e.g., the

TABLE 7.1. Selected guidelines applicable to toxicity studies and drug development.

ICH Guidance	
S1A	Need for carcinogenicity studies of pharmaceuticals
S1B	Testing for carcinogenicity of pharmaceuticals
S1C (R2)	Dose selection for carcinogenicity studies of pharmaceuticals
S3A	Note for guidance on toxicokinetics: The assessment of systemic exposure in toxicity studies
	Single-dose toxicity tests
S4A	Duration of chronic toxicity testing in animals (rodent and nonrodent toxicity testing)
S6	Preclinical safety evaluation of biotechnology-derived pharmaceuticals
S8	Immunotoxicity studies for human pharmaceuticals
S9	Nonclinical evaluation for anticancer pharmaceuticals
M3(R2)	Guidance on nonclinical safety studies for the conduct of human clinical trials for pharmaceuticals and marketing authorizations for pharmaceuticals

National Guidelines		
FDA	EMEA	
✓		Carcinogenicity study protocol submissions
✓		Content and format of INDs* for Phase 1 studies of drugs, including well-characterized, therapeutic, biotechnology-derived products
✓		Exploratory IND* studies
✓		Immunotoxicology evaluation of INDs*
✓		Nonclinical studies for the safety evaluation of pharmaceutical excipients
✓	✓	Photosafety testing
✓		Safety testing of drug metabolites
✓		Nonclinical safety evaluation of drug or biologic combinations
✓		Nonclinical studies for the safety evaluation of pharmaceutical excipients
✓		Safety testing of drug metabolites
✓	✓	Single-dose toxicity
✓	✓	Nonclinical development of combination drugs
✓	✓	Nonclinical guideline on drug-induced hepatotoxicity (draft)
	✓	Repeated dose toxicity
	✓	CHMP SWP conclusions and recommendations on the use of genetically modified animal models for carcinogenicity assessment
	✓	Carcinogenic potential
	✓	Nonclinical local tolerance testing of medicinal products
	✓	Nonclinical studies required before first clinical use of gene therapy medicinal products
	✓	Preclinical evaluation of anti-cancer medicinal products
	✓	Preclinical pharmacological and toxicological testing of vaccines
	✓	Note for guidance on the preclinical evaluation of anticancer medicinal product

* IND: investigational new drug.

current interest in antisense oligonucleotides or nanotechnologies). In these instances, the application of basic principles allows key toxicological issues to be identified, and the current guidelines provide baseline recommendations that can be adapted to address these issues.

TOXICOLOGY STRATEGY DEVELOPMENT

There is no single "right" general toxicology strategy for all compounds; however, a good starting point in deciding which studies are needed is the ICH M3(R2) guideline [14]. It must be borne in mind that in developing a strategy, the interests of a number of development partners must be protected [15]: clinical volunteers, patients, the pharmaceutical company, the scientific community, and regulatory authorities. A strategy should be developed on a case-by-case basis, taking the physicochemical characteristics of the test compound, its pharmacological profile, the target therapeutic indication, and clinical dosing regimen into account [16, 17]. Strategies developed for compounds that have similar structures and/or pharmacological activity to the compound to be tested is a useful source of (often-underexploited) information. In most cases, the strategy decided upon must ensure that:

1. ICH and national guidelines are met,
2. the toxicology data needed to support clinical trials are produced
3. all the toxicity data needed to support the drug marketing application are produced
4. target organ/s of toxicity are identified,
5. the toxicity-dose response is characterized,
6. the NOAEL is determined.

Only points relating to regulatory compliance are an absolute requirement (points 1–3). With respect to the toxicological endpoints (points 4–6), there are instances in which the data are not required, as when testing drugs derived from biotechnology or due to dosing issues [18–21], for example. Ideally, the studies in the toxicology strategy should also do the following:

- identify biomarkers of toxicity for use in clinical studies,
- ensure that the availability of toxicity data is not rate limiting in reaching key project milestones and decision points, and
- provide sufficient data to support the development of a risk management strategy for humans.

Three major categories of studies must be considered for inclusion in any well-thought-out strategy that we shall call core studies, bridging studies, and investigative/

TABLE 7.2. Toxicology studies included in a benchmark strategy* for drug development.

	Species	
	Rodent	Nonrodent
Core Toxicology Studies		
Escalating dose	√	√
7- to 14-day repeat-dose range finding	√	√
14- or 28-day repeat dose*	√	√
6-month repeat dose*	√	
9-month repeat dose*		√
3-month range-finding study	√	
2-year carcinogenicity*	√	
Bridging Studies	As necessary	As necessary
Investigative/Mechanistic	As necessary	As necessary

* Regulatory toxicology studies.
* Typical studies that form part of a benchmark strategy. Nonregulatory studies are conducted to assist dose selection in regulatory studies. Regulatory studies are consistent with international regulatory guidelines and support the conduct of clinical trials. Bridging and mechanistic studies should be designed on an as-needed basis to address specific issues.

mechanistic studies. A benchmark toxicology strategy would be based on the core studies shown in Table 7.2; these are studies of increasing duration and complexity and usually run sequentially. Data from the preceding study are used to establish the doses and to refine the study design for follow-up studies. Core studies can be run in parallel; however, this is a high-risk strategy and is often only warranted if there is a high level of understanding of the structural and pharmacological class of the compound under study. It is useful at this point to make a distinction between so-called "regulatory studies" and "nonregulatory studies." Regulatory studies are mandated by the regulatory authorities to support clinical trials and product registration; all other studies (even though they provide useful and at times critical supporting data) are nonregulatory. Drug development is a dynamic process. As the toxicology program unfolds, changes are often made to the development program. For example, the test formulation may be revised, the synthetic pathway for the test compound may be modified, or the clinical route of administration may change. To avoid unnecessary repetition of core studies, bridging studies are conducted. These studies are designed to investigate the impact of the change in the development program on the toxicological profile of the test compound. They provide a bridge between the toxicology data generated using the new formulation, route of administration, or test compound derived from the new synthetic route with the toxicology data already in hand. Ideally, a bridging toxicology study should be a repeat of one of the core studies (usually the 1-month study) in one species (usually the rat) and use the same doses tested in the core study. If there is no significant difference between the original toxicology data and that from the bridging study, then the change is "qualified" and a "bridge" has been established to the data available. If there is a significant difference, a bridging study should be conducted in a nonrodent species. Then, in the light of all data from both bridging studies, a decision is made as to the effect of the new findings on the overall nonclinical risk assessment. If necessary, the need for additional studies and/or the need to repeat core studies are decided. To better understand and manage findings in a core study, a more detailed characterization of the toxicities observed may be needed (e.g., time to onset of the lesion, refinement of the dose–response curve, or to investigate the underlying pathogenic mechanism for production of a lesion). These aims could be achieved by incorporating additional endpoints into a core study. Although this aspect is superficially attractive because there is an apparent saving in time and resources, it is not the best strategy to adopt in our view. The increased complexity of the studies can compromise the primary objectives of the core study. In addition, there is limited flexibility in dose selection, dosing regimen, and the range, type, and timing of samples that are collected in core studies. It is much better to design and conduct specific investigative/mechanistic studies to address these concerns. The design of an investigative study is flexible and can be tailored to the specific treatment and sampling needs required to meet study objectives. In the end, this is the most cost-effective approach.

Drug development is a long, often-slow process, and there is always pressure to reduce nonclinical use of the test compound or to speed up the nonclinical development program. One way to achieve these goals is to develop a strategy in which preliminary studies are shorter than usual or even omitted altogether. For example, escalating dose and range-finding studies are reduced in duration or omitted altogether; the high dose is set as a function of test compound availability or as a small multiple of projected clinical doses. In some cases, studies are conducted in only one gender of test animals. The decision to use these modified approaches must be made in the light of the available data; also, the project team and management must understand, and be prepared to accept, the risks involved in these approaches. If the test compound is from a well-characterized pharmacological class, or if there are extensive toxicity data for a close structural analog, then the benefits of such an abbreviated toxicology program may outweigh the risks. We have found that this is rarely the case. Given the high attrition rate of drug candidates [22], due in many cases to toxicity, it is important to develop a solid understanding of the potential toxicity of the test compound as soon as possible. Olson et al. [23] have shown that in the majority of cases, it is possible to identify the principal toxicities of a test compound in 1-month toxicity studies in two species. The most effective way to do achieve this is by conducting a robust series of toxicity studies in male and female animals; this saves time, money, and test compound in the end.

TOXICITY STUDIES NEEDED TO SUPPORT CLINICAL STUDIES

The type and duration of toxicology studies needed to support clinical trials (and marketing approval) is mandated by the regulatory authorities and discussed in detail in the ICH M3(R2) guideline [14]. As might be expected, the longer the duration of the clinical trial, the more animal toxicology data are needed. We have summarized current (core) study requirements in Table 7.3. The studies listed apply directly to the development

TABLE 7.3. General requirements for nonclinical studies in support of clinical studies and marketing [14].

	Repeat-Dose Toxicity Studies	
	Rodent	Nonrodent
To Support Clinical Trials		
Duration of Clinical trial		
≤2 weeks	2 weeks	2 weeks
2 weeks to 6 months	Same Duration as Clinical Trial	
>6 months	6 months	9 months
To Support Marketing		
Treatment duration	Rodent	Nonrodent
≤ 2 weeks	1 month	1 month
>2 weeks to 1 month	3 months	3 months
>1 month to 3 months	6 months	3 months
> 3 months	6 months	9 months

General guidance on duration of repeat-dose toxicity studies are needed to support clinical trials in the ICH regions. Requirements are discussed in detail in ICH M3(R2) guideline [2].

of NCEs; however; the full range of studies is often not appropriate [24] for NBEs; for example, studies of long duration with protein drugs are usually not possible due to the development of antibodies. In addition, drugs under development for the treatment of life threatening or serious diseases without current and or effective therapy may warrant an expedited nonclinical development program. In these cases, studies may be abbreviated, deferred, or omitted (18, 19, 25, 26). In addition, the EMEA has developed guidelines for combination drugs, vaccines, anticancer drugs, and gene-therapy medicinal products. It is best to develop a nonclinical strategy on a case-by-case basis, even for an NCE. In cases where there is significant regulatory or scientific ambiguity (e.g., in developing a drug derived from biotechnology), it is possible to customize the study list given in Table 7.3 to the needs of the compound under development. This is based on the accepted objectives of toxicity studies, the guidelines that are available, and the data needed to develop a risk–benefit assessment. It is worth noting that if ambiguity exists for the toxicologist, it probably also exists for the regulatory authorities; as a result, the underlying rationale for the proposed strategy must be clearly described and discussed and finalized after consulting the regulatory authorities whenever possible.

In recent years, approaches that are more experimental have emerged regarding the type of early clinical studies being conducted. With these new approaches, Phase 1 clinical studies can be started much earlier than with a "classical" approach, and less supporting toxicity data are needed. For example, in an exploratory Investigational New Drug (IND) [27, 28], the duration of clinical dosing is limited (e.g., 7 days). However, unlike a normal IND, the exploratory IND is designed to investigate pharmacodynamic

TABLE 7.4. Main design and features of core toxicology studies.

Type of Study	No. of Doses	Species	No. of Dose Groups	Animals/Sex/Group R	Animals/Sex/Group NR	Study Groups R and NR Main	Study Groups R and NR Rev	Study Groups R TK
Escalating dose	Single	R and NR	≥1	≤2	1	√		
Up to 1 month	Repeat	R and NR	≥4	5	3	√	√	√
Up to 3 months	Repeat	R and NR	≥4	10	4	√	√	√
Up to 12 months	Repeat	R and NR	≥4	20	4	√		√
2 years*	Repeat	R	≥4	50		√		√

* Carcinogencity studies.

Typical design feature of core toxicology studies. Reversibility studies can either be conducted as part of a 1-month or 3-month toxicity study. Because blood samples for toxicokinetics analysis are usually taken from main study animals, there are no toxicokinetics groups in nonrodent studies.

Abbreviations: TK = toxicokinetics; R = rodent; NR = nonrodent; Rev = reversibility.

endpoints, not tolerability. Three types of clinical studies are allowed under an exploratory IND:

- *Microdose trials to evaluate pharmacokinetics or imaging of specific targets*
  - Extended single-dose toxicity studies in a single mammalian species are used to support this clinical study if justified by *in vitro* metabolism data and by comparative data on *in vitro* pharmacodynamic effects.
- *Clinical trials designed to study pharmacologic effects of candidate products*
  - Repeat-dose clinical trials lasting up to 7 days can be supported by a 2-week repeat-dose toxicology study in a sensitive species, accompanied by toxicokinetic evaluations.
- *Clinical studies intended to evaluate mechanisms of action*

CONDUCT OF TOXICOLOGY STUDIES: OVERVIEW OF STUDY DESIGN

A well-designed toxicity study should produce adverse effects, at the highest dose, in the test species with the exceptions discussed below. It is also essential that all those involved in conducting toxicology studies recognize that one of their responsibilities is to ensure that animal suffering is kept to a minimum. Not only does this ensure ethical (and legal) experimentation, but it is also good science, as excessive toxicity will cause unnecessary suffering for the test animal and, in many instances, will probably confound assessment of the toxicity of the test molecule. The degree of systemic or local exposure to the test compound must be determined, and, at some stage, the reversibility or otherwise of adverse effects must also be determined. To achieve this, a standardized study design is used in core studies, the main features of which we have summarized in Table 7.4. Detailed descriptions of toxicology study design are provided by the Organisation for Economic Co-operation and Development (OECD) [29], the National

TABLE 7.5. Typical data collected in toxicology studies.

	Single Dose		Repeat Dose	
Parameter	R	NR	R	NR
In-Life Parameters				
Mortality	✓	✓	✓	✓
Clinical signs	✓	✓	✓	✓
Body weight	✓	✓	✓	✓
Food and water consumption	✓	✓	✓	✓
Ophthalmology			✓	✓
Blood Pressure				✓
ECG				✓
Laboratory Analysis				
Toxicokinetics			✓	✓
Hematology			✓	✓
Clinical Chemistry			✓	✓
Urinalysis			✓	✓
Postmortem				
Necropsy	✓	✓	✓	✓
Organ weights			✓	✓
Histopathology of tissue			✓	✓

Abbreviations: R: Rodent; NR: nonrodent.

Toxicology Program [30], and the FDA's *Redbook* [31]. These study descriptions should be used as baseline designs and tailored to the needs of the compound being studied, taking account of any specific project-related issue. Studies are usually conducted with rodents and nonrodents. For carcinogenicity studies, only rodents are used. In 1-day toxicity studies, groups of animals are treated once and then observed for clinical signs for up to 14 days; in escalating dose studies, the dose is increased or decreased in the light of the effects produced by the previous dose. Animals in repeat-dose studies are treated each day of the study; there are usually at least four main study groups per gender (control, low, mid, and high dose). Additional rodent groups (so-called toxicokinetic groups) are added for monitoring systemic exposure. In nonrodent studies, blood samples for toxicokinetics are taken from the main study animals. When the reversibility of treatment-induced lesions is assessed, additional groups of animals (usually at least one additional control and high-dose group/sex) are added to the study. At the end of the treatment, the main study animals are sacrificed and animals in the reversibility groups are maintained without further treatment for a time that is sufficient to allow partial or complete reversal of lesion prior to the animals being sacrificed.

A wide range of parameters is monitored in studies; the most commonly collected data are summarized in Table 7.5. The objectives of a single-dose study can be met by collecting a limited set of data; this simplified design also allows rapid completion of these studies. A wider range of parameters is monitored in repeat-dose toxicity studies.

The in-life data provide information about the general health of animals and the effects of treatment on physiological functions. Blood pressure and ECG data are usually not collected for rodents, as they are highly variable and unreliable. These data are collected in nonrodents, but the data will be more variable in toxicity studies (these studies use animals that are unaccustomed to the data-gathering procedure) as compared with data obtained from specialized studies using animals that are accustomed to this type of procedure. Blood is sampled for laboratory analysis and at the end of the study, all animals are sacrificed; the main study animals are necropsied and their tissues harvested for histopathological assessment.

Regulatory studies must be conducted in accordance with Good Laboratory Practice (GLP) regulations. We do not discuss these requirements here, as they have been described comprehensively elsewhere [32]. It is sufficient to say that these regulations define operational requirements that must be met so that technical data are acceptable to the regulatory authorities. Nonregulatory studies are not required to follow GLP guidelines; however, they are not necessarily poorer in quality than GLP studies. In our experience, in a high-quality facility, all toxicology studies are conducted to the same exacting standards and GLP studies are differentiated from non-GLP studies only by the range of supporting documentation and the inspection of key study phases by the quality assurance department. Non-GLP studies merely adopt simplified administrative and record-keeping procedures. GLP regulations require that a detailed outline of a study be documented in a comprehensive study plan referred to as the study protocol. We list the key headings for a typical regulatory study protocol in Table 7.6, and discuss key operational aspects of toxicology study conduct drawn from this outline. The protocol describes the nature and timing of all experimental steps, administrative procedures that must be followed, key study personnel, and their responsibilities. We recommend using a simplified study protocol modeled on that used for GLP studies for all non-GLP studies. This ensures a consistent approach, facilitates communication with the study team, and enables incorporation of data into regulatory documents.

In recent years, significant effort has been focused on the development of *in vitro* alternatives [33–35] to animals and *in silico* toxicology (the use of computational toxicology, computer-assisted toxicology; e-tox; i-drug discovery; predictive absorption, distribution, metabolism, and excretion (ADME), etc.) for predicting nonclinical toxicological endpoints; clinical adverse effects; and metabolism of test substances [36–39]. An additional significant change has been the application of the "3R concept" [40, 41], an initiative to replace animals in studies (i.e., adopt *ex vivo* approaches), reduce the numbers of animals used in studies, and the refinement of studies [42]. Overall, despite the significant progress made in *ex vivo* approaches, toxicology assessments still rely primarily on the use of laboratory animals.

Test Species Selection

The choice of test species is conditioned by a number of practical and scientific factors [43, 44]:

- availability of a reproducible population of test animals,
- well-developed husbandry techniques to ensure a good supply of animals,

TABLE 7.6. Outline of a typical toxicology study protocol.

Cover Sheet
    Study title
    Product name
    Study director
    Approval signatures
    Distribution list
Table of Contents
Introduction and Study Objectives
Study Sponsor
Address of Test Facility and Additional Test Sites
Regulatory Status and Requirements of the Study
Study Schedule
Materials and Methods
    Vehicle
    Test item, formulation, and stability
    Formulation analysis
Experimental Design
    Animals and housing
    Allocation to test groups
    Test groups and identification of test groups
    Method of administration
    Justification of route
    Blood-sampling schedule and method/s
    Schedule for mortality and clinical observations, body weight, food consumption
    Ophthalmology, blood pressure, ECG observations/measurements
    Hematology and clinical chemistry measurements
    Urine collection methods; schedule and measurements
Postmortem Examinations
    Unscheduled deaths
    Scheduled necropsy
    Method and conditions of sacrifice
    Tissue collection
    Tissue preservation
    Tissue weighing list
    Tissues examined microscopically list
Toxicokinetics
    Sample collection method and schedule
    Storage and analysis of samples
    Disposition of animals
Data Acquisition
Statistical Analysis
Report Preparation
Quality Assurance
Archiving of Data and Samples
List of Key Study Personnel

The study protocol summarizes key activities, timing, and responsibilities for a study. There is no set format for such a document, this example of a protocol format should be adapted to the format preferred by individual sponsors and the needs of individual studies.

- animals of a size that is adapted to the housing conditions of studies,
- growth and maturation characteristics consistent with the duration of studies,
- presence of the pharmacological target in the test animal,
- absorption, distribution, metabolism, and excretion of the test compound similar to that of humans, and
- treatment by the same route as that planned for humans is possible.

Ideally, there should be two test species, one rodent and one nonrodent, that meet these conditions. In practice, this is not always possible; for example, the test species may not express or has low expression of the target pharmacological receptor/s, the target receptor/s may have a lower affinity than in humans, and there may be low tolerance to the test compound [19]. In these cases, a pragmatic approach must be adopted: in light of the data the best possible choice should be made of test species. Usually, the rat is the rodent species used, and the dog is the nonrodent species. Nonhuman primates can be used instead of dogs; however, given the high sensitivity (public and governmental) to their use for experimentation, strict in-house procedures should be in place to ensure that their use is justified. There should be extensive historical data, particularly for histopathology, for the strain of animal chosen. Young, healthy animals are obtained from registered breeders or suppliers; females must be nulliparous and not pregnant. At the start of the study, rodents should be 6–8 weeks old and dogs about 9 months old. Rats infected with the ialodacryoadenitis virus are avoided, as this can affect the quality of studies [45]. If wild-caught nonhuman primates are used, transmission of infections to study personnel may also be an issue [46].

Allocation of Animals to Studies and Animal Care

More animals than needed (about 10% is adequate) for the study should be obtained. This way, unsuitable animals are not entered into the study, and, if it is deemed necessary, dead or moribund animals can be replaced early in the study. Animals are randomized to their study cage at least 5 days prior to the start of the study to allow for acclimation to the study conditions and so that prestudy reference data can be generated. At the start of the study, the individual bodyweight of animals should be within at least ±20% of the group mean body weight and the mean body weight of each test group as nearly identical as possible. The housing, feeding, and general welfare of experimental animals is governed by regulations and laws in principal ICH zones. The study team should be aware of, and ensure compliance with, national and international animal care regulations. In the European Union, the Council of Europe has adopted a convention to protect vertebrate animals used for experimental and scientific purposes [47]. This convention applies to any animal used in any experimental or other scientific procedure, including the safety testing of "drugs, substances, or products." The provision of a minimum degree of freedom of movement, food, water, and care appropriate to the health and well-being of animals is required. In an appendix to the document, a detailed guideline covers all aspects of the accommodation and care of experimental animals. Laws, regulations, and federal policies that apply in the United States are available from the Web site of the Office of Laboratory Animal Welfare of the U.S. Department of Health and Human Services [48]. In Japan, the only guidance and regulation covering the use of animals in experiments is provided by the Law for the Protection and Management of Animals in 1973 (Law No. 105, October 1, 1973) and Standards Relating to the Care and Management of Experimental Animals (Notice No. 6 of the Prime Minister's office, March 27, 1980). Additionally, the Science Council of Japan; the Ministry of Education, Science, and Culture; and the Japanese Association for Laboratory Animal Science have published guidelines on the use of animals for experimentation [49]. Fillman-Holliday and Landi [50] have reviewed best practices in animal care, and the Association for Assessment and Accreditation of Laboratory Animal Care International (AAALAC), a nonprofit organization that promotes the humane treatment of animals in science, has a voluntary accreditation scheme [51]. Accreditation involves an internal review of policies, animal housing and management, veterinary care, and facilities by the institution applying for accreditation. AAALAC evaluators then review the findings and conduct an on-site assessment. If deficiencies are found and corrected, accreditation is awarded.

Rodents are housed in either wire or solid-bottomed cages, singly or in groups. Group housing has advantages in terms of reduced workload for technical staff, allows socialization between animals, and presents a more "natural" habitat. However, it is more difficult to monitor clinical signs in individual animals. Dealing with aggressive behavior is also a problem and can result in some animals not getting adequate access to food and water, which may then affect the quality of the study. Dogs and primates are usually housed individually, but cages should be arranged so that animals can socialize. Dogs must have regular exercise outside their cage and in groups. To avoid confusion and possible cross-contamination, dogs from the same dosage group are exercised together; males should be kept separate from females.

Animal diets are strictly controlled. Only commercially certified diets should be used, which guarantee both the nutritional contents of the diet <u>and</u> the absence, or minimization, of contaminants. Rodents are fed *ad libitum*, whereas dogs and monkeys receive a fixed ration. Take care to ensure that the ration provided meets the animals' nutritional needs. The drinking water is usually town water and should be periodically analyzed to ensure its quality and consistency.

Compound Administration

The administration route should be the same as the intended clinical route whenever possible, for example, oral (gavage, in-diet, capsule, or drinking water), parenteral (intravenous, intramuscular, intraperitoneal, subcutaneous or continuous infusion), inhalation, dermal, ocular, or sublingual. Occasionally dosing of animals using the clinical route is not possible for a number of reasons:

- bioavailability by the clinical route may be insufficient to produced systemic exposure levels that produce adverse effects
- The maximum achievable concentration of the test solution used for dosing animals may be insufficient to reach target doses.

TABLE 7.7. Proposed dosing volumes in toxicity studies (adapted from Diehl et al. [52]).

| | Route and Volume | | | | | |
| | mL/kg | | | | | mL/Site |
	Oral (gavage)	sc	ip	iv-Bolus	iv-Slow Injection	im
Mouse	10(50)	10(40)	20(80)	5	(25)	0.05 (0.1)
Rat	10(40)	5(10)	10(20)	5	(20)	0.1(0.2)
Dog	5(15)	1(2)	1(20)	2.5	(5)	0.25(0.5)
Monkey	5(15)	2(5)	10	2	—	0.25(0.5)

Abbreviations: sc = subcutaneous; ip = intraperitoneal; iv = intravenous; im = intramuscular.
Dosing volumes in a toxicity study vary as a function of the test species and the route of administration. Routine volumes and, in parentheses, maximal dosing volumes, ensure the health and welfare of test animals.

- The clinical route may not be practical for long-term toxicity studies. For example, repeated intramuscular administration produces localized tissue damage, even when a number of different sites of administration are used in rotation. Cumulative damage and the limited number of sites available, especially in rodents, limit the maximum duration of studies.
- The physicochemical properties of the test compound may exclude a given route of administration. For IV dosing, a solution of the test compound is needed. If this not available, an alternate route of administration should be used.

Regardless of the route of administration, it is important to ensure that the volume of dosing solution/suspension administered to animals is consistent with good scientific practice and the welfare of the test animals. Diehl et al. [52] have proposed acceptable treatment volumes for test animals via different routes of administration, based on a literature review and the practices of a number of pharmaceutical laboratories. Their proposals are summarized in Table 7.7. The proposed volumes are regarded by the authors as best practice. The volume of administration should be the smallest possible consistent with achieving the target doses for the study; however, it should not be so small as to introduce experimental error due to measuring mistakes. If necessary, a preliminary or exploratory study can be used to determine the optimal volume to use. Use of maximum volumes should only be considered when there are problems of solubility and/or bioavailability. In these instances, it is worthwhile to consider using a divided dosing regimen to reduce the volume of each individual administration while achieving the desired final dose. If the volume needed to achieve target doses is so great that it affects the test animals' welfare, an alternate route of administration should be considered.

It is usual to dose animals once daily. The principal factor to be considered when deciding on the frequency of test compound administration is the systemic exposure that results. The dosing frequency must produce sufficient systemic exposure to the test compound to reach toxic doses and/or provide a sufficiently large multiple of (expected) human exposure to allow a meaningful hazard assessment to be made. If the molecule under test has a very short half-life, then twice-a-day or three-times-a-day dosing may be needed to achieve the target systemic exposure. If the human dosing regimen involves repeat cycles of treatment interspersed with a rest from treatment (as is often the case for anticancer drugs), a similar dosing regimen can be adopted in toxicology studies (see the EMEA guideline for preclinical studies of anticancer drugs). If the test compound has a very long half-life, the frequency of treatment or doses is adapted to avoid excessive systemic accumulation of the test compound. Sometimes adverse events induced by treatment are more severe than expected. For example, single, high doses of antihypertensive drugs can induce a profound and life-threatening decrease in blood pressure in test animals [53]. In such instances, the dose can be fractionated by increasing the frequency of treatment and attenuating the severity of adverse effects. If adverse effects remain unacceptably severe, that dose should be reduced or abandoned.

Choice of Vehicle

The vehicle used is at the discretion of the investigator. As a rule, the vehicle should be well characterized and have no or low toxicity [54]. Where there is little or no knowledge of the toxicity of the vehicle, it may be necessary to conduct separate studies in advance of the toxicology studies to ensure its suitability for use. In part, choice of vehicle is driven by the route of administration, and it should meet several requirements with respect to the final formulation:

- Steps needed to prepare the dosing formulation should not result in chemical or physical alteration of the test substance,
- The test substance should be stable in the vehicle,
- The concentration of test substance in the vehicle should be sufficient to allow use of acceptable dosing volumes,
- The pH of the final formulation should be within an acceptable range for the route of administration, and
- Parenteral formulations should have acceptable levels of sterility and controlled levels of endotoxins.

There is an extensive choice of vehicles available to the experimenter; however, not all of them are suitable for all routes of administration. In addition, there are significant differences in the degree to which different species tolerate the same vehicle. Gad et al. [55] has reviewed the vehicles that are available for toxicology studies. In our experience, there is rarely a customized vehicle for the test compound in the early stages of drug development when toxicology studies start. In these cases, we have found it is best to be pragmatic when choosing the vehicle for administering the test compound. In oral studies for example, methylcellulose–Tween is a good, all-purpose vehicle for producing test article solutions or suspensions with adequate bioavailability and is well tolerated by rodents and nonrodents. As with other aspects of toxicology study conduct, there will always be instances where the ideal requirements cannot be met. In these cases, a pragmatic approach must be adopted once more. On completion of a robust, well-documented program of studies to find a vehicle to use in toxicology studies, the vehicle with the best overall profile is adopted, even if this limits the choice of doses for studies.

Dose Selection

The doses selected are dependent on the physicochemical, pharmacological, and toxicological properties of the test compound. Ideally, a range of effects should be produced (e.g., adverse effects at a high dose, moderate adverse effects at middose, and few or no effects at a low dose. The toxicity induced by test compound is related to dose, dosing frequency (i.e., exposure to the test chemical), and duration of treatment [27]; however, it should be remembered that adverse effects may also be attenuated with treatment. For example, in studies of vasodilators, there may be an attenuation of the effects on blood pressure and/or heart rate with increased duration of treatment due to resetting of blood pressure receptors in test animals. There is a temptation, particularly with inexperienced toxicologists, to overinterpret the meaning of "adverse effects," which can result in poor dose selection (particularly the high dose), the need to repeat need to repeat studies, and result in delays to project timelines. However, in some cases, a study may fulfill its regulatory and scientific objectives even if no toxicity is produced. There is no set formula or approach for selecting a dose. However, an approach that we have found valuable is as follows: the starting dose for single-dose escalating toxicity studies can be set as a multiple ($\times 1$–$\times 10$) of the highest dose used in the safety pharmacology studies, the multiple being determined by the type and severity of effects in the safety pharmacology study. Based on the effects produced by the first dose, subsequent doses are increased by two- or threefold increments. Ideally, after three or four doses the MTD should be reached; if necessary, a lower dose/s can then be tested to refine the MTD. The first repeat-dose studies are usually range-finding studies. Unlike regulatory studies, it is not necessary or even advisable to have a NOAEL dose in these studies because the principal objective of this study is to identify the high dose for the follow-up regulatory study. In this instance, the single-dose MTD (and data from two or three repeat doses if available) is used to set the high dose; the low and middoses are fractions of the high dose (say $1/2$ and $1/4$). Dose selection for the first repeat-dose studies is based on limited data; it is empirical and benefits greatly from input from experienced toxicologists to a certain extent. For subsequent repeat-dose studies, dose selection is based on data from the range-finding studies and is more rationally based.

A wide range of data is collected in toxicity studies (see Table 7.5) and indicate the response of animals to treatment. Changes in any parameter can indicate an adverse effect and can be used to set the high dose. Some effects are readily apparent during the course of the study: for example, effects on mortality, clinical signs, food consumption, body weight, ophthalmology, blood pressure, and ECG. Data for other parameters only become available some days after sample collection or even after the in-life phase of the study is complete, including hematology, clinical chemistry, necropsy, and histopathology. Several factors must be considered when deciding on the severity and impact of effects induced by treatment:

- type of finding or associated findings,
- severity,
- incidence, and
- test species.

All these factors determine whether a finding is severe enough to limit the high dose; moreover, the criteria applied to nonrodents, particularly nonhuman primates, are more conservative than those applied to rodents. Although a detailed discussion of all possible causes for high-dose limitation is not possible, following are general examples to guide the reader through the dose selection process. In many cases, deciding on the significance of a treatment-related finding is a judgment call. In these cases, the inexperienced toxicologist is well advised to consult a more experienced colleague.

Mortality. Treatment-related mortality is unequivocally an adverse event. Thus, the death of all animals is a clear indication that the dose involved is excessive. The death of one or two animals in a rodent study is not, in our view, sufficient reason to abandon the dose at which death occurred. This is with the proviso that any agonal clinical signs were not indicative of severe suffering and/or that surviving animals at the same dose do not have severe clinical signs. However, in nonrodent studies, a single treatment-related death is sufficient reason to consider that dose unsuitable for use in subsequent studies regardless of the nature of concurrent clinical signs.

Clinical signs. Some clinical signs are nonspecific indicators of toxicity: reduced activity and hunched posture, for example. In a rodent study, if all animals present with these signs for the greater part of the day, the dose is adverse in our view. If only a few animals are affected for a short period this may not be the case. In contrast, if one animal in a nonrodent study is affected, this can be dose limiting. Single or repeat episodes of vomiting in one or two dogs over a few days of the study are not necessarily of concern, particularly in the absence of collateral effects on body weight and the hydration state of the animals. However, if episodes of vomiting occur throughout the study, this should be of concern. Other clinical signs are clear indicators of toxicity: treatment-induced convulsions are dose limiting but depend on incidence, frequency, whether animals recover, and test species. Because the interpretation of the severity and impact of clinical signs is a question of judgment, the advice of an experienced toxicological scientist/veterinarian should be used whenever possible in using these effects to set the high dose of a study or in deciding the necessity of reducing or abandoning a dose.

Body weight. A modest decrease in body weight gain, linked or not to an effect on food consumption, is not adverse. However, a decrease in body weight gain of about 10% is accepted as dose limiting. Once again, changes of this magnitude in a few rodents per group, or a sporadic decrease, is not problematic; there should be an effect on the group mean body weight. For nonrodents, given the smaller number of animals used, a biologically significant loss of body weight in even one animal is significant.

Clinical pathology. A wide range of clinical pathology parameters are monitored in studies. A treatment-related, biologically significant change in any of these parameters can be used to limit the high dose. Thus, a small increase in serum liver enzyme activity (e.g.,, alanine aminotransferase, aspartate aminotransferase, and alkaline phosphatase) or changes in blood cell parameters in all animals would not necessarily limit the high dose. Marked changes, which are significantly outside the range of values for concurrent control animals, from historical data and which are also biologically significant probably would be dose limiting even in the absence of concurrent histopathological findings.

Histopathology. Any histopathological change can potentially be used to set the high dose. This relies on an evaluation of the incidence, severity, and significance of the change (e.g., not adverse, marginal/borderline, adverse) by study pathologists. The advice of an experienced pathologist is invaluable when dealing with marginal/borderline effects. For example, a finding of "slight hepatic hypertrophy" in all animals is not necessarily a reason to limit the high dose, as this could be part of an adaptive repose to treatment [56], particularly in the absence of elevated liver enzymes. However, multifocal hepatic necrosis even when limited to a few animals could be dose limiting.

Pharmacological effects. Pharmacological effects within the normal range expected of the test compound cannot be used to limit the high dose. However, exaggerated pharmacological effects can be considered adverse if they affect the well-being of the test animal. Consider an antihypertensive compound. A dose producing a decrease in blood pressure within the pharmacological range is not suitable as a high dose in a toxicity study, whereas a dose that produces profound hypotension is suitable, as this would be a possibly life-threatening effect.

Toxicokinetics. In some circumstances, toxicokinetic or formulation considerations can be used to limit the high dose. It is important to bear in mind that when toxicokinetic considerations are used to limit the high dose, there must be robust toxicokinetic data, and it is advisable to test alternate routes of administration (e.g., switching from dermal to oral or from oral to IV dosing) and different formulations to try to overcome this problem.

- *Saturation of absorption*: If a compound's absorption becomes saturated as the oral dose of a test compound is increased, and systemic exposure does not reach toxic levels, the high dose can be set to the "saturation" dose.
- *Bioavailability*: If the test compound has low oral bioavailability, even very high doses of the test compound produce low systemic exposure. In these cases, the

high dose can be limited to the maximum ethically acceptable dose for the test species, considering maximum recommended administration volumes.

- *Maximum feasible dose (MFD)*: If the test compound is poorly soluble, then toxic dose levels may not be reached at the maximum acceptable dosing volume and regimen. In this case, the high dose is limited by the maximum concentration of the dosing solution and the maximum acceptable administration volume.

Use of limit doses. In acute, subchronic, and chronic studies, a limiting dose of 1000 mg/kg/day for rodents and nonrodents is considered appropriate (see the ICH(M3) guideline) except in specific cases:

- where a dose of 1000 mg/kg/day does not produce a 10-fold mean exposure margin of the clinical exposure and the clinical dose exceeds 1 g/day. In this instance, the high dose is limited to a 10-fold exposure multiple, or a dose of 2000 mg/kg/day or the MFD. If a dose of 2000 mg/kg/day is less than the clinical exposure, a higher dose up to the MFD should be considered.
- A 50-fold exposure to the parent drug or the pharmacologically active moiety of a prodrug is acceptable.
- In the United States, dose-limiting toxicity generally should be identified in at least one species when using the 50-fold margin of exposure as the limit dose to support Phase III clinical trials. If this is not the case, a study of 1 month or longer duration in one species should be conducted using a high dose of 1000 mg/kg—the MFD or the MTD, whichever is lowest.

Selecting doses for carcinogenicity studies is broadly similar to that for shorter studies. Additionally, the high dose can be set using endpoints defined in the ICH S1C(R2) guideline [57]:

- *Exposure multiple:* A high dose that produces systemic exposure that is a 25-fold multiple of the anticipated maximum human AUC can be used. This is an apparently simple approach. However, it should be borne in mind that factors such as the degree of protein binding of the drug (rodent as compared with human), and the effects of study duration on AUC must be considered.
- *Limit dose:* A limit dose of 1500 mg/kg/day applies where the maximum recommended human dose does not exceed 500 mg/day. However, a limit dose does not apply if it cannot be demonstrated that animal exposure after treatment with 1500 mg/kg/day is high compared to the exposure achieved in humans.

A specificity of carcinogenicity studies is that proposed study doses, with an accompanying rationale, can be submitted to the FDA's Carcinogenicity Assessment Committee (CAC) [57] for comment. This committee considers and comments on the suitability of doses selected for study. Although submitting a dose proposal to the CAC is not obligatory, and although the comments of the committee are not binding, failing to consult with or ignoring comments from the CAC is done at the investigator's peril.

Once the high dose has been set, selection of the low and middoses is relatively straightforward. The low dose should produce no or slight toxicity and, in some instances, this dose will overlap with the highest doses used in safety pharmacological studies. In practical terms, the low dose is a small multiple of the expected clinical dose or the highest dose used in pharmacology studies that produced only slight pharmacological effects. The mid dose should be positioned between the low and high doses to optimize characterization of the toxicity–dose response. A useful starting point for setting the mid dose is as follows:

$$\text{Mid dose} = (\text{low dose} \times \text{high dose})^{1/2}$$

The final choice of the mid dose is then made in light of data from previous studies.

In-Life Observations

We have summarized a typical set of data collected in Table 7.8. Note that blood pressure and ECG data are not usually collected in rodents. In general, about five days before animal dosing begins, collection of in-life data starts. Animals are observed daily for clinical signs; blood pressure measurement, ECG monitoring, and/or ophthalmological examination, which are performed at least once prior to the start of the study. These are baseline data used as part of the selection process to ensure that only healthy animals are entered into the study. In large animals, one or two pretest blood samples are collected to establish a baseline for comparison with samples collected during the study. Clinical observations should be made at the same time/s each day. Initially, the general condition of the animals should be assessed once daily, and morbidity and mortality at least twice daily. Once animal dosing starts, the frequency of observation is determined by the effects of treatment; the more serious the effects, the more frequently the animals are observed. The nature and incidence, severity, and frequency of occurrence of the clinical signs are recorded.

Body weight is a good general indicator of the health status of test animals. Test animals should be weighed as part of the selection process for entry into the study and then at least once during the prestudy phase. If body weight changes rapidly, the frequency with which animals are weighed can be increased. Once animal dosing has started, each animal should be weighed at least once a week; at the end of the study animals are weighed prior to sacrifice. When animals are treated in-diet with the test compound, it is important to verify that any loss of body weight is not due to reduced food consumption resulting from low palatability of the food. If poor palatability is an issue, then food and possibly water consumption data are of limited value. For rodents, food and water consumption can be determined from the weight change in food and water containers relative to their starting weight. Some food spillage (particularly when a powdered diet is used) is inevitable; however, excess spillage should be noted (it may reflect a palatability problem). For nonrodents, the amount of the food ration

TABLE 7.8. Typical range of in-life data collected in toxicity studies.

| | Study Type | | | | |
| | Single Dose | | Repeat Dose | | Carcinogenicity |
Parameter	R	NR	R	NR	R
Signs of morbidity	✓	✓	✓	✓	✓
Mortality	✓	✓	✓	✓	✓
Detailed clinical observations	✓	✓	✓	✓	✓
Skin	✓	✓	✓	✓	✓
Fur	✓	✓	✓	✓	✓
Eyes	✓	✓	✓	✓	✓
Mucous membranes	✓	✓	✓	✓	✓
Occurrence of secretions and excretions	✓	✓	✓	✓	✓
Lacrimation	✓	✓	✓	✓	✓
Piloerection	✓	✓	✓	✓	✓
Unusual respiratory pattern	✓	✓	✓	✓	✓
Changes in gait and posture and response to handling	✓	✓	✓	✓	✓
Presence of clonic or tonic movements	✓	✓	✓	✓	✓
Body weight	✓	✓	✓	✓	✓
Food consumption	✓	✓	✓	✓	✓
Water consumption	✓		✓	✓	✓
Ophthalmological examination			✓	✓	✓
ECG				✓	
Blood pressure				✓	

This baseline list of study parameters is adapted from the OECD guidelines for the conduct of toxicity studies [7]. The data collected in a toxicity study should be adapted to the needs of the study in question.
Abbreviations: R = rodents; NR = nonrodents; ECG = electrocardiograph.

consumed by each animal is graded semiquantitatively (all of the ration, most of the ration, or none of the ration); the hydration state of the test animal may also indicate reduced water consumption. Blood pressure and ECG measurements should be taken immediately before treatment and then post-treatment when blood levels of the test compound reach about C_{max}. Additional measurements are made as a function of the rate of elimination of the test compound. The scope for multiple measurements is clearly greater in longer-term studies than in short-term studies. An additional constraint is that to reduce the level of stress in animals, and thereby improve the quality of the data collected, it is advisable to obtain blood pressure measurements and ECG recordings on separate days of the study. There should be at least one ophthalmological examination once steady-state systemic levels of the compound have been achieved. For long-term studies, an additional examination should be performed near the end of the study. Experienced technical staff usually collect and record in-life data. Some of the data collected are numerical (blood pressure, incidence, and ECG waveform intervals, for

TABLE 7.9. Commonly used blood sampling sites in toxicology studies.*

	Mouse	Rat	Dog	Monkey
Without Anesthesia				
Jugular		√	√	
Cephalic			√	√
Saphenous/lateral tarsal	√	√	√	√
Femoral				√
Lateral tail	√	√		
With Anesthesia				
Sublingual		√		
Retrobulbar plexus	√	√		

* Adapted from Diehl et al. [52].

example), whereas other data are qualitative (clinical signs, severity of findings, and ECG waveform anomaly, for example). The quality of the numerical data is relatively easy to control by using rigorous data capture and recording procedures. Additional measures are needed to ensure the quality and reproducibility of the qualitative data. We have found the following steps to be essential:

- data capture should be descriptive; interpretation and diagnosis can be made at a later stage,
- diagnoses should be made under the direction of an experienced and expert scientist, and
- standardized lexicons from which the technicians/scientists who are gathering the data can select appropriate descriptions should be available for clinical signs, ophthalmology, and ECG waveform anomalies. This facilitates harmonization, and the lexicons can be regularly updated to include any new observations or changes to existing terms that are agreed upon by an experienced peer review group.

BLOOD SAMPLING

Diehl et al. [52] have discussed good practice for blood sampling. Typically about 0.5 ml of blood is needed for hematology and about 1 ml of blood for clinical chemistry analysis. The volume of blood needed for TK, or special analysis, is a function of the sensitivity of the analytical method. Blood may be sampled from a variety of sites; the sites most commonly used in toxicology studies are listed in Table 7.9. Choice of sampling site is based on the expertise and preference of the laboratory conducting the study. If possible, a single sampling site should be used throughout the study, as well as across multiple studies performed in a given species with a single compound, and is best without the complicating factors due to anesthesia use. Repeated blood sampling is routine in toxicology studies; however, this can be a major problem in rodent studies given the limited number of sampling sites available and small total blood volume of the animals. Diehl et al. [52] proposed limit volumes and re-covery periods for multiple blood sampling based on a review of the literature and the experience of a number of pharmaceutical laboratories. They suggest the following schedule:

- 7.5% of total blood volume sampled in 24 hours with a frequency of once per week,
- 10%–15% of total blood volume sample in 24 hours with a frequency of once every 2 weeks and
- 20% of total blood volume sample in 24 hours with a frequency of once every 3 weeks

Blood samples should be collected to minimize introducing bias with regard to sampling time. Animals should be randomized for blood collection, and samples should be collected as quickly as possible and analyzed in the order in which they were collected. If a large number of animals must be sampled, such that blood collection occurs over a 2-day period, it is advisable to collect and analyze samples from males on one day and from females on the other day.

Laboratory Measurements

Blood is collected in various tubes for analysis. Whether whole blood, plasma, or serum is used depends on the analysis to be performed. Samples for hematology (whole blood) are generally collected in tubes containing an anticoagulant (EDTA), whereas samples used to evaluate coagulation parameters are collected in tubes containing citrate. For clinical chemistry evaluation, clot tubes or tubes containing heparin are used to collect serum or plasma, respectively.

The laboratory data that are routinely collected during toxicology studies are sum-marized in Table 7.10. Analyzers should be programmed to report absolute reticulo-cyte and differential white blood cell counts, as these values are more meaningful for interpreting hematology changes than relative (%) counts. Although not routinely eval-uated, the following parameters are easily programmed on today's automated analyz-ers and can be useful in interpreting hematology findings: red cell distribution width (RDW), mean platelet volume (MPV), platelet distribution width (PDW), and plateletcrit. Samples of blood and urine are obtained from nonrodents prior to the start of the study. Animals should be allowed to acclimate to their new surroundings prior to taking pretest samples. Pretest blood sampling in rodents is not recommended. The reasons include the possibility of adversely affecting the health of the animals due to their relatively small blood volume or from the trauma induced by blood collection, the homogene-ity of the values of the parameters evaluated, and the rapid changes that are expected to occur in evaluated parameters between pretest sampling time and the end of the study.

The sampling frequency during the study is determined by the type and severity of anticipated and/or treatment-induced effects. In a 2- or 4-week rodent study, blood is

TABLE 7.10. Laboratory measurements in toxicity studies.

Blood		Urine
Hematology	Clinical chemistry	
Red blood cells	Urea	Total volume
Hemoglobin	Glucose	pH
Hematocrit	Creatinine	White blood cells
Mean corpuscular volume	Triglycerides	Nitrites
Mean corpuscular hemoglobin	Aspartate aminotransferase	Proteins
Mean corpuscular hemoglobin	Total cholesterol	Glucose
concentration	Alanine aminotransferase	Ketone bodies
Red cell distribution width	Albumin/globulin ratio	Uroglobin
Hemoglobin distribution width	Alkaline phosphatase	Bilirubin
Platelets	Calcium	Hemoglobin/red blood cells
Platelet hematocrit	Total bilirubin	Specific gravity
Mean platelet volume	Inorganic phosphorous	Microscopic examination
Platelet distribution width	Total proteins	
White blood cells	Potassium	
Differential white blood cells	Albumin	
	Sodium globin	
	Chloride	
	Gamma-glutamyl transferase	

A wide range of clinical chemistry, hematological, and urinalysis parameters are available for inclusion in ion toxicity studies. The final choice of parameters should be tailored to the study in question and to regulatory requirements [7–9].

generally taken pretrial and once at the end of the study. In longer studies, an interim blood sample, and in rare instances, two interim blood samples, should also be considered; this is often the case for anticancer drug development when evaluating the toxic and rebound effects of treatment on bone marrow. The last samples for hematology and clinical pathology analysis are usually taken at sacrifice. Blood smears are routinely prepared for analysis in the event that there is a problem with the automated analyzer or a need for further investigation of results reported by the analyzer.

Urine collection can be a problem, as urine may be contaminated with feces and/or other foreign material [58]. To overcome this problem, urine is collected from animals housed in specially adapted cages that exclude foreign matter (metabolism cages for rodents, for example) or by direct sampling [59, 60]. Spillage of water into the urine sample from the water source in the cage can confound urinalysis results. To avoid bacterial contamination, a preservative such as thimerosal or azide should be added to samples.

Generally, there are no laboratory measurements in single-dose studies unless there is a specific need for it. However, all the parameters described in Table 7.10 are monitored in repeat-dose studies. Single-dose studies often use small numbers of animals, which increases the already high variability of the laboratory parameters. Adding these parameters to such a study would produce data, which are of limited value at best. This being said, if one (or more) of these parameters is a biomarker for an anticipated toxic effect, it can be included in single-dose studies to provide an early assessment of an adverse effect. The advantage gained from this would justify increasing the number of animals in the study. In carcinogenicity studies, laboratory samples are generally limited to differential blood counts performed at intervals (possibly beginning as early as 6 months) and/or at the end of the study. No chemistry or urinalysis evaluations are undertaken.

NECROPSY, TISSUE COLLECTION, AND HISTOPATHOLOGY

Necropsy marks the beginning of the postmortem phase of the toxicology study. It is a critical phase of the study because errors committed during macroscopic evaluation and tissue collection are seldom correctable later. Therefore, it is important that skilled technical staff and well-documented procedures are in place prior to undertaking this process. The method of anesthesia/euthanasia selected should be carefully considered for its impact on animal welfare and on the interpretation of organ weight and histopathology findings [61]. In most cases, animals are anesthetized, then exsanguinated and necropsied as soon after death as possible. Principal study animals that die prematurely, that are sacrificed during the study, or that are sacrificed at the end of the study are subject to gross necropsy. There is an examination of external surfaces; all orifices; cranial, thoracic, and abdominal cavities; the carcass; and all organs. A bone marrow smear is prepared for each animal in the event that cytologic evaluation of this tissue is required, and a range of organs is collected. The range of tissues collected is at the discretion of the investigator. Satellite animals, such as those used for evaluating toxicokinetics, are usually not necropsied.

    In the interest of time and economy, no tissues are collected in acute studies. Only a limited range of tissues is collected in range-finding studies—usually major organs, any known target organs of toxicity, and all tissues that have macroscopic findings. The tissues listed in Table 7.11 are recovered at necropsy in a regulatory toxicology study. Tissues samples from all gross lesions should be examined microscopically, regardless of the treatment group in which the lesions were observed. In investigative studies, the choice of tissues to be collected is determined by the objectives of the study. Fresh tissues should be handled with great care to avoid producing artifacts that may confound histopathologic evaluation. The tissues should be rinsed and kept hydrated with saline during the necropsy procedure. Fat and/or contiguous tissue and blood clots should be removed from organs prior to weighing; routinely weighed tissues are indicated in bold in Table 7.11. Macroscopic findings are recorded using standardized nomenclature that describes the size, number, shape, color, and consistency of the changes observed. Small pieces of tissue are recovered from each organ and preserved in an appropriate fixative. Care is taken to preserve sections of all tissues with macroscopic findings in addition to sections that are normally taken according to standard operating procedures. Ten percent-buffered formalin is a generally acceptable fixative for most tissues, but eyes and testes are better preserved in modified Davidson's solution [62]. Most tissues are fixed by immersion, but some, such as lungs, urinary bladder, stomach, and intestines, benefit from inflation

TABLE 7.11. Tissues usually collected in regulatory toxicology studies.

Adrenals	Nasal turbinates
Aorta	**Ovaries and Fallopian tubes**
Bone (femur)	Pancreas
Bone marrow (sternum)	Pituitary
Brain	Prostate
Cecum	Rectum
Colon	Salivary gland
Duodenum	Sciatic nerve
Epididymis	Seminal vesicle
Esophagus	Skeletal muscle
Eyes	Skin
Gall bladder (nonrodents)	Spinal cord
Harderian gland (rodents)	**Spleen**
Heart	Stomach
Ileum	**Testes**
Jejunum	**Thyroid/parathyroid**
Kidneys	**Thymus**
Liver	Urinary bladder
Lymph nodes	**Uterus**
Mammary glands	Vagina
	Zymbal's gland

A wide range of tissues is collected for histopathological analysis. The final tissue list for a study should be tailored to the study in question and to regulatory requirements [7–9].

with fixative. The fixed tissue samples are trimmed and embedded in paraffin wax prior to being sectioned (traditionally at 4 to 6 microns) and stained with hematoxylin and eosin or another suitable stain prior to microscopic evaluation and assessment.

Histopathologic evaluation is generally performed by a single pathologist. The study pathologist should use standardized nomenclature when making diagnoses and strive to record findings in a way that is suitable for tabular evaluation. Severity grading is generally used to qualify the diagnoses made. The study pathologist should have the in-life laboratory macroscopic evaluation and organ weight data available when he or she is evaluating any given study so that the chances of drawing meaningful conclusions from histopathology findings are maximized. Peer review of the pathologist's work is highly desirable. In most cases, it is from the microscopic evaluation of tissues that evidence of toxicity is obtained. Tissues samples from all gross lesions should be examined microscopically regardless of the treatment group from which the samples were taken. Ideally, all tissues from all animals in the study should be examined; in our view, this provides a comprehensive view of the effects of treatment. However, it is not uncommon for tissues from only control and high-dose animals to be examined in repeat-dose studies. Then, any tissue that has been affected by the treatment is also examined in samples from the next lowest dose level. This continues until the no-effect level is reached. If treatment produces effects in only one gender and/or only at higher doses, this stepped approach may save resources and reduce the time needed to complete a study. However, in carcinogenicity studies, all tissues from all dose groups should routinely be examined.

CONCLUSION

A wide range of molecules (e.g., chemicals, proteins, vaccines, oligonucleotides) undergoes nonclinical investigation as part of a drug development program. In terms of toxicological characterization, the information needed to progress to clinical trials and to support a marketing application should be tailored to individual molecules, taking the therapeutic area involved, the prognosis of patients, and the effectiveness and availability of competitor compounds into account. To achieve this, a baseline toxicology strategy is established using the study sequence described in regulatory guidelines. This strategy is then tailored to the molecule being tested considering the specific needs of the molecule. Rapid advancement of projects at the smallest cost is a legitimate goal; however, it is critical that speed is not confused with haste The most cost-effective resource-sparing toxicology strategies are usually those that involve a robust series of studies, with clear adverse events at the high dose, focused on regulatory toxicology needs. If required, additional studies can then be conducted to investigate the pathogenesis of a lesion or to bridge to the main study program in cases where key project variables change (e.g., impurities profile, route of administration). All regulatory studies must be conducted to GLP standards; however, all studies should be held to the same high scientific standard. Although baseline study designs are available from a number of sources (the OECD, for example), it is essential to adapt the design of the study to the type of molecule under development. Finally, given the uncertainty that is an inescapable part of any toxicology program, and the need to make decisions based on often-incomplete information, the inexperienced toxicologist is advised to seek help and counsel from more experienced colleagues.

REFERENCES

1. Sneader W, 2005. *Drug Discovery: A History*. Hoboken, NJ Wiley
2. Ostrove JM, 1994. Safety testing programs for gene therapy viral vectors. *Cancer Gene Ther* *1*:125–131
3. Buckel P, ed., 2001. *Recombinant Protein Drugs*. New York: Birkhauser
4. Buchwald UK and Pirofski L, 2003. Immune therapy for infectious diseases at the dawn of the 21st century: The past, present and future role of antibody therapy, therapeutic vaccination and biological response modifiers. *Curr Pharm Des* *9*:945–968
5. Adachi Y, Yoshio-Hoshino N, and Nishimoto N, 2008. Gene therapy for multiple myeloma. *Curr Gene Ther* *8*:247–255
6. Spizzo R, Rushworth D, Guerrero M, and Calin GA, 2009. RNA inhibition, microRNAs, and new therapeutic agents for cancer treatment. *Clin Lymphoma Myeloma* *9*:S313–S318

7. Dorato MA and Engelhardt JA, 2005. The no-observed-adverse-effect-level in drug safety evaluations: Use, issues, and definition(s). *Regul Toxicol Pharmacol* **42**:265–274

8. Travis KZ, Pate I, and Welsh ZK, 2005. The role of the benchmark dose in a regulatory context. *Regul Toxicol Pharmacol* **43**:280–291

9. Haseman JK, 1985. Issues in carcinogenicity testing: Dose selection. *Fundam Appl Toxicol* **5**:66–78

10. U.S. Food and Drug Administration, 2002a. Guidance for industry and reviewers: estimating the safe starting dose in clinical trials for therapeutics in adult healthy volunteers. http://www.fda.gov/cber/gdlns/dose.htm

11. Fielden MR and Kolaja KL, 2008. The role of early *in vivo* toxicity testing in drug discovery toxicology. *Expert Opin Drug Saf* **7**:107–110

12. Stevens JL and Baker TK, 2009. The future of drug safety testing: Expanding the view and narrowing the focus. *Drug Discov Today* **14**:162–167

13. Chalmers AA, ed., 2000. *International Pharmaceutical Registration*. St. Helier, Jersey, UK: Informa HealthCare

14. International Conference on Harmonization, 2009. Guidance on nonclinical safety studies for the conduct of human clinical trials and marketing authorization for pharmaceuticals M3(R2). http://www.ich.org/cache/compo/276-254-1.html

15. Olejniczak, K, Gunzel, P, and Bass, R, 2001. Preclinical testing strategies. *Drug Inf J* **33**:321–336

16. Baldrick P, 2008. Safety evaluation to support First-In-Man investigations II: Toxicology studies. *Regul Toxicol Pharmacol* **51**:237–243

17. Sistare FD and DeGeorge JJ, 2007. Preclinical predictors of clinical safety: Opportunities for improvement. *Clin Pharmacol Ther* **82**:210–214

18. International Conference on Harmonization, 1997. S6 Guideline. Preclinical safety evaluation of biotechnology-derived pharmaceuticals. http://www.ich.org/LOB/media/MEDIA503.pdf

19. International Conference on Harmonization, 2009. S6(R1)Draft consensus guideline. Addendum to ICH 6: Preclinical safety evaluation of biotechnology-derived pharmaceuticals. http://www.ich.org/LOB/media/MEDIA5784.pdf

20. Black LE, Bendele AM, Bendele RA et al., 1999. Regulatory decision strategy for entry of a novel biological therapeutic with a clinically unmonitorable toxicity into clinical trials: Pre-IND meetings and a case example. *Toxicol Pathol* **27**:22–6

21. Serabian MA and Pilaro AM, 1999. Safety assessment of biotechnology-derived pharmaceuticals: ICH and beyond. *Toxicol Pathol* **27**:27–31

22. Gad, CS, 2002. *Drug Safety Evaluation. Strategy and Phasing for Drug Safety Evaluation in the Discovery and Development of Pharmaceuticals*. Hoboken, NJ: John Wiley and Sons. pp 1–29

23. Olson, H, Betton, G, Robinson, DE et al., 2000. Concordance of the toxicity of pharmaceuticals in humans and animals *Regul Toxicol Pharmacol* **32**:56–67

24. Brennan FR, Shaw L, Wing MG, and Robinson C, 2004. Preclinical" safety testing of biotechnology-derived pharmaceuticals: understanding the issues and addressing the challenges. *Mol Biotechnol* **27**: 59–74

25. Nakazawa T, Kai S, Kawai M et al., 2004. "Points to consider" regarding safety assessment of biotechnology-derived pharmaceuticals in non-clinical studies (English translation). *J Toxicol Sci* **29**:497–504

26. Snodin DJ and Ryle PR, 2006. Understanding and applying regulatory guidance on the nonclinical development of biotechnology-derived pharmaceuticals. *BioDrugs* **20**:25–52

27. U.S. Food and Drug Administration, 2006. Guidance for industry, investigators, and reviewers. Exploratory IND studies. http://www.fda.gov/cder/guidance/7086fnl.htm

28. Sarapa N, 2007. Exploratory IND: A new regulatory strategy for early clinical drug development in the United States. In: J. Venitz and W. Sittner, editors. *Appropriate Dose Selection—How to Optimize Clinical Drug Development*, Ernst Schering Research Foundation Workshop 59. New York: Springer. pp. 151–163

29. Organisation for Economic Co-operation and Development, 2009. http://www.oecd.org/home

30. National Toxicology Program, 2009. http://ntp-server.niehs.nih.gov/

31. U.S. Food and Drug Administration, 2009. Toxicological principles for the safety assessment of food ingredients, *Redbook 2000*. http://vm.cfsan.fda.gov/~redbook/red-toca.html

32. U.S. Food and Drug Administration, 2001. Bioresearch monitoring good laboratory practice, Compliance Program 7348.808 (Nonclinical Laboratories). http://www.fda.gov/ora/compliance_ref/bimo/7348_808/default.htm.

33. Daston GP and McNamee P, 2005. Alternatives to toxicity testing in animals: Challenges and opportunities. *Environ Health Perspect*. http://ehp.niehs.nih.gov/docs/2005/7723/7723.html

34. European Centre for the Validation of Alternative Methods, 2010. Validated methods. http://ecvam.jrc.it/index.htm

35. Center for Alternatives to Animal Testing (Johns Hopkins School of Hygiene and Public Health), 2010. http://caat.jhsph.edu/programs/index.htm

36. Valerio LG Jr, Arvidson KB, Chanderbhan RF, and Contrera JF, 2007. Prediction of rodent carcinogenic potential of naturally occurring chemicals in the human diet using high-throughput QSAR predictive modeling. *Toxicol Appl Pharmacol* **222**:1–16

37. Muster W, Breidenbach A, Fischer H et al., 2008. Computational toxicology in drug development. *Drug Discov Today* **13**: 303–310

38. Merlot C, 2008. In silico methods for early toxicity assessment. *Curr Opin Drug Discov Devel* **11**: 80–85

39. Valerio LG, 2009. In silico toxicology for the pharmaceutical sciences. *Toxicol Appl Pharmacol* **241**:356–370

40. Schechtman LM, 2002. Implementation of the 3Rs (refinement, reduction, and replacement): Validation and regulatory acceptance considerations for alternative toxicological test methods. *ILAR J* **43**:S85–S94

41. Rusche B, 2003. The 3Rs and animal welfare—Conflict or the way forward? *ALTEX* **20**:63–76

42. Balls M, 2009. The origins and early days of the three Rs concept. *Altern Lab Anim* **37**:255–265

43. Phalen RF, Oldham MJ, and Wolff RK, 2008. The relevance of animal models for aerosol studies. *J Aerosol Med Pulm Drug Deliv* **21**:113–124

44. Festing MF, 1980. The choice of animals in toxicological screening: Inbred strains and the factorial design of experiment. *Acta Zool Pathol Antverp* **75**:117–131

45. Nicklas, W, Homberger, FR, Illgen-Wilcke, B et al., 1999. Implications of infectious agents on results of animal experiments. GV-SOLAS Working Group on Hygiene. Lab Animals *33*:S1:39–S1:87

46. Hankenson FC, Johnston NA, Weigler BJ, and Giacomo RF, 2003. Zoonoses of occupational health importance in contemporary laboratory animal research. *Comp Med 53*:579–601

47. Sauer, UG, 2004. The revision of European housing guidelines for laboratory animals: Expectations from the point of view of animal welfare. *Altern Lab Anim 32*:187-190

48. Office of Laboratory Animals Welfare, 2009. http://grants.nih.gov/grants/olaw/links.htm#GOV

49. Nomura, TI, 1995. Laboratory animal care policies and regulations: Japan. *ILAR J 37*:60–61

50. Fillman-Holliday D and Landi MS, 2002. Animal care best practices for regulatory testing. *ILAR J 43*:S49–S58

51. Association for Assessment and Accreditation of Laboratory Animal Care International, 2009. http://www.aaalac.org/

52. Diehl K-H, Hull R, Morton D, Pfister et al., 2001. A good practice guide to the administration of substances and removal of blood, including routes and volumes. *J Appl Toxicol 21*:15–23

53. Greaves, P, 2000. Patterns of cardiovascular pathology induced by diverse cardioactive drug. *Toxicol Lett 15*:547–552

54. Neervannan S, 2006. Preclinical formulations for discovery and toxicology: Physicochemical challenges. *Expert Opin Drug Metab Toxicol 2*: 715–731

55. Gad, SC, Cassidy, CD, Aubert, N et al., 2006. Nonclinical vehicle use in studies by multiple routes in multiple species. *Int J Toxicol 25*:499–521

56. Williams GM and Iatropoulos MJ, 2002. Alteration of liver cell function and proliferation: Differentiation between adaptation and toxicity. *Toxicol Pathol 30*:41–53

57. U.S. Food and Drug Administration, 2002b. Guidance for industry. Carcinogenicity study protocol submissions. http://www.fda.gov/cder/guidance/4804fnl.htm.

58. Jackson AJ and Sutherland JC, 1984. Novel device for quantitatively collecting small volumes of urine from laboratory rats. *J Pharm Sci 73*:816–818

59. Horst PJ, Bauer M, Veelken R, and Unger T, 1988. A new method for collecting urine directly from the ureter in conscious unrestrained rats. *Ren Physiol Biochem 11*:325–231

60. Mandavilli U, Schmidt J, Rattner DW et al., 1991. Continuous complete collection of uncontaminated urine in conscious rodents. *Lab Anim Sci 41*:258–261

61. Institute for Laboratory Animal Research, 2010. *Guide for the Care and Use of Laboratory Animals*. At http://dels.nas.edu/ilar_n/ilarhome/guide.shtml

62. Cox ML, Schray CL, Luster CN et al., 2006. Assessment of fixatives, fixation, and tissue processing on morphology and RNA integrity. *Exp Mol Pathol 80*:183–191

8

GENETIC TOXICOLOGY

Peggy Guzzie-Peck, Jennifer C. Sasaki, and Sandy K. Weiner

INTRODUCTION

Genetic toxicology is a specialty field within toxicology that studies the toxic effects of agents on DNA. The primary purpose of genetic toxicology testing of chemicals, some of which are pharmaceutical candidates, is to identify the hazards of potential genotoxic risks to humans, which includes the potential to induce heritable changes to DNA that could lead to increased risks for developing cancer and/or birth defects. These DNA changes can occur as alterations to single base pairs, chromosome structure, and/or chromosome number either directly or indirectly following exposure to a genotoxicant and can contribute to multistep molecular processes involved in carcinogenicity. Similar heritable effects that lead to germ cell mutations can result in decreased fertility, increased spontaneous abortions, and/or the potential for birth defects. Although these germ cell changes are difficult to assess in routine testing, the same type of changes occur in somatic cells at the molecular level and can be easily assessed using standard genotoxicity testing, which is conducted using somatic cells. Another complicating factor in studying genetic toxicology is DNA repair systems. These systems need to be considered when evaluating DNA changes using genetic toxicology testing, as DNA repair systems themselves may contribute to adverse DNA changes because of incorrect or lack of repair.

DNA alterations can occur as changes to single base pairs (called point mutations) through deletion, addition, or substitution of one or more base pairs. If a single base is

Pharmaceutical Toxicology in Practice: A Guide for Non-Clinical Development, Edited by Alberto Lodola and Jeanne Stadler
© 2011 John Wiley & Sons, Inc.

deleted or added in a gene, every codon downstream from this point is altered, resulting in a "frameshift" mutation. Frameshift mutations will usually result in no functioning protein being made by the genes past the deletion or insertion point. Depending on the size of the damage, location within a gene(s), and the function of the gene or mutated cell, mutational events can produce effects ranging from no, or minimal, adverse effects to lethality to the cell. Substituting one base pair for another "substitution mutation" may have minimal to no adverse effect on the organism, as there is a built-in redundancy within the coding sequence for most amino acids (i.e., the third base in a codon can change in many cases but still code for the same amino acid). However, with some genes, even a small substitution of one or two base pairs may result in what is termed a "missense mutation" when it results in an amino acid alteration that is sufficient to affect the ultimate structure and/or function of the protein or enzyme.

Changes in chromosome structure, referred to as chromosome breakage or clastogenesis, occurs when segments of chromosomes containing many base pairs of DNA are added, deleted, or rearranged. Chromosome breakage (both chromatid arms) and single chromatid damage are the most frequently observed types of damage. Chromosome rearrangements are rare and can occur as the result of multiple chromatid breakage in severely damaged cells that have attempted to repair the damage, or in less severely damaged cells, that remained capable of dividing. Most types of chromosome damage are unstable, usually leading to the death of the aberrant cell, and thus are not of significant long-term consequence to a somatic cell. However, reduced fertility may be observed as an indirect consequence of chromosome damage if a significant number of germ cells are affected, or birth defects may result if the aberration is not lethal. Some types of aberrations can survive multiple cell divisions and have been associated with tumorigenesis in somatic stem cells.

Non–DNA-reactive mechanisms can affect DNA synthesis, the integrity of chromosomes, and gene expression. For example, aneugenicity is one way that the normal chromosome number is altered from what is typically denoted as the normal number for the organism. This occurs when the cell division apparatus (associated with chromosomal segregation and division of the cytoplasm) is damaged, resulting in intact chromosomes being either added or deleted. Other indirect mechanisms of genotoxicity may be the result of effects on transcription, translation, and the result of direct pharmacologic activity of the drug. These types of events, like other forms of toxicity that do not involve direct damage to DNA, are thought to have clear threshold concentrations below which there is minimal cause for concern.

THE REGULATORY ENVIRONMENT

Harmonized guidance, approved by the three major pharmaceutical registration regions of the United States, Western Europe, and Japan, have been issued by the International Conference on Harmonization (ICH). The standard core test battery for assessing genotoxicity has been defined in the ICH S2B [1] guideline and includes, among other things:

- an assessment of mutagenicity in a bacterial reverse mutation test,
- a mammalian *in vitro* test for chromosome damage, and
- an *in vivo* test for chromosome damage.

The ICH M3 guideline [2] describes the staging of these tests as they relate to traditional clinical development programs such that two *in vitro* tests—one for gene mutations and one for chromosome damage—be conducted prior to the first human exposure (Phase I clinical trials). In addition, additional testing should be performed if there are any equivocal or positive findings in the tests. Abbreviated genotoxicity evaluation is possible in support of exploratory clinical trial designs, depending on the total dose and number of administrations given.

Recent changes to the S2A [3] and S2B genotoxicity testing guidances have resulted in revision and combination of the two guidances into a single S2(R1) document [4]. At this time, the proposed updates to S2(R1) include the following:

1. Lowering the maximum concentration of test compound for use in an *in vitro* chromosome damage assay when not limited by solubility or cytotoxicity to 1 mM.

2. The possibility of using the *in vitro* micronucleus test as a test for *in vitro* chromosome damage (using automated analysis such as image analysis and flow cytometry if appropriately validated).

3. An option to eliminate the requirement for an *in vitro* mammalian test for chromosome damage by performing *in vivo* assessment of genotoxicity in two tissues (typically a micronucleus and a second *in vivo* assay).

4. An option that allows for one or more genetic toxicity endpoints to be added onto pivotal rodent toxicity tests of ≤4 weeks' duration as long as appropriate dose levels are reached.

The reader is encouraged to consult the current version of the S2(R1) guideline to confirm the regulatory acceptability of these proposed revisions, as health authority representatives have expressed caution in the adoption of new genotoxicity strategies and approaches to testing [5].

PROTOCOL DESIGN AND ASSAY CONDUCT

The core battery of genotoxicity tests conducted to support clinical trials should be performed under conditions of good laboratory practice (GLP) guidelines using protocols that reflect ICH and Organization for Economic Development (OECD) recommendations specific for each test. These protocols define requirements that must be met in order for an assay to be considered acceptable by regulatory agencies. General information regarding GLP requirements are described by the OECD [6, 7]. Figure 8.1 shows some of the general features that are common to most *in vitro* and *in vivo* protocols for genotoxicity testing. Typically, two to five grams of a well-characterized test compound, preferably synthesized under the conditions of good manufacturing practice, are

In Vitro Tests	*In Vivo* Tests

• Preliminary Cytotoxicity test for dose selection
• Direct Tests (-S9 metabolic conditions)
  • 3-6 hr exposure
  • Continuous exposure
• Metabolic Tests (+S9)
  • 3-6 hr exposure, 24 hr exposure
• At least 5 Treated Concentrations
  – High dose- cytotoxic,
  insoluble or 5 mg/ml (plate)
• Negative (solvent) controls
  • Vehicle and untreated
• Positive controls- direct acting and requiring S9 activation
	• Range-finder (MTD) for dose selection
	• Male/Female Rats (or mice)
	• Single day dosing with multiple cell harvest times; or
	• Multiple days of dosing with single harvest time
	  – At least 3 dose groups (low, mid, high)
	  – High dose- MTD; target cell toxicity or 2 g/kg limit dose
	• Negative control
	  • Vehicle control
	• Positive control

Figure 8.1. General test protocol designs for *in vitro* and *in vivo* tests for genotoxicity

sufficient to conduct all phases of *in vitro* tests. The *in vivo* test will require substantially more of the test compound. Exact amounts depend on the inherent toxicity or solubility of the compound, steepness of the toxicity dose–response curve, and the need for repeat or confirmatory tests. It is preferable that the active pharmaceutical ingredient (API) used in the standard battery be representative of that to be used in clinical testing when possible and that any impurities be present at levels similar or higher than impurities present in the API that is used in clinical trials.

TESTING FOR A GENE MUTATION IN BACTERIA

Typically, the first *in vitro* assay conducted as part of the genetic toxicology standard battery is the bacterial reverse mutation test, also known as the "Ames assay" or the "Ames test," which was developed by Dr. Bruce Ames in the early 1970s. The test has been validated extensively and has the longest history of use in a regulatory testing environment [8,9]. The purpose of the Ames assay is to evaluate a chemical's genotoxicity by measuring its ability to induce reverse mutations at selected loci in several bacterial strains. This assay has been shown to detect genetic changes that predict rodent and human carcinogenesis, but the correlation is not absolute. There are classes of chemical carcinogens that are not detected by the Ames test, possibly due to mechanisms that do not produce a response in this test system. A very large database exists for many structures associated with genotoxic activity in the Ames test [10]. Well-established variants of this test have been developed for testing chemicals with different physical and chemical properties [11].

The overall conduct of the Ames test should follow OECD guideline 471 for the bacterial reverse mutation test [12] and the International Workshop on Genotoxicity Testing (IWGT) report [13]. The Ames assay measures genetic damage at the single base level in DNA using as least five strains of bacteria. The *Salmonella typhimurium* and *Escherichia coli* strains used in the assay each have a unique mutation that has turned off histidine or tryptophan biosynthesis, respectively [9]. Because of these unique mutations, the bacteria require exogenous histidine or tryptophan to survive. However, in the presence of a mutagen, the bacteria can undergo a reverse mutation turning the essential gene back on permitting the cell to grow in the absence of these amino acids, thereby serving as a beacon that a mutagenic event occurred. These bacterial strains were created to have specific mutations, either a base–pair substitution or a frameshift mutation. These mutations can be reversed by varying mechanisms, thus potentially providing some useful insights as to the types of mutations that are induced by the chemical.

The Ames assay protocol includes a range-finding test, which may also include mutational analysis, followed by a definitive mutation test. Each test includes exposing the individual bacterial strains to either:

- a buffer or a metabolic activation system (consisting of a cofactor supplemented postmitochondrial fraction (S9) typically prepared from the livers of rats treated with Aroclor 1254; most laboratories purchase commercially prepared S9 homogenates),
- a negative (solvent) control, a strain-specific positive control or the test chemical up to a maximum dose level of 5000 μg/plate when not limited by solubility or cytotoxicity.

A trace of histidine or tryptophan is also added to the agar support layer. Following a minimum of 2 days incubation, the bacteria use trace amounts of histidine or tryptophan to undergo a few cell divisions, resulting in a distinctive background lawn, whereas the bacteria that had undergone a reverse mutation have grown into a visible colony. The background lawn density is evaluated followed by enumeration of revertant colonies. Mutational results are reported as revertants per plate. Each of the specific bacterial strains has an expected (historic) spontaneous and a positive control revertant per plate background, which should be observed to consider the test acceptable. A chemically induced dose-related increase (typically two- to three fold increase) in revertants per plate over that obtained with the vehicle control for a specific strain is considered a positive response. Equivocal or weak positive results may indicate the need to repeat the test, possibly with a modified protocol such as altered spacing of dose levels. Because the majority of bacterial mutagens are rodent carcinogens, a robust positive response should be followed up with additional *in vitro* and *in vivo* tests for mutagenicity and carcinogenicity. Assessment of DNA adducts (covalent binding) can be a useful approach to rule out the potential of direct DNA damage of the drug or its metabolites, particularly if the molecule contains structural components associated with mutagenicity.

Cytogenetic Testing for Chromosomal Damage

The *in vitro* mouse lymphoma *tk* gene mutation assay, also known as the mouse lymphoma L5178Y *tk±* assay (or the MLA assay), can be used to measure chemically induced forward gene mutations at the thymidine kinase (TK) locus in mouse lymphoma cells caused by base pair changes, frameshift, and small deletions [14]. There is some evidence that the mouse lymphoma assay can also detect chromosome loss. Although mutations may be induced at multiple gene loci, only those induced at the reporter loci, thymidine kinase (tk) are detected in the MLA. The MLA assay can detect both point mutations and larger scale chromosomal anomalies that can be differentiated through colony sizing, fulfilling the ICH requirement for chromosome damage testing. Although the MLA is a very sensitive assay and detects a large proportion of known mutagens, under the test conditions that have been historically used, it lacks specificity and therefore produces a high rate of false positive results. Thus, a positive finding in the MLA could indicate either a false positive response or an increased risk of gene mutations, chromosome damage, and/or a change in chromosome number.

Thymidine monophosphate (TMP), as one of the four nucleotides found in DNA, is highly conversed and serves as a regulator for DNA synthesis. Thymidine kinase (TK) mediates phosphorylation of thymidine to TMP. Because the *tk* gene is a heterozygous (*tk±*) autosomal gene in MLA cells, only one chromosome needs to be mutated to produce the mutant phenotype. Thus, functionally the heterozygous state is important for the sensitivity of this assay. The basis for selection within the MLA assay lies with the fact that the normal *tk±* karyotypes require the addition of thymidine to the culture medium to survive. In this assay, the thymidine is replaced by trifluorothymidine (TFT) that is phosphorylated by the TK to a toxic nucleotide analogue. The MLA assay uses TK (with *tk±*)-competent cells. These cells, following treatment with chemicals and an expression period in thymidine-containing media, are ultimately grown in media containing only TFT. The normal "wild-type" cells with functional *tk* genes will incorporate the TFT in place of thymidine, resulting in death of the normal cells. Cells that grow to form colonies in the presence of TFT are therefore assumed to have mutated, either spontaneously or as induced by the test article, at the *tk±* locus.

The overall conduct of the MLA Assay test should follow OECD guideline 476 for the in vitro mammalian cell–gene mutation test [15] and IWGT report [16]. The MLA assay protocol includes a range-finding test, which may also include mutational analysis, followed by a definitive mutation test. The cells are prepared as clonal suspension cultures. Cells are exposed to either media or a metabolic activation system (consisting of a cofactor-supplemented postmitochondrial fraction (S9) typically prepared from rat treated with Aroclor 1254; test laboratories purchase commercially prepared S9 homogenates) or a negative (solvent) control, a positive control, or the chemical up to a maximum dose level of 1 mM or 0.5 mg/ml, whichever is lower, when not limited by solubility or cytotoxicity.

Three treatment regimens are required: 3–4 hours treatment with and without a metabolic activation system and 24 hours without metabolic activation. The media containing the chemical treatment is replaced with fresh media either with or without the TFT; an expression period for formation of the newly induced mutants is then required. Appropriate sensitivity is achieved in the MLA assay by limiting the chemical dose level to one that results in close to 20% relative total growth (RTG). Colonies are enumerated and sized as appropriate. Large colonies have been associated with small-scale point mutational events, and small colonies correlate with larger chromosomal breaks or aneuploidy. Small and large colony mutants result from differences in growth rate. Mutant cells with extensive genetic damage have prolonged doubling times and thus form small colonies. Induction of small colony mutants has been associated with drugs that induce large-scale chromosomal aberrations. Mutant cells resulting from small point mutations will more often grow at rates similar to the parental cells and thus form large colonies. The mutational results are reported as mutant frequencies per culture. The expected (historic) spontaneous and positive control mutant frequencies per culture, treatment, and condition should be observed to consider the test acceptable. A chemical dose-related increase in mutant frequency over that obtained with the vehicle control would be considered a positive response. If there is a positive treatment-related increase in mutants in the MLA, it is necessary and required by regulatory guidelines to size the colonies and classify the counts by large versus small colonies for positive control cultures and for at least one positive test compound dose, preferably at the concentration that produced the highest mutant response. Equivocal or weak positive results may indicate the need to repeat the test, possibly with a modified protocol such as altered spacing of dose levels. For some mutagens, a mammalian mutation assay may be less sensitive than the bacterial mutation tests for detecting a mutagenic response since mammalian cell lines have some proficiency for DNA repair and since mammalian DNA is afforded some protection by chromosomal proteins that are not present in bacteria.

IN VITRO METAPHASE CHROMOSOME ABERRATION TEST

The *in vitro* chromosome aberration assay, also known as the *in vitro* cytogenetic assay, is used to detect chromosome damage by evaluating the induction of chromosome aberrations in metaphase spreads in either cell lines or primary cell cultures following chemical treatment. Chromosome damage (clastogenicity) is defined in this test system as microscopically visible structural alterations of metaphase chromosomes. Changes in chromosome structure offer morphological evidence of damage to the genetic material [17] and is considered essential for heritable effects and in the multistep process of malignancy. The *in vitro* chromosome aberration assay can also be used to detect polyploidy, which indicates the potential of a test compound to induce changes in chromosome number.

The overall conduct of the i*n vitro* chromosome aberration assay should follow the OECD guideline 473 [17]. The *in vitro* chromosome–aberration assay protocol includes a range-finding test, which includes a mitotic index analysis for toxicity microscopically or via flow cytometry [18] followed by a definitive aberration analysis test. Each test includes the following:

- exposing actively dividing cells (mitogen-stimulated human or rodent peripheral blood lymphocytes or karyotypically stable cell line such as CHO or mouse lymphoma cells) to either media or a metabolic activation system (consisting of a cofactor supplemented postmitochondrial fraction (S9) typically prepared from rats treated with Aroclor 1254; test laboratories purchase commercially prepared S9 homogenates),

- a negative (solvent) control, a positive control, or the test chemical up to a maximum dose level of 1 mM or 0.5 mg/ml, whichever is lower, when not limited by solubility or cytotoxicity.

Three treatment regimens are required, 3–6 hours treatment with and without a metabolic activation system and 24 hours without metabolic activation. The media containing the test chemical is replaced with fresh media, and depending on the treatment regimen is allowed a recovery period prior to cells being harvested. Mitotic spindle inhibitors such as colchicine or synthetic colcemid should be added during the final 2–3 hours of culture to arrest the cells during division and is used to achieve a sufficient number of cells in metaphase for analysis. Cells are harvested at a sample time that allows approximately 1.5 normal cell cycles (typically 18–24 hours for most mammalian cell lines and primary cultures) from the beginning of treatment. Slides of cells in metaphase are prepared and analyzed for the mitotic index, chromosome aberrations, rearrangements, and changes in chromosome number (ploidy). Tests for chromosome aberrations are labor-intensive assays and can take up to a few months to complete. Slide evaluation is technically demanding and time consuming. Chromosomal aberrations results are reported as the number of aberrant cells per treatment with differentiation made between chromosome or chromatid gaps, breaks, and rearrangements. The expected (historic) spontaneous and positive control number of aberrant cells per treatment and condition should be observed to consider the test acceptable. A test chemical dose-related increase in the number of aberrant cells per treatment over that induced with the vehicle control is considered a positive response; however, statistical analysis is required to determine the significance. Equivocal or weak positive results may indicate the need to repeat the test, possibly with a modified testing protocol such as altered spacing of dose levels. Drug-induced toxicity can cause indirect DNA damage. Careful consideration should be taken with respect to dose selection and the evaluation of aberration frequencies around these dose levels to prevent these types of indirect responses [5, 19].

IN VITRO MICRONUCLEUS TEST

The *in vitro* micronucleus assay is used to detect chromosome damage by evaluating the induction of micronuclei within cell lines or primary cell cultures following treatment with the test chemical. Chromosome damage is visible as microscopic pieces of DNA that appear to be a small nucleus, also known as micronuclei. Micronuclei (small nuclei) are formed from acentric fragments of chromosomes (clastogenic mechanism) or whole chromosome losses (aneugenic mechanism) that are not included in the main nucleus of the interphase cell. There may be more than one micronuclei induced per cell; however, this occurrence is considered as a single event. This assay, using secondary staining techniques, can be used to detect aneugenicity (loss or gain of chromosomes). Drug-induced aneugenicity, for the most part, occurs as a result of cytotoxicity to the spindle apparatus involved in cell division rather than as direct DNA damage. Therefore, a threshold level and "no-effect level" can usually be defined.

The *in vitro* micronucleus assay has been widely evaluated in international collaborative studies [20] and is validated by the European Centre for the Validation of Alternative Methods (ECVAM) [21] and should follow the draft of OECD guideline 481. This assay is currently part of the draft ICH S2 (R1) guideline [4]. The *in vitro* micronucleus assay uses the same actively dividing cells from primary cultures or established cell lines as is used in mammalian assays for gene mutation and chromosome damage. It can be similarly treated with the test compound both in the presence and absence of metabolic activation as described previously. The testing protocol can be conducted with or without a cytokinesis-blocking agent (e.g., cytochalasin B), and it includes both range-finding and definitive testing legs. Each test includes the following:

- exposing actively dividing cells to either media or a metabolic activation system (consisting of a cofactor-supplemented postmitochondrial fraction (S9) typically prepared from rats treated with Acroclor 1254; test laboratories purchase commercially prepared S9 homogenates),
- a negative (solvent) control, a positive control, or the test chemical up to a maximum dose level of 1 mM or 0.5 mg/ml, whichever is lower, when not limited by solubility or cytotoxicity.

The assessment of micronuclei is typically conducted microscopically or via automated methods and is quantitated in the first interphase after exposure, as this is the most sensitive time to detect chromosome damage and aneugenicity (lagging chromosomes). The expected (historic) spontaneous and positive control number of micronucleated cells per condition should be observed to consider the test acceptable. A test chemical dose-related increase in the number of micronucleated cells per treatment over that induced with the vehicle control would be considered a positive response. Equivocal or weak positive results may indicate the need to repeat the test, possibly with a modified protocol such as altered spacing of dose levels. Drug-induced toxicity can cause indirect DNA damage, and careful consideration should be taken with dose selection and evaluation of micronucleated cells around these dose levels to prevent these types of response [19, 22]. Micronuclei can be quantified faster, more objectively, and with less technical training than the assessment of chromosome damage in metaphase cells. Because a substantially larger portion of cells are in interphase compared to metaphase, more cells can be scored, which further increases the sensitivity of the assay thereby making this an attractive alternative to the *in vitro* chromosome aberration assay or the mouse lymphoma assay [23].

IN VIVO RODENT MICRONUCLEUS TEST

The third test of the standard ICH S2B [1] guideline battery for genotoxicity is a rodent micronucleus test for chromosomal damage. The *in vivo* rodent micronucleus assay is used to detect chromosome damage by evaluating the induction of micronuclei within immature erythrocytes from either bone marrow or peripheral blood [24] following *in vivo* chemical treatment [25, 26]. As mentioned previously, chromosome damage is visible as microscopic pieces of DNA that appear as micronuclei. Micronuclei are first seen *in vivo* in bone marrow and peripheral blood smears as small acentric (without centromeres) fragments of nuclear material that are not integrated with the main nucleus after cell division.

The overall conduct of the *in vivo* rodent micronucleus assay should follow OECD guideline 474 for the mammalian erythrocyte micronucleus test [27]. The *in vivo* micronucleus assay involves dosing either mice or rats with a negative (solvent) control, a positive control, or the chemical up to a maximum tolerated dose (MTD). The high dose should demonstrate significant adverse clinical signs, body weight loss, and bone marrow effects; is limited by lethality; or is the highest technically deliverable dose of the test chemical. However, it is recognized that drugs with specific biological activities at low nontoxic doses (such as hormones and mitogens) may pose exceptions to the dose-setting criteria as defined by guidance, and alternative dose selection criteria can be used on a case-by-case basis if scientifically justified. *In vivo* exposure information is required for this test. In the absence of compound-induced toxicity, a limit dose of 2000 mg/kg/day (for acute exposure) is acceptable. Lower doses may also be acceptable if there are technical or solubility limitations, or if the toxicokinetic profile (TK) indicates saturation of absorption and distribution at lower doses. Cells from either bone marrow or peripheral blood may also be collected and assessed for micronuclei from animals used for a general toxicity (2–4 weeks) study as long as the bone marrow or peripheral blood is collected within 24 hours of the final dosing. Bone marrow or peripheral blood is collected, smears are prepared and analyzed, or fixed samples of these tissues are analyzed by flow cytometry. The expected (historic) spontaneous and positive control number of micronucleated cells should be observed to consider the test acceptable. A test chemical dose-related increase in the number of micronucleated cells per treatment over that induced with the vehicle control would be considered a positive response. Equivocal or weak positive results may indicate the need to repeat the test, possibly with a modified protocol such as altered spacing of dose levels. The *in vivo* micronucleus test conducted with newly formed erythrocytes can be subject to artificially elevated increases in micronuclei because of the stimulation of erythropoiesis through a variety of mechanisms including excessive blood loss, test compound- induced anemia, or a pharmacological response that activates erythropoiesis. Furthermore, accelerating the multiplication of erythroblasts by administering erythropoietin prior to dosing, or inducing erythropoiesis by bleeding the animals, will increase the frequency of micronuclei [28, 29]. The rapid generation of new red blood cells (RBCs) can lead to error-prone synthesis and the release of imperfect RBCs that escape normal repair and/or surveillance systems that typically limit the background frequency of micronuclei in the RBCs of the bone marrow and peripheral blood. Thus, a potential confounding factor of micronucleus assays, particularly in repeat-dose toxicity studies, is disturbance of erythropoiesis such as extramedullary hematopoiesis or increased reticulocyte production. Prolonged conditions of chemical-induced hypothermia, hyperthermia [30,31], and hypoxia-induced hypothermia [32] have been associated with increases in micronuclei, even in untreated animals.

IN VIVO RODENT CHROMOSOMAL ABERRATION TEST

Artifactual increases in micronuclei can occur with test compounds that stimulate erythropoietin (anemia induced) resulting in substantial increases in immature erythrocytes (e.g., drug-induced temperature changes). In addition, chemical-induced erythrocyte bodies such as siderocytes or Heinz bodies may affect micronuclei analysis. Therefore, it may be necessary to test these compounds for induction of chromosome damage through the cytogenetic evaluation of metaphase cells in the bone marrow rather than the erythrocytes used for micronucleus evaluation. Traditionally, the *in vivo* rodent chromosomal aberration test, also called the *in vivo* cytogenetics assay, is conducted as per OECD guideline 475 for the mammalian bone marrow chromosome aberration test [33]. For this test, rodents are treated with either a negative (solvent) control, a positive control, or the test compound up to the MTD as is done with the *in vivo* rodent micronucleus test or, alternatively, the highest dose may be defined as a dose that produces toxicity in the bone marrow (e.g., a significant reduction in mitotic index). As with most *in vivo* tests, exposure information (TK) is a requirement for this test. Although either bone marrow metaphase analysis or micronucleus evaluation are acceptable *in vivo* tests per ICH guidelines, the micronucleus test is generally the preferred test system, as it is less technically demanding and requires substantially less time to evaluate slides. For either test, chromosome aberrations or micronuclei are typically quantified in the first metaphase or interphase after dosing, respectively, as this is the most sensitive time for their detection. For the *in vivo* chromosome aberration test in rodents, the first sampling interval is 1.5 times the normal cell–cycle length (12–18 hours) following treatment. When a single dose protocol design is used, a second set of animals is required to collect bone marrow 24 hours after the first sample time to allow for uptake and potential metabolism of the test substance as well as potential delays in the cell–cycle kinetics that can affect the optimum time for detecting chromosome damage. Animals should be injected intraperitoneally (ip) with an appropriate dose of Colcemid or colchicine, approximately 3–5 hours prior to the collection of bone marrow cells, to enhance the numbers of bone marrow stem cells in metaphase. Cells are harvested, fixed, and prepared for microscopic analysis for mitotic index and chromosome abnormalities. For the chromosome aberration study, the number of aberrant cells with one or more aberrations should be calculated for each animal as well as the mitotic index and the frequencies for each animal in all treated and control groups. Polyploidy is rarely seen *in vivo* and should be noted and counted while scoring. A polyploidy index should be undertaken if there is an increase in polyploid cells. As in the *in vitro* chromosome aberration assay, an increase in polyploidy in the *in vivo* assay may indicate that the test compound is capable of inhibiting the processes involved in chromosome segregation. Although an *in vivo* increase in polyploidy is viewed to be of greater concern and biological significance, a clear no-observed adverse effect level (NOAEL) can be defined and used to assess the risk of numerical changes at doses intended for clinical usage. In addition, an *in vivo* evaluation of micronucleus induction potential would be desirable to rule out the potential for aneuploidy (chromosome loss) at similar or even lower levels than those at which polyploidy was seen in the *in vivo* metaphase assay.

APPROACHES TO EARLY GENOTOXICITY SCREENING

Historically, most genotoxic effects are mediated via direct, nonthreshold mechanisms resulting from direct DNA damage. Nonthreshold mechanisms have been demonstrated for several chemical classes [34]; however, the burden of proof for such arguments generally rests with the investigator. Strategies to determine the risk and relevance of positive genotoxicity findings are discussed in the following sections. However, investigators should be aware that positive genotoxicity findings uncovered during nonclinical or clinical development might nonetheless result in onerous genotoxicity follow-up testing and costly program delays. Therefore, pharmaceutical companies should have genotoxicity screening assays in place to identify potential genotoxic liabilities as early as possible, typically before the acceptance of a compound into early development

Screening approaches allow for earlier identification of potential genotoxicity hazards and enable additional follow-up testing to identify potential mechanisms and understand the relevance of the finding, or pursuit, of alternative structural chemotypes. Screening assays may range from *in silico* approaches to bacterial mutagenicity assays, clastogenic screening assays, and DNA damage assays.

Computational *in silico* analyses can yield useful predictions for toxicology endpoints without the need for experimental testing [35–37]. In most cases, however, small amounts (milligram to subgram quantities) of a test compound can readily be obtained during lead optimization or late lead optimization phases, allowing for experimental testing in screening-format genotoxicity assays, thus evaluating genotoxicity responses before the commitment of more extensive drug development resources. At this stage, a drug substance may be obtained from early routes of synthesis coming directly from drug discovery laboratories. Therefore, it is important to consider confounding factors such as impurities and residual solvents, which may not be fully characterized at this early stage of testing (discussed further in Chapter 6).

Most pharmaceutical companies will run a modified, high-throughput bacterial mutation assay using a minimum of two bacterial strains (TA98 and TA100). Additionally, an early screen for chromosomal damage such as the *in vitro* micronucleus test, which is useful for predicting the behavior of a compound in *in vitro* mammalian cell assays (e.g., chromosomal aberration, *in vitro* mammalian mutation, and/or the *in vitro* micronucleus assay), may also be conducted. Despite the high sensitivity/low specificity of *in vitro* mammalian cell assays, early prediction of these endpoints can provide a valuable early warning for positive genotoxicity results that can arise in the course of early drug development [38].

Screening can also be a valuable tool for collecting structure–activity response data. Depending on the size and scope of the training data set and the variability of biological

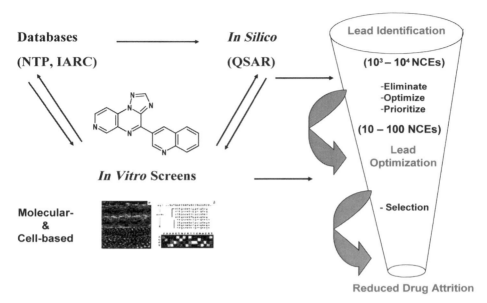

Figure 8.2. Data from screening assays can be used during "Lead Optimization" and "Candidate Selection to enhance selection of better drug candidates. Screening data can then be feedback to computerized predictive QSAR systems to improve future predictivity at "Lead Identification"

Figure taken from Nonclinical Drug Safety Assessment, 2007, FDAnews, 300 N; Washington St., Suite 300, Falls Church, VA 22046. 703-538-760, www.fdanews.com

response, generation, and genotoxicity screening structural analogues may enable the discovery chemist to "design out" problematic chemical motifs that confer genotoxic liability (see Fig. 8.2) while preserving efficacy and potency.

DATA INTERPRETATION AND EVALUATION OF RISK AND RELEVANCE TO HUMANS

Regulatory guidance outlines the use of the "three test battery" for genotoxicity testing. In addition, many pharmaceutical companies have an in-house strategy for staging these assays, data interpretation of these assays, plus decision points and follow-up strategies in the case of positive genotoxicity results. Examples of such schemes can be found in Kirkland et al. [39] and Lorge et al. [40].

Assessment of Biological Relevance and Weight of Evidence

False positive tests are commonplace for assays such as the mouse lymphoma mammalian mutation assay and the *in vitro* chromosome aberration assay, which have been shown to be highly sensitive, and exhibit a high positive outcome rate among both marketed pharmaceuticals and new chemical entities in preclinical and clinical development [41].

Generally, a weight of evidence (WOE) approach is taken to assess risk of these findings. At the 2006 IWGT workshop (San Francisco, CA), the following conditions were listed as criteria that could be used for establishing that a finding is of low significance based on insufficient WOE and/or weak or irrelevant *in vitro* findings as follows:

- The effect is weak, of low magnitude relative to controls, and not dose related,
- Positive increases are only seen at high concentrations of a test compound but not at lower concentrations that are moderately toxic (e.g., >50% in the chromosome aberration assay or >80% in the mouse lymphoma assay),
- The response is within the spontaneous historical control range, with a probability similar to a response that can occur by chance alone (random biological variation),
- The result is not repeatable under similar conditions, at similar concentrations or levels of cytotoxicity.

The U.S. Food and Drug Administration/*Center for Drug Evaluation and Research* (FDA/CDER) Guidance for Industry on Integration of Genetic Toxicology Study Results [42] similarly recommends using a WOE approach and/or establishing a mechanism of action for assessing the risk and relevance of genotoxic findings. Equivocal studies should be repeated to establish reproducibility of the results and, if the results are reproducibly positive, an additional fourth test should be conducted as is consistent with the ICH guidelines. Examples of *in vitro* conditions that can produce nonphysiological changes include pH and osmolarity fluctuations or unreasonably high concentration levels of the test compound [43]. The FDA/CDER also recognizes that even if the test compound has produced a positive result in an *in vitro* genetic toxicology assay, the finding may have resulted from a number of differences between cultured cells and intact animals. This includes "differing metabolic pathways occurring *in vitro* and *in vivo*; metabolic inactivation in the intact animal; failure of the parent compound or active metabolite to reach the target cell; or simply an inability to achieve plasma levels *in vivo* comparable to concentrations that generated positive responses in the *in vitro* assays." Strategies for addressing positive results due to metabolic considerations was addressed by a 2005 IWGT working group and can be found in Ku et al. [44].

In addition to IWGT efforts, workshops sponsored by ECVAM and the ongoing International Life Sciences Institute–Health and Environmental Sciences Institute (ILSI-HESI) "Relevance and Follow-up of Positive Results in *in vitro* Genetic Toxicity Testing" (IVGT) Project Committee efforts have produced complementary publications to address the interpretation and management of positive genotoxicity results [41, 45].

Potential Reactive Metabolites

A positive response seen only in the presence of metabolic activation suggests that a reactive metabolite may have been generated. In this case, one could monitor metabolites in general toxicity studies, in addition to conducting a parallel assessment of mutagenicity of the potential metabolites using *in vitro* mammalian genetic toxicology assays. Using human metabolic activation may be a useful tool to evaluate whether reactive metabolites would be formed under clinical exposure conditions [44,46].

Impurities

A reproducible, weak increase in a genotoxicity signal may be indicative of a true genotoxic hazard or could suggest the presence of a low-level mutagenic impurity. To rule out a genotoxic impurity, investigators should conduct a thorough review of the synthetic pathway for potential reactive intermediates and process reagents and, if possible, conduct additional analytical testing to rule out the presence of potential mutagenic impurities [47 and Chapter 6].

Indirect Mechanisms of Genotoxicity

In addition to direct DNA-reactive mechanisms of genotoxicity, *in vitro* and *in vivo* tests for detecting gene mutations and chromosome damage can respond via indirect mechanisms [48] and be detected as genotoxic activity. These mechanisms may demonstrate a threshold effect, as in the case of aneuploidy, which can result from perturbation of the mitotic spindle. Mueller et al. [49] describe several examples of pharmaceutical classes that exhibit genotoxicity responses that are well understood. If the genotoxic response of a new pharmaceutical substance can be clearly attributed to an established indirect mechanism, it may be possible to define a NOAEL, below which the risk would be considered acceptably low. Follow-up testing strategies may include testing for direct DNA interaction to rule out direct covalent interaction with DNA, as well as pharmacological and pharmacokinetic information that can determine the biological relevance of a finding under therapeutic exposure conditions. In addition, complementary methodologies such as toxicogenomics may be helpful in identifying and supporting a particular mechanism of action. For compounds that produce genotoxicity though indirect mechanisms, the FDA recommends presenting evidence of a mechanism that is not expected to occur *in vivo* or a threshold that would otherwise not be attainable during clinical tails. If a positive response has a clear indirect mechanism or is not achievable under clinical conditions, the FDA may allow clinical studies in normal volunteers or in patients to proceed without additional studies [42].

ASSAYS USEFUL FOR FOLLOW-UP OF POSITIVE GENOTOXICITY FINDINGS

When data from the three-assay genotoxicity battery are not sufficient, additional assays can be undertaken to better understand and interpret the results of positive genotoxicity findings. DNA damage can be assessed in potential target tissues using tests for DNA adducts (^{32}P postlabeling or ^{14}C-labeled toxicophore) and DNA strand breakage (alkaline elution assays and Comet assays) and through direct assessment of mutation induction in potential target tissues of transgenic mice (MutaMouse, Big Blue® mouse). These tests can all be used to either support or rule out a direct DNA-reactive mechanism for an *in vitro* or *in vivo* finding.

Unscheduled DNA Synthesis Assay (UDS)

The *in vivo/in vitro* version of the unscheduled DNA synthesis (UDS) test was initially cited in the original ICH S2 guidance as a preferred second *in vivo* assay for following up positive *in vitro* findings as it was well validated [50]. A large data base existed for the liver UDS assay at that time [51], and a comprehensive literature review by Tweats [52] showed that a combination of the liver UDS test and the bone marrow micronucleus test was able to detect most genotoxic carcinogens with few false positive results. However, false negative results with this combination of assays have been seen with some genotoxic compounds that are unstable and some aromatic amines that are difficult to detect in most *in vivo* screens [52]. DNA damage assays such as the *in vivo* Comet assay, DNA covalent binding assays, and *in vivo* transgenic mouse mutation assays should be considered when conducting an *in vivo* genotoxicity assay for follow-up purposes (see the draft ICH S2(R1) guideline).

DNA Binding/Interaction Assays

DNA binding and interaction studies are particularly useful when it is not clear if genotoxicity resulted from direct DNA damaging mechanisms or from indirect effects related to excessive cytotoxicity or other mechanisms that can be amenable to risk management by establishing a threshold. Because it can often be difficult and time consuming to establish a definitive indirect mechanism, a reverse approach is to rule out or confirm a direct DNA-reactive mechanism by assessing the ability of the molecule to covalently bind or interact with DNA. Typically, these binding assays are conducted using radiolabeled (^{14}C) drug substance; however, creating this labeled compound is very costly and time consuming, which may limit the application of this assay to routine follow-up studies [53].

DNA Adduct Analysis: ^{32}P Postlabeling Assay

Detection and analysis of DNA adducts using the ^{32}P postlabeling technique is a sensitive method that is particularly useful when it is difficult or impossible to synthesize the ^{14}C radiolabeled test compound. The postlabeling procedure as developed by Randerath et al. [54] has been applied extensively to quantify DNA adducts in different cellular systems. However, the method is best applied when the structure of the adducted molecule is known or can be predicted, as different extraction techniques may be necessary depending on various properties including size, charge, and potential sites of adduction. This technique will detect most types of adducts including those formed directly by the covalent binding of carcinogens and mutagens to nucleotide bases in DNA, plus other DNA lesions resulting from modification of bases by endogenous or exogenous agents (e.g., oxidative damage). The 32P postlabeling technique requires less than 10 μg of

DNA and is capable of detecting certain types of adducts at levels as low as one adduct in 10^{-9} to 10^{-10} normal nucleotides [55]. The disadvantage of the 32P postlabeling technique is that it does not detect all classes of DNA adducts, requires the use of high levels of gamma radiation, and once DNA adducts have been detected, their conclusive chemical identification requires further analytical testing by mass spectrometry. In addition, the experimental conditions to resolve adducts are unique to a particular drug and, in most cases, adducts are easily missed due to such a degree that one almost needs to know the expected adducts prior to selecting the experimental conditions.

Adduct Analysis: Mass Spectrometry Techniques

Various mass spectrometry methods exist for measuring the levels of chemical adducts *in vivo* including conventional mass spectrometry and accelerator mass spectrometry (AMS) [56, 57]. The maximum sensitivity and cost and availability of the technology are the driving factors when selecting the appropriate platform [58]. The measurement of hemoglobin adducts is a sensitive and accessible approach by which to monitor exposure of reactive species in peripheral blood. Recently, measurement of ethyl valine adducts was used to quantify exposure of ethyl methanesulfonate (EMS), as related to response in *in vivo* transgenic mutagenicity and micronucleus assays [59]. In this example, a sensitive method to determine exposures accurately at low levels was necessary to demonstrate the existence of a threshold-mediated effect [60].

AMS is a highly sensitive technique for measuring concentrations of low levels of radiolabeled isotopes in small samples of less than a milligram. Principles and detailed methodology regarding the approach can be found in recent reviews [61, 62]. AMS differs from other forms of mass spectrometry in that it accelerates ions to extraordinarily high kinetic energies before mass analysis and is exceptional in its ability to analyze elemental and isotopic compositions sensitively and accurately and can yield quantitative data regarding adduct formation, with sensitivities at the level of $1/10^{12}$ adducts/nucleotide [58]. In practice, this approach requires costly instrumentation. However, growing interest in applications in pharmacokinetic Phase 0 "microdosing" studies have led to the availability of commercial vendors for this technology [63].

In vitro and *in vivo* Comet Assay

Using electrophoresis, a cell expressing DNA damage in the Comet assay takes on the appearance of a "comet" with the head of the comet representing the nuclear region of the cell and the tail containing DNA fragments of various size and charge. The Comet assay can detect multiple classes of DNA damage provided they result in strand breaks at alkaline pH. This assay is capable of measuring damage at the level of a single cell. Comet assays conducted either *in vitro* or *in vivo* are relatively simple compared to their analogous UDS assays, as they do not require difficult perfusions to acquire cell samples, or the use of radiolabeling, autoradiography, or scintillation techniques to detect damage. However, a primary advantage of the *in vivo* Comet assay is that it can be used to assess damage in any target tissue, regardless of whether the tissue is capable of dividing or not. This advantage is particularly important when one wants to assess potential damage at the sites of highest contact of the test drug and its metabolites, particularly when a bone marrow assay is inadequate due to poor systemic exposure.

In recent years, the *in vivo* Comet test has become a favored test for following up positive findings or assessing genotoxicity at potentially high sites of contact that might not be amenable to detection using other *in vivo* test systems. The recommended standardized protocol for this assay, as developed by Singh et al. [64] and Tice et al. [65], is to use an alkaline buffer (pH >13). Standardization of the *in vivo* Comet assay has evolved from various working groups and intralaboratory validation studies [66]. The basic steps involved in processing the tissue and conducting the assay are described in detail in Hartmann et al. [67]. Briefly, animals are treated once with the test substance and tissue/organ samples are obtained at 2–6 and 16–26 hours postdosing, respectively. The shorter sampling time is required to detect rapidly absorbed, as well as unstable or direct acting, compounds; and the longer sampling time is used to detect compounds that require time to be absorbed, distributed, and metabolized. Alternative sampling times may be used when justified based on TK data.

Selection of the tissue(s) to be evaluated should be based on absorption, distribution, metabolism, and excretion data and/or toxicological information to support that the tissue is a relevant target tissue for toxicity or exposure of the test compound and/or its metabolite(s). In the absence of tissue-specific TK information, the liver typically is assessed for comet induction, as it is the major organ for metabolizing compounds and is often the tissue of first site of contact for orally administered drugs taken up through the portal circulation. Care must be taken to avoid conditions that would lead to positive results that do not reflect genotoxicity but that might arise from DNA damage (double-strand breaks) associated with apoptosis or necrosis.

Syrian Hamster Embryo (SHE) Cell Transformation Assay

Syrian hamster embryo (SHE) cells have been used to assess cell transformation [68–72] and to assess the carcinogenic potential of pharmaceuticals and chemicals [73, 74]. Cell transformation assays such as the SHE assay have been shown to be useful for studying the mechanisms and processes of morphological cell transformation that potentially lead up to carcinogenesis. The assay uses frozen SHE cells prepared at gestation day 13. Target cells are seeded onto a layer of feeder cells (X-ray irradiated SHE cells) and treated with a test article for 24 hours or 7 days. After a growth period of 7 days, the cells are fixed, stained, and evaluated for morphological cell transformation. The SHE assay has been previously suggested as a follow-up assay for positive *in vitro* genotoxicity results. The literature suggests that the SHE assay correlates well with rodent carcinogenicity results for chemicals in general [75]. However, results from an ILSI collaborative validation study on human pharmaceuticals indicated that the SHE assay is less predictive for human carcinogenic risk [75] for some human pharmaceuticals. In this study, the SHE assay had high sensitivity (83%) for detection of human carcinogens but a low specificity (15%) for predicting noncarcinogens, resulting in a low overall concordance of 37%. Thus, caution should be used in stopping development of a test compound based on a positive outcome in this assay without further follow-up, unless the compound is of a class that has previously been shown to induce tumors in standard bioassays.

Nonetheless, for some classes of chemicals and drugs, negative results from an *in vitro* cell transformation assay such as the SHE assay may be a useful approach for risk managing an *in vitro* finding and continuing development of the drug in question. The assay analysis has inherent problems in colony transformation interpretation due to colony reader bias, thus the confidence in the outcome is sometimes questionable [76].

Transgenic Rodent Bioassays

To address a genotoxic response, on a case-by-case basis, it may be necessary to carry out early oncogenicity tests including short-term transgenic studies using p53± knock-out mice or ras H2 transgenic mice. Both assays are suitable for detecting genotoxic carcinogens, and the ras H2 test model can detect nongenotoxic carcinogens. Factors that may influence the decision to discontinue development or expedite oncogenicity studies include target population, disease indication, duration of exposure, and safety profile of other drugs in the class or other drugs serving the same medical need [77–80].

Toxicogenomic Approaches

Toxicogenomics, proteomics, and other tests for gene expression may provide useful insights regarding genetic toxicity outcome. Although toxicogenomics is less sensitive than the traditional genotoxicity battery assays, it can contribute to mechanistic understanding, for instance, discriminating nongenotoxic vs genotoxic modes and mechanisms of action [81]. Toxicogenomic approaches have been shown to identify particular classes of genotoxicants, such as mitotic spindle inhibitors, or can signal the critical importance of metabolizing enzymes in metabolic activation [82]. Follow-up testing of a test compound with positive genotoxicity findings can be designed using information obtained from toxicogenomic signatures and complement mode of action hypothesis, for instance, when explaining the irrelevance of an *in vitro* or preclinical finding in regards to assessing human health risks.

RISK–BENEFIT CONSIDERATIONS—SYNTHESIS OF THE DATA

Not all positive genetic toxicology findings will result in an increased cancer risk or require the early termination of clinical development. As for other potentially adverse effects, the risk and relevance of findings must be weighed against the cost–benefit that the new drug may afford the patient population. Regulatory agencies consider multiple factors including the risks vs benefits of the drug, availability of other drugs that are not genotoxic, duration of treatment, treatment population, and total weight of evidence to support the validity and relevance of the finding. Additional factors considered in the "approvability" of a potentially genotoxic compound include whether or not there are other nongenotoxic drugs available, or if there is any suggestion of an increase in tumorigenicity. Exceptions would be if the mechanism were clearly established to be nonrelevant to humans, or if the drug was for a life-threatening condition (e.g., anticancer therapy with no nongenotoxic alternative). In the latter case, usage might be restricted to short-duration therapy or in a restricted patient population that is unlikely to include juvenile subjects. Differences in safety labeling profiles, including mutagenicity endpoints, can also be used to a competitive advantage in marketing by selectively differentiating a nongenotoxic pharmaceutical agent from ones with a similar therapeutic efficacy profile but having no statements on positive genotoxicity in the label.

Reconsidering Threshold Concepts and Dose–Response Assessments in Genotoxicity: The Case of EMS

Genotoxicity assays have historically been designed to identify potential hazards. However, a growing movement has emphasized the need to move the field in a direction to address human risk and relevance of genotoxicity assay results [45, 83]. Notably, the recent case of EMS in the antitretroviral drug Viracept has advanced thinking regarding thresholded mechanisms of genotoxicity and acceptable human exposures to genotoxicants [84]. Due to an unforeseen exposure of thousands of patients to the genotoxic impurity EMS, the pharmaceutical sponsor rapidly proposed follow-up measures that presented a body of evidence demonstrating "significant thresholds" between determined patient exposures and exposure levels, which induced genotoxic changes [84]. Although this effort has demonstrated the possibility for threshold response among direct DNA-acting agents, it is important to realize the cost, resources, and substantial body of data and literature on EMS that were available to the sponsor at the time that genotoxicity threshold investigations were initiated [59]. Nonetheless, investigations by academic and industrial groups have challenged the previous dogma of nonthresholded direct-acting genotoxicants [85, 86]. These developments suggest that future genotoxicity analyses methods may include tools for quantitative dose-response assessment could support low-level exposures in humans, resulting in low an/or acceptable risk.

Assessment of Active Pharmaceutical Ingredient (API) Impurities and Degradation Products

ICH guidelines (Q3A for drug substances [87] and Q3B for drug products [88]) require an *in vitro* assessment of mutagenicity and clastogenicity once an impurity or degradant exceeds a 0.15% level of the drug or at lower levels if genotoxicity is suspected through structural alerts or through the literature. Although the ICH Q3 guideline indicates, "lower thresholds (for reporting, identifying, and qualifying) can be appropriate if the impurity is unusually toxic," the guidance does not specify how "unusually toxic" should be defined, does not consider the total daily intake of the drug, or specify how to perform the qualification testing.

Guidances that specifically address management of genotoxic impurities should also be followed [89–91]. Identifying and monitoring such impurities should be performed throughout early- and late-drug development stages to ensure compliance with recommended exposure limits. Managing genotoxic impurities are typically performed in a staged manner, with both *in silico* and experimental approaches used. Testing the suspected genotoxic impurity may confidently be carried out as a spiked impurity of API test article, as the Ames assay has been shown to have sensitivity to pick up mutagens at or above 250 μg/plate dose levels [92]. The European Medicines Agency Question and Answers document on genotoxic impurities also indicates the acceptability of a spiked testing approach [91]. However, the recent FDA draft guidance on genotoxic impurities notes that the sponsor is obligated to demonstrate that testing of neat impurity is not feasible before resorting to testing a spiked test article [89].

Default total daily maximum allowable doses of genotoxic impurities are generally based on the analysis of Kroes et al. [93] of Gold's database that showed a *de minimus* dietary consumption of 0.15 μg/day of a potent genotoxic carcinogen present in food would provide a negligible risk ($<10^{-6}$) of cancer over a lifetime of exposure. This limit dose for pharmaceutical impurities was based on risk data that shows a threshold of toxicological concern (TTC) below which there would be an insignificant (less than 10^{-5}) increase in relative risk for excess cancers in the clinical population. "Staged" TTC approaches account for shorter durations of clinical exposure, allowing up to a maximum of 120 μg/day daily dose of genotoxic impurity. However, this may need to be considered if an additive nature of other genotoxic impurities is present in the drug substance.

REFERENCES

1. International Conference on Harmonization, 1997. A standard battery for genotoxicity testing for pharmaceuticals (ICH Harmonized Tripartite Guideline S2B). http://www.ich.org/LOB/media/MEDIA494.pdf

2. International Conference on Harmonization, 2009. M3(R2): Guidance on nonclinical safety studies for the conduct of human clinical trials and marketing authorization for pharmaceuticals. http://www.ich.org/LOB/media/MEDIA5544.pdf

3. International Conference on Harmonization, 1995. Guidance on specific aspects of regulatory genotoxicity tests for pharmaceuticals (ICH Harmonized Tripartite Guideline S2A). http://www.ich.org/LOB/media/MEDIA493.pdf

4. International Conference on Harmonization, 2008. Guidance on genotoxicity testing and data interpretation for pharmaceuticals intended for human use, Current Step 2 version http://www.ich.org/LOB/media/MEDIA4474.pdf

5. Elespuru RK, Agarwal R, Atrakchi AH et al., 2009. Current and future application of genetic toxicity assays: The role and value of in vitro mammalian assays. *Toxicol Sci* **109(2)**: 172–179

6. Organization for Economic Development, 1997. No. 1, *OECD Principles of Good Laboratory Practice*, Revised 1997. http://www.olis.oecd.org/olis/1998doc.nsf/LinkTo/NT00000C5A/$FILE/01E88455.PDF

7. Organization for Economic Development, 2004. OECD series on principles of good laboratory practice and compliance monitoring, number 14, Advisory document of the working group on good laboratory practice, The application of the principles of GLP to in vitro studies. http://www.olis.oecd.org/olis/2004doc.nsf/LinkTo/NT00008FEE/$FILE/JT00174939.PDF

8. Ames BN, Lee FD, and Durston WE, 1973. An improved bacterial test system for the detection and classification of mutagens and carcinogens. *Proc Natl Acad Sci U S A* **70(3)**:782–786

9. Ames BN, McCann J, and Yamasaki E, 1975. Methods for detecting carcinogens and mutagens with the Salmonella/mammalian-microsome mutagenicity test. Mutat Res *31*:347–364

10. Mortelmans K and Zeiger E, 2000. The Ames *Salmonella*/microsome mutagenicity assay. *Mutat Res 455(1–2)*: 29–60

11. Maron DM and Ames BN, 1983. Revised methods for the salmonella mutagenicity test. *Mutat Res 113*:173–215

12. Organization for Economic Development, 1997. Test No. 471: Bacterial reverse mutation test. http://lysander.sourceoecd.org/vl=351133/cl=40/nw=1/rpsv/cgi-bin/fulltextew.pl?prpsv=/ij/oecdjournals/1607310x/v1n4/s37/p1.idx

13. Gatehouse D, Haworth S, Cebula T et al., 1994. Report from the working group on bacterial mutation assays: International workshop on standardisation of genotoxicity test procedures. *Mutat Res 312*:217–233

14. Clive D and Spector JFS, 1975. Laboratory procedure for assessing specific locus mutations at the TK locus in cultured L5178Y mouse lymphoma cells. *Mutat Res 31*:17–29

15. Organization for Economic Development, 1997. Test No. 476: In vitro mammalian cell gene mutation test. http://lysander.sourceoecd.org/vl=921109/cl=12/nw=1/rpsv/cgi-bin/fulltextew.pl?prpsv=/ij/oecdjournals/1607310x/v1n4/s41/p1.idx

16. Moore MM, Honma M, Clements J et al., 2006. Mouse lymphoma thymidine kinase gene mutation assay: Follow-up meeting of the International Workshop on Genotoxicity Tests, Aberdeen, Scotland, 2003—Assay acceptance criteria, positive controls, and data evaluation. *Environ Mol Mutagen 47*:1–5

17. Evans HJ, 1976. Cytological methods for detecting chemical mutagens. In: A Hollaender, editor. *Chemical Mutagens, Principles and Methods for their Detection*, vol. 4. New York and London: Plenum Press. pp. 1–29

18. Muehlbauer PA and Schuler MJ, 2003. Measuring the mitotic index in chemically treated human lymphocyte cultures by flow cytometry. *Mutat Res 537*:117–130

19. Kirkland D, Pfuhler S, Tweats D et al., 2007B. How to reduce false positive results when undertaking in vitro genotoxicity testing and thus avoid unnecessary follow-up animal tests: Report of an ECVAM workshop. Mutat Res *628*:31–55

20. Kirsch-Volders M, Sofuni T, Aardema M, Albertini S et al., 2003B. IWGT Report from the in vitro micronucleus assay working group. *Mutat Res 540*:153–163

21. Corvi R, Albertine S, Hartung T et al., 2008. ECVAM retrospective validation of in vitro micronucleus test (MNT). *Mutagenesis 23*:271–283

22. Lorge E, Hayashi M, Albertini S, and Kirkland D, 2008. Comparison of different methods for an accurate assessment of cytotoxicity in the in vitro micronucleus test. I. Theoretical aspects. *Mutat Res 655*:1–3

23. Lorge E, Lambert C, Gervais V et al., 2007. Genetic toxicity assessment: employing the best science for human safety evaluation. Part II: Performances of the in vitro micronucleus test compared to the mouse lymphoma assay and the in vitro chromosome aberration assay. *Toxicol Sci 96*:214–217

24. Wakata A, Miyamae Y, Sato S-I, Suzuki T, Morita T, Asano N, Awogi T, Kondo K, and Hayashi M, 1998. Evaluation of the rat micronucleus test with bone marrow and peripheral blood: Summary of the 9th collaborative study by SGMT/JEMS.MMS. *Environ Mol Mutagen 32*:84–100

25. Heddle JA, 1973. A rapid *in vivo* test for chromosomal damage, *Mutat Res 18*:187–190

26. Schmid W, 1975. The micronucleus test. *Mutat Res 31*:9–15

27. Organisation for Economic Co-operation and Development, 1997. Test No. 474: Mammalian erythrocyte micronucleus test. http://titania.sourceoecd.org/vl=1133448/cl=22/nw=1/rpsv/cgi-bin/fulltextew.pl?prpsv=/ij/oecdjournals/1607310x/v1n4/s39/p1.idx

28. Suzuki Y, Nagae Y, Ishikawa T, Watanabe Y, Nagashima T, Matsukubo K, and Shimizu H, 1989. Effect of erythropoietin on the micronucleus test. *Environ Mol Mutagen 13*: 314–318

29. Hirai O, Miyamae Y, Fujino Y et al., 1991. Prior bleeding enhances the sensitivity of the in vivo micronucleus test. *Mutat Res 264*:109–114

30. Asanami S and Shimono K, 1997. Hypothermia induces micronuclei in mouse bone marrow cells. *Mutat Res 393*:91–8.

31. Asanami S and Shimono K, 1999. The effect of hyperthermia on micronucleus induction by mutagens in mice. *Mutat Res 446*:149–154.

32. Snyder RD and Diehl MS, 2005. Hypoxia-induced micronucleus formation in mice. Drug Chem Toxicol *28(4)*:373–378

33. Organisation for Economic Co-operation and Development, 1997. Test No. 475: Mammalian bone marrow chromosome aberration test. http://titania.sourceoecd.org/vl=1133448/cl=22/nw=1/rpsv/cgi-bin/fulltextew.pl?prpsv=/ij/oecdjournals/1607310x/v1n4/s40/p1.idx

34. Kirkland DJ and Muller L, 2000. Interpretation of the biological relevance of genotoxicity test results: The importance of thresholds. *Mutat Res 464*:137–147

35. Snyder RD, Pearl GS, Mandakas G et al., 2006. Assessment of the sensitivity of the computational programs DEREK, TOPKAT, and MCASE in the prediction of the genotoxicity of pharmaceutical molecules. *Environ Mol Mutagen 43*:143–158.

36. Matthews EJ, Kruhlak NL, Cimino MC et al., 2006. An analysis of genetic toxicity, reproductive and developmental toxicity, and carcinogenicity data: I. Identification of carcinogens using surrogate endpoints. *Regul Toxicol Pharmacol 44*:83–96

37. Yang C, Benz Rd and Cheeseman MA, 2006. Landscape of current toxicity databases and database standards. *Curr Opin Drug Discov Devel 9*:124–133

38. Jacobson-Kram D, and Contrera JF, 2007. Genetic toxicity assessment: Employing the best science for human safety evaluation. Part I: Early screening for potential human mutagens. *Toxicol Sci 96*:16–20

39. Kirkland D, Aardema M, Henderson L, and Müller L, 2005. Evaluation of the ability of a battery of three in vitro genotoxicity tests to discriminate rodent carcinogens and noncarcinogens I. Sensitivity, specificity and relative predictivity. *Mutat Res 584*:1–256

40. Lorge E, Gervais V, Becourt-Lhote N et al., 2007. Genetic toxicity assessment: employing the best science for human safety evaluation part IV: A strategy in genotoxicity testing in drug development: some examples. *Toxicol Sci 98*:39–42

41. Kirkland DJ, Aardema M, Banduhn N et al., 2007. In vitro approaches to develop weight of evidence (WoE) and mode of action (MoA) discussions with positive in vitro genotoxicity results. *Mutagenesis 22*:161–175

42. U.S. Food and Drug Administration, 2006. Guidance for industry on integration of genetic toxicology study results. http://www.fda.gov/downloads/Drugs/GuidanceCompliance RegulatoryInformation/Guidances/ucm079257.pdf

43. Scott D, Galloway SM, Marshall RR et al., 1991. Genotoxicity under extreme culture conditions. A report from ICPEMC Task Group 9. *Mutat Res 257*:147–204

44. Ku WW, Bigger A, Brambilla G et al., 2007. Strategy for genotoxicity testing-metabolic considerations. Strategy Expert Group, IWGT. Mutat Res *627*:59–77.

45. Thybaud V, Aardema M, Clements J et al., 2007C. Expert working group on hazard identification and risk assessment in relation to in vitro testing. Strategy for genotoxicity testing: hazard identification and risk assessment in relation to in vitro testing. *Mutat Res 627*:41–58

46. Dobo KL, Obach RS, Luffer-Atlas D, and Bercu JP, 2009. A strategy for the risk assessment of human genotoxic metabolites. *Chem Res Toxicol 22*:348–356

47. Dobo KL, Greene N, Cyr MO et al., 2006. The application of structure-based assessment to support safety and chemistry diligence to manage genotoxic impurities in active pharmaceutical ingredients during drug development. *Regul Toxicol Pharmacol 44*:282–293

48. Kirsch-Volders M, Vanhauwaert A, Eichenlaub-Ritter U, and Decordier I, 2003A. Indirect mechanisms of genotoxicity. *Toxicol Lett 140–141*:63–74

49. Muller L and Kasper P, 2000. Human biological relevance and the use of threshold-arguments in regulatory genotoxicity assessment: experience with pharmaceuticals. *Mutat Res 464*:19–34

50. Mitchell AD, Casciano DA, Meltz et al., 1983. Unscheduled DNA synthesis tests. A report of the U.S. Environmental Protection Agency Gene-Tox Program. *Mutat Res 123*:363–410

51. Madle S, Dean SW, Andrae U et al., 1994. Recommendations for the performance of UDS tests in vitro and in vivo. *Mutat Res 312*:263–285

52. Tweats DJ, 1994. Follow-up of in vitro positive results. In: PF D'Arcy and DWG Harron, editors. *Proceedings of the Second International Conference on Harmonisation (ICH).* Antrim, Northern Ireland: Greystoke Books Ltd. pp. 240–244

53. Hah SS, Sumbad RA, de Vere White RW et al., 2007. Characterization of oxaliplatin-DNA adduct formation in DNA and differentiation of cancer cell drug sensitivity at microdose concentrations. *Chem Res Toxicol 20(12)*:1745–1751

54. Randerath K, Reddy MV, and Gupta RC, 1981. ^{32}P-labeling test for DNA damage. *Proc Natl Acad Sci U S A 78*:6126–6129

55. Reddy MV, 1992. ^{32}P-Postlabeling analysis of small aromatic and bulky nonaromatic DNA adducts. In: DH Phillips, M Castegnaro, and H Bartsch, editors. *Postlabeling Methods for Detection of DNA Adducts.* Lyon, France: IARC Scientific Publications. pp. 25–34

56. Du HF, Xu LH, Wang HF et al., 2005. Formation of MTBE-DNA adducts in mice measured with accelerator mass spectrometry. Environ Toxi*col 20(4)*:397–401

57. Yuan Y, Wang HF, Sun HF et al., 2007. Adduction of DNA with MTBE and TBA in mice studied by accelerator mass spectrometry. *Environ Toxicol 22*:630–635

58. Farmer PB, Brown K, Tompkins E et al., 2005. DNA adducts: mass spectrometry methods and future prospects. *Toxicol Appl Pharmacol 207(2)*:293–301

59. Gocke E, Ballantyne M, Whitwell J, and Mueller L, 2009. MNT and MutaMouse studies to define the *in vivo* dose response relations of the genotoxicity of EMS and ENU. *Toxicol Lett 190(3)*:286–297

60. Gocke E, Bürgin H, Müeller L, and Pfister T, 2009. Literature review on the genotoxicity, reproductive toxicity and carcinogenicity of ethyl methanesulfonate. Toxicol Lett *190(3)*: 254–265

61. Brown K, Dingley KH, and Turteltaub KW, 2005. Accelerator mass spectrometry for biomedical research. *Methods Enzymol 402*:423–443

62. Brown K, Tompkins EM, and White IN, 2006. Applications of accelerator mass spectrometry for pharmacological and toxicological research. *Mass Spectrom Rev 25*:127–145

63. Lappin G and Garner RC, 2008. The utility of microdosing over the past 5 years. *Expert Opin Drug Metab Toxicol* **4**:1499–506

64. Singh NP, McCoy MT, Tice RR, and Schneider EL, 1988. A simple technique for quantitation of low levels of DNA damage in individual cells. *Exp Cell Res* **175**:184–191

65. Tice RR, Agurell E, Anderson D et al., 2000. Single cell gel/Comet assay: Guidelines for in vitro and in vivo genetic toxicology testing. *Environ Mol Mutagen* **35**:206–221

66. Lovell DP and Omori T, 2008. Statistical issues in the use of the comet assay. *Mutagenesis* **23**:171–82

67. Hartmann A, Agurell E, Beevers C et al., 2003. Recommendations for conducting the *in vivo* alkaline Comet assay. *Mutagenesis* **18**:45–51

68. Berwald Y and Sachs L, 1965. In vitro transformation of normal cells to tumor cells by carcinogenic hydrocarbons. J Natl Cancer Inst **35**:641–661

69. LeBoeuf RA and Kerckaert GA, 1986. The induction of transformed-like morphology and enhanced growth in Syrian hamster embryo cells grown at acidic pH. *Carcinogenesis* **7**:1431–1440

70. LeBoeuf RA and Kerckaert G, 1987. Enhanced morphological transformation and early passage Syrian hamster embryo cells cultured in medium with a reduced bicarbonate concentration and pH. *Carcinogenesis* **8**:689–697

71. LeBoeuf RA, Kerckaert GA, Aardema MJ, and Gibson DP, 1990. Multistage neoplastic transformation of Syrian hamster embryo cells cultured at pH 6.70. *Cancer Res* **50**:3722–3729

72. Kerckaert GA, Isfort RJ, Carr GJ et al., 1996. A comprehensive protocol for conducting the Syrian hamster embryo cell transformation assay at pH 6.70. *Mutat Res* **356**:65–84

73. Huberman E, Salzberg S, and Sachs L, 1968. The *in vitro* induction of an increase in cell multiplication and cellular life span by the water soluble carcinogen dimethylnitrosamine. *Proc Nat Acad Sci U S A* **59**:7782

74. Isfort RJ, Kerckaert GA, and LeBoeuf RA, 1996. Comparison of the standard and reduced pH Syrian hamster embryo (SHE) cell transformation assays in predicting the carcinogenic potential of chemicals. *Mutat Res* **356**:11–63

75. Mauthe RJ, Gibson DP, Bunch RT, and Custer L, 2001. The Syrian hamster embryo (SHE) cell transformation assay: Review of the methods and results. *Toxicol Pathol* **29**:138–146

76. Walsh MJ, Bruce SW, Pant K et al., 2009. Discrimination of a transformation phenotype in Syrian golden hamster embryo (SHE) cells using ATR-FTIR spectroscopy. *Toxicology* **258**:33–38

77. Jacobson-Kram D, Sistare FD, and Jacobs AC, 2004. Use of transgenic mice in carcinogenicity hazard assessment. *Toxicol Pathol* **32**:49–52

78. MacDonald J, French J E, Gerson RJ et al., 2004. The utility of transgenic mouse assays for identifying human carcinogens: A basic understanding and path forward. *Toxicol Sci* **77**:188–194

79. Tennant RW, Stasiewicz S, Mennear J et al., 1999. Genetically altered mouse models for identifying carcinogens. *IARC Sci Publ* **146**:123–150

80. Pritchard JB, French JE, Davis BJ, and Haseman JK, 2003. The role of transgenic mouse models in carcinogen identification. *Environ Health Perspect* **111**:444–454

81. Thybaud V, Le Fevre AC, and Boitier E, 2007A. Application of toxicogenomics to genetic toxicology risk assessment. *Environ Mol Mutagen* **48**:369–379

82. Ellinger-Ziegelbauer H, Aubrecht J, Kleinjans JC and Ahr HJ, 2009. Application of toxicogenomics to study mechanisms of genotoxicity and carcinogenicity. *Toxicol Lett 186*:36–44

83. Thybaud V, Aardema M, Casciano DR et al., 2007B. Relevance and follow-up of positive results in in vitro genetic toxicity assays: An ILSI-HESI initiative. *Mutat Res 633*:67–79

84. Walker VE, Casciano DA, and Tweats DJ, 2009. The Viracept EMS case: Impact and outlook. Toxicol Lett *190(3)*: 333–339

85. Doak SH, Jenkins GJ, Johnson GE, Quick E, Parry EM and Parry JM, 2007. Mechanistic influences for mutation induction curves after exposure to DNA-reactive carcinogens. *Cancer Res 67(8)*:3904–3911.

86. Johnson GE, Doak SH, Griffiths SM et al., 2007B. Relevance and follow-up of positive results in in vitro genetic toxicity assays: an ILSI 2009. Non-linear dose-response of DNA-reactive genotoxins: Recommendations for data analysis. *Mutat Res 678*:95–100

87. International Conference on Harmonisation, 2002. Q3A(R2): Impurities in new drug substances. http://www.ich.org/LOB/media/MEDIA422.pdf

88. International Conference on Harmonisation, 2006. Q3B(R2): Impurities in New Drug Products. http://www.ich.org/LOB/media/MEDIA421.pdf

89. U.S. Food and Drug Administration, 2008. Guidance for Industry: Genotoxic and carcinogenic impurities in drug substances and products: Recommended approaches. http://www.fda.gov/cder/guidance/7834dft.pdf

90. European Medicines Agency, 2006. Guideline on the limits of genotoxic impurities. CPMP/SWP/5199/02 EMEA/CHMP/QWP/ 251344/2006. http://www.emea.europa.eu/pdfs/human/swp/519902en.pdf

91. European Medicines Agency, 2008. Question & answers on the CHMP Guideline on the limits of genotoxic impurities. EMEA/CHMP/SWP/431994/2007 http://www.emea.europa.eu/pdfs/human/swp/43199407en.pdf

92. Kenyon MO, Cheung JR, Dobo KL, and Ku WW, 2007. An evaluation of the sensitivity of the Ames assay to discern low-level mutagenic impurities. *Regul Toxicol Pharmacol 48*:75–86

93. Kroes R, Renwick AG, Cheeseman M et al., 2004. Structure-based thresholds of toxicological concern (TTC): guidance for application to substances present at low levels in the diet. Food Chem Toxicol *42*: 65–83

9

DEVELOPMENTAL AND REPRODUCTIVE TOXICOLOGY

Jeanne Stadler

INTRODUCTION

Toxicological evaluation of pharmaceuticals must include a specific assessment of their potential effects on reproduction and development, which is to evaluate the effects of the test compound on reproductive function from conception to adulthood. The life cycle of animals is defined as "a series of changes that the members of a species undergo as they pass from the beginning of a given developmental stage to the inception of that same developmental stage in a subsequent generation" [1]. This cycle starts when adult (diploid) animals produce haploid gametes through gametogenesis. Gametes from males and females fuse during mating to produce a diploid cell, which, in mammalian species, progressively goes through embryonic then fetal developmental phases *in utero* until birth. The neonate will then continue to develop until adulthood, going through critical steps such as weaning and puberty.

At any given time in their development cycle, humans can be exposed to one or more of the 500,000–600,000 chemical entities that currently exist (and that increase by about 600 new entities per year). In many instances, exposure to these chemicals is not intentional and is part of daily life. Exposure to pharmaceuticals is voluntary and linked to the medical benefits of this exposure. Whether voluntary of involuntary, exposure to chemical entities can result in developmental and reproductive toxicology (DART). Thus, understanding potential adverse effects of chemical entities on reproduction is essential

Pharmaceutical Toxicology in Practice: A Guide for Non-Clinical Development, Edited by Alberto Lodola and Jeanne Stadler
© 2011 John Wiley & Sons, Inc.

from an environmental/worker safety perspective and forms part of the risk/benefit assessment for pharmaceuticals. In this chapter, we discuss the DART studies that are needed to support the nonclinical development of novel pharmaceuticals.

REPRODUCTIVE TOXICITY

The adverse effects of chemicals on reproductive function can involve altered endocrine function, effects on spermatogenesis and/or oogenesis, fertilization, implantation, and/or the development of the conceptus.

A well-documented example of reproductive toxicity is that provided by the study of endocrine disruptors. In 1991, the term "endocrine disruptor" was coined and first appeared in the scientific literature in 1993 [2]; the author stated that "environmental chemicals disrupt the development of the endocrine system, and that effects of exposure during development are permanent." The endocrine disruption hypothesis is based on the theory that exposure to a low dose of a chemical/s that interact with hormone receptors can interfere with reproduction, development and other hormonally mediated processes. Given that endogenous hormones are present in the body at low concentrations, exposure to relatively small amounts of exogenous hormonally active chemicals can disrupt the normal function of the endocrine system. As a result, adverse effects could be produced at much lower doses than a toxicant acting through a different mechanism. Many chemicals, among them some drugs, have been shown to be hormonally active. When animals are exposed to these compounds, the extent of endocrine disruption varies with the route of administration and the age of the individual. For example, during prenatal and postnatal development, interference with hormonal signaling can result in adverse effects, which are often irreversible and which do not occur in adults exposed to the same dose for the same duration [3–5]. Furthermore, three phases of pre- and postnatal development have been identified when exposure to chemicals with endocrine disrupting potential produces adverse and/or permanent changes to the reproductive system [4, 6–8]. Disruption of thyroid function early in development may cause abnormal sexual development in males [9] and females [10], impairment of early motor development [11], and learning disabilities [12]. An example of endocrine disruption caused by pharmaceuticals is the effects of diethylstilbestrol (DES), a synthetic estrogen. DES was prescribed to about 5 million pregnant women to prevent miscarriage and promote fetal growth. In a large number of children born to mothers who had been treated with DES, there was an abnormal development of their reproductive system sometimes associated with tumors. DES is now considered a teratogen, which can induce adenocarcinoma of the vagina and cervix, infertility, autoimmune disorders, epididymal cysts, feminization of the male fetus, and hypospadias [13–16]; it was withdrawn from the market in the early 1970s. The evaluation of the potential endocrine disruption properties of novel pharmaceuticals was reinforced by additional regulatory testing requirements following the DES disaster. In addition to *in vivo* animal studies, this issue should be addressed in juvenile toxicity studies on a case-by-case basis.

TABLE 9.1. Milestones in our understanding of teratogenesis.

Time	Event
Middle Ages/ Renaissance	Occurrence of malformations attributed to "nature" (i.e., environmental causes)
	Malformation shown to result from an interruption, or disruption, in embryonic or fetal development
Nineteenth century	Foundation of descriptive and fundamental teratology
Twentieth century	Establishment of relationship between the critical period of exposure and the occurrence of birth defects
	Shown that the Vitamin A deficiency produced ocular agenesis in the pig fetus
	Demonstration that rat fetuses born to dams that have a Vitamin A deficiency presented a malformative syndrome consisting of various malformations of the eyes, the diaphragm, the lungs, the urogenital system, the heart, and the great vessel
	One in six children of mothers exposed to the Rubella virus during the first trimester of pregnancy shown to have a malformative syndrome consisting of cataracts, cardiac malformations, and deafness

DEVELOPMENTAL TOXICOLOGY

Prenatal manifestations of developmental toxicity are usually known as teratogenesis, derived from the ancient Greek, *teras*, for monster. Teratology is the study of structural malformations or deviations from the normal organism. It is also the discipline concerned with experimental production and development, anatomy, and classification of malformed fetuses. A teratogen is a substance that induces birth defects in a developing organism. There are four main types of prenatal manifestations of teratogenesis:

- structural malformations,
- growth retardation,
- functional impairment, and
- death of developing organism.

A fifth category is transplacental carcinogenesis in which exposure of the pregnant female to a xenobiotic initiates cancer development in the embryo or the fetus and results in a cancer later in an individual's life [1]. This is a manifestation of "delayed teratogenesis" or "transgenerational teratogenesis." Table 9.1 summarizes key milestones in the development of our understanding of teratogenesis. As a result, a series of principles were elaborated that govern modern teratology [17] and that we list as follows:

1. Susceptibility to teratogenesis depends on the genotype of the conceptus and the manner in which this susceptibility interacts with environmental factors.

2. Susceptibility to teratogenic agents varies with the developmental stage at time of exposure.

3. Teratogenic agents act in specific ways (mechanisms) on developing cells and tissues to initiate abnormal embryogenesis.

4. Final manifestations of abnormal development are death, malformation, growth retardation, and functional disorder.

5. Access of adverse environmental influences to developing tissue depends on the nature of the influences (agent).

6. Manifestations of deviant development increase in degree as dosage increases from the no-effect to the totally lethal level.

Although we focus on the potential adverse effects of novel pharmaceuticals on the developing embryo/fetus in this chapter, we also note that there is also a significant incidence of "spontaneous" adverse outcomes in pregnancy:

- 50% to 60% of pregnancies do not develop into a durable clinically detectable pregnancy,
- about 20% of recognizable pregnancies end in a spontaneous abortion, mostly during the first trimester of pregnancy,
- after the 20th week of pregnancy, 1% to 3% of all pregnancies end in miscarriages, and
- about 2% of neonates carry a major malformation, and 3% of children carry a malformation that will be detected only during the five first years of life.

Most spontaneous malformations are functional, affecting mainly the urinary system, vision, hearing, and the central nervous system. There are many origins of these birth defects; however, less than 1% of them are due to xenobiotics, 15% are a genetic in origin, and 65% are of an unknown cause. It is sobering to consider that of the thousands of chemicals, including drugs, which have been tested for developmental toxicity, only 50–60 chemicals are recognized as human teratogens. Examples are given in Table 9.2.

REGULATORY GUIDELINES

Prior to 1962, the effects of chemicals on general reproductive function, and to a lesser extent on development, was evaluated in chronic toxicity studies in rats, involving two or three generations of animals (F_0, F_1, and F_2). The main study endpoints were the effects of treatment on reproductive organs and the incidence of mortality for concepti. These tests were required for food additives and chemicals that could act on reproductive organs but were not routinely required for pharmaceuticals. The thalidomide tragedy provided the impetus for the revision of regulatory requirements for DART testing of novel pharmaceuticals. Despite the nonclinical tests that had been performed, thousands of malformed babies were born to women who had been treated with thalidomide,

TABLE 9.2. Examples of drugs recognized as teratogenic and drugs that induce birth defects in humans.

Category	Example
Strictly contraindicated during pregnancy	Isotretinoin Acitretin
Contraindicated when a therapeutic alternative exists	Valproic acid
Tolerated exceptional use depending on severity of the mother's pathology	Methotrexate Cyclophosphamide
Tolerated use in the absence of therapeutic alternatives and under strict medical surveillance (benefit > risk)	Carbamazepine Phenobarbital Phenytoin
Drugs highly suspected to be teratogenic	Mycophenolate Misoprostol
Drugs contraindicated for fetal exposure	Ibuprofen Ketoprofen Nimesulide Captopril
Drug known to induce birth defects	Pyrimidone Trimethadione Carbamazepine Busulfan Cyclophosphamide Chlorambucil Mechlorethamine Aminopterin Cytarabine Danazol Lovastatin Atorvastatin Diethystilbestrol Thalidomide Penicillamine Fluconazole Misoprostol
Other factors	Cocaine Alcohol Tobacco smoke

an antiemetic, when they were pregnant. The children involved had characteristic limb malformations. This tragedy revealed the limits of the developmental toxicity assessment requirements that were in place at the time. The absence of malformations in a single test species did not extrapolate to safe use for humans because, as for any other type of toxicity, this extrapolation depends on the sensitivity of the test species, doses (level of exposure) tested, frequency and duration (period) of administration, and differences in

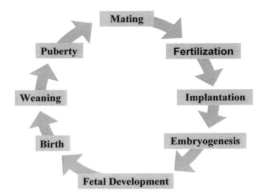

Figure 9.1. Stages of mammalian reproductive cycle

metabolism between species, among others. As a result, the regulatory requirements for developmental toxicity testing were reinforced and required the nonclinical testing of novel pharmaceuticals in two animal species: a rodent and a nonrodent.

In 1966, the U.S. Food and Drugs Administration (FDA) was the first regulatory authority to issue a series of guidelines for evaluating novel pharmaceuticals for their effects on reproductive function and development. These guidelines described three studies:

- Segment 1 study (effects on mating and fertility),
- Segment 2 study (effects on embryofetal development, i.e., teratology) and
- Segment 3 study (effects on peri- and postnatal development).

Since then, internationally harmonized regulations for evaluating potential toxic effects of drugs on reproductive function have been developed. As for other, nonclinical studies (see Chapters 5–8), reproductive and developmental study requirements for novel pharmaceuticals are defined by International Conference on Harmonization (ICH) guidelines. The first version of the core guidance, the S5A guideline (Detection of Toxicity to Reproduction for Medicinal Products) was issued in 1993 and an amendment, the S5B guideline (Toxicity to Male Fertility), was released in 1995 with a revision in 2000. In 2005, both guidance documents were revised and combined in the S5(R2) guideline, "Detection of Toxicity to Reproduction for Medicinal Products & Toxicity to Male Fertility" [18]. The S5(R2) guideline describes recommended strategies, study protocols, and practices to be used to evaluate the potential effects of pharmaceuticals on the different steps of the reproductive life cycle (Fig. 9.1). Note that vaccines intended for pregnant women or women of childbearing age require embryofetal and postnatal studies with a design adapted to obtain appropriate fetal and maternal exposure during gestation and the postnatal period. With respect to the ICH guidelines, the six main steps of the reproductive life cycle that need to be investigated nonclinically are as follows:

1. A: Premating to conception (adult male and female reproductive functions, development and maturation of gametes, mating behavior, fertilization),

2. B: Conception to implantation (adult female reproductive functions, preimplantation development, implantation),

3. C: Implantation to closure of the hard palate (adult female reproductive functions, embryonic development, major organ formation),

4. D: Closure of the hard palate to the end of pregnancy (adult female reproductive functions, fetal development and growth, organ development, and growth),

5. E: Birth to weaning (adult female reproductive functions, neonate adaptation to extrauterine life, preweaning development and growth), and

6. F: Weaning to sexual maturity (postweaning development and growth, adaptation to independent life, attainment of full sexual function).

The recommended studies outline in the S5(R2) guideline are equivalent to the series of studies previously called Segment 1, Segment 2, and Segment 3. In these studies, the effect of test compound on reproductive function and development are evaluated in the parents and the progeny. However, the effects of the test compound on juvenile animals (from birth to puberty) have not been evaluated. Recently, the need for specific regulations dealing with evaluating the toxic potential of pharmaceuticals prescribed to pediatric populations has emerged because a child should be regarded as "a work in progress" rather than a miniature adult. Although this led to new United States and European Union requirements for the inclusion of juvenile toxicity data in the final submission dossier [19, 20], most of the pharmaceutical companies involved in developing drugs for pediatric use had been testing novel drugs in juvenile animals for many years before the new regulation [21–23] was implemented. However, the results of these studies were rarely included in international marketing submissions. The reason is that it was commonly accepted and part of the regulatory guidance of the time that data collected from humans were more relevant than data coming from assays in juvenile animals [24]. Therefore, it was expected that the human data, whether from adult use or from off-label pediatric use, should be reviewed and considered before deciding to conduct additional juvenile animal studies. This strategy is relevant when human data are available, but animal experiments become essential when human data are lacking. Animal studies are also useful to explore whether, and how, a toxic effect in adult animals translates into juveniles and, therefore, by extrapolation to children. Both the FDA and the European Medicines Agency (EMA) have developed specific guidance documents on the need for juvenile toxicity studies to test whether the juvenile is more susceptible than the adult to the general organ toxicity of the drug and testing the drug for adverse effects on postnatal development. Although the ICH S5(R2) guideline describes the strategies to be used to evaluate the potential effects of pharmaceuticals on the different steps of the reproductive life cycle, there must be flexibility in the design of testing strategies. Although the strategies outlined in the guideline represent the most widely applicable option, they cannot address all the problems raised by all test compounds. There are occasions, for example, when using a one- or two-generation study design is more appropriate than segmenting the assessment of reproductive effects into the three studies recommended in the S5(R2) guideline.

PROTOCOL DESIGN AND ASSAY CONDUCT

Reproductive and Developmental Toxicity Studies

There are many points common to each of the three core DART studies, and these are discussed here before we address the specificities of each study protocol and assay separately.

Choice of Species. As for the other nonclinical studies, a key point is the choice of the species. ICH guidelines recommend use of the species and strains used for the general toxicity studies. The rat is the rodent species of choice, as it allows comparison with the general toxicology studies already conducted and for which a large amount of background data on reproductive function are available in a variety of strains. For embryofetal studies, the rabbit is the nonrodent of choice because gestation of rabbits is of short duration, its litters are large, there are numerous background data on reproductive function, and it has economic advantages when compared to the dog. The use of primates as the nonrodent species is in practice limited to rare, specific occasions such as mechanistic complementary studies. Other mammalian species are rarely used (and then primarily for mechanistic studies), as the available historical information/data on physiological and reproductive parameters are extremely limited.

Use of the rat presents some disadvantages, however. The rat is highly sensitive to sexual hormones and therefore cannot be used to test dopamine agonists, for example. Treatment with such compounds will compromise the establishment and the maintenance of pregnancy, which is highly dependent on the prolactin level in this species. Caution should be also exercised using the rat to test nonsteroidal anti-inflammatory drugs (NSAIDs), as they interfere with the prostaglandin pathway and with the normal parturition process. NSAIDs prolong gestation leading to death of the females and/or a high rate of pup mortality. Using the mouse also presents problems, as this species often manifests cluster of malformations that makes interpretation of data from embryofetal studies difficult. The mouse is also highly susceptible to stress, another confounding factor for data interpretation in maternal and progeny toxicity studies. Moreover, given the small size of fetuses and pups, it is sometimes difficult to evaluate fetal adverse effects (e.g., effects on body weight and difficulties in interpretation of visceral findings). For the rabbit, there is often a lack of toxicokinetic (TK) data and data from general toxicity studies. Additionally, the rabbit can show disturbances of the digestive tract due to stress, to variations in the food ration or composition, and to the test compound. These disturbances induce weight loss, absence of food consumption, and modification of fecal output that, when severe, can lead to death of the females. An example of drug-induced toxicity of this type is that produced by oral administration of antibiotics to rabbits. Antibiotics kill the intestinal flora, and, consequently, production of the soft fecal pellets containing the Vitamins B and K and the volatile fatty acids, essential to the rabbit (and usually reingested via the caecotrophy process), is reduced, or even stopped. This enterotoxemia most often leads to death of the females. A way to overcome this problem is to use a "sequential treatment scheme" where animals are treated for only two or three days at a time. However, this type of study has a significant impact on the study design. For example, a Segment 2 evaluation requires using three to four times more animals than usual, each treated group being divided into three to five subgroups to cover the complete period of organogenesis.

Dose Levels. Using three dose levels and a vehicle control group is usual in studies. However, there are exceptions: for example, when testing vaccines, only the dose administered to humans and, when necessary, a low multiple of the clinical dose will be tested. As a rule of thumb, and recommended by the ICH, the high dose should induce minimal toxicity to the adults. This does not mean a minimum of toxicity but that the toxic effect should be clearly evidenced without impairing the survival of progeny or modifying animal behavior. For example, toxicity should not be as severe as that produced in general toxicity studies (see Chapter 7) or so severe that mating becomes impossible or lactation does not take place. The low dose should, whenever possible, be the no-observed adverse effect level (NOAEL) or better still the no-observed effect level (NOEL). However, particular attention should be paid to these dose intervals, as the dose–response curve can be very steep with this type of study. When this happens, for example, in an embryofetal development study, there can be minor fetal effects at middose and a high incidence of fetal deaths at the high dose. Therefore, it is advisable when a steep dose–response curve is expected, to add a fourth dosage group to the study to reduce the dose interval and avoid missing key effects in the progeny. The need to add a fourth dosage group can be determined from a preliminary study.

ICH guidelines give several examples of acceptable signs of maternal (parental) toxicity. It is commonly accepted, based on the Organisation for Economic Cooperation and Development (OECD) guidelines for chemicals, that a 10% reduction in body weight gain (when compared to the control group) is a good marker of maternal toxicity. Caution should be used, however. A reduction in body weight gain is meaningful only if it is calculated using the body weight at the beginning of gestation (or first day of treatment) and the corrected body weight (carcass weight) at the end of the study. Maternal toxicity can also be established using clinical chemistry or histopathology parameters (see Chapter 7). Because evaluating clinical chemistry and histopathology is not routinely part of DART studies, a preliminary study may be required, in which these parameters are included. Finally, we emphasize that the severity of maternal toxicity should remain moderate in all cases. If maternal toxicity is too high, fetal findings become difficult, or even impossible, to evaluate. If toxicity is too low, extrapolating the results to humans is impossible.

Toxicokinetics. Metabolism is modified during pregnancy and lactation. Consequently, the distribution of a xenobiotic within the tissues and/or plasma of a pregnant/ lactating animal may be different to that of a nonpregnant animal. For example, nonpregnant rats excrete gentamicin faster than pregnant rats do [25] and plasma levels of primidone, but not phenobarbitone, are much lower in pregnant mice than in nonpregnant animals [26]. Apart from the direct consequence on the expression of toxicity in the dam, these differences may be key factors governing the onset and/or severity of adverse effects in fetuses or pups. Because drug metabolism and kinetics are primarily evaluated in nonpregnant animals, it is necessary to verify potential modifications of the TK profile of a test compound in pregnant animals. The TK profile of a test compound can be assessed in a preliminary (range-finding) study, if done; a more complete profile can be obtained in the definitive study. Assessing only maternal exposure to a test compound is valuable but insufficient to the needs of a rigorous evaluation. Fetal (or pup) exposure to a test compound should also be evaluated as well as concentrations in the amniotic fluid when necessary. This will allow discrimination between direct and indirect effects on the progeny to take place. TKs in DART are discussed in detail in Chapter 6.

Segment 1 Study (ICH 4.1.1: General Fertility and Reproductive Performance Study)

In the ICH female fertility study, females are treated at least 2 weeks prior to mating, during the mating period, and until implantation (i.e., day 6-postcoitum in rats). Animals are then sacrificed, submitted to a Cesarean section at midpregnancy and reproduction parameters and embryo status recorded. Table 9.3 gives details of the data collected. The ICH S5(R2) guideline requires an evaluation of the effects of treatment on the estrus cycle, tubal transport, implantation, and early development (i.e., the preimplantation stages) of the conceptus. The maturation of gametes, mating behavior, fertility, preimplantation stages of the embryo, and the implantation process/status must also be assessed. For the males, the study should detect functional effects (e.g., effects on libido, epididymal maturation) that may not be detected by histological examination of the male reproductive organs. Maturation of gametes, mating behavior, and fertility must be assessed in the females. Monitoring the estrus cycle is a key parameter used in assessing the possible adverse impact of a test substance on fertility and should be monitored at least during the mating period. However, monitoring this cycle during the premating period to establish baseline data helps in detecting a perturbation of the cycle as early as possible, thus allowing a better estimation of the time to positive copulation. Staging the estrus cycle and detecting spermatozoa are achieved by examining vaginal smears. Caution is needed when taking smears; vaginal lavage with saline is preferable to taking vaginal smears with a cotton tip. The latter provokes a local reaction (stimulation) that may induce a cascade of hormonal events leading to a pseudo-pregnancy, accompanied by a blockade of the estrus cycle in metestrus (typified by a cornified aspect of the vaginal cells on the smears). Only freshly prepared vaginal smears should be analyzed to avoid storage-induced artifacts that can lead to errors in interpreting the stage of the estrus cycle. From vaginal smears, an estimate can be made of the effects of treatment on the mating process and behavior; however, there are cases where a more precise evaluation of mating behavior is needed. For example, when there is suspicion of a hormonal disturbance, it may be useful to monitor the mating process directly by continuous observation of selected mating couples in specific racks of cages or in arenas equipped with cameras to record their behavior. Then a precise analysis of the behavior can be performed, evaluating the different phases of the mating process: precopulatory behavior of both animals, lordosis of the female, number of intromissions, refractory time, number of mounts, and time to the first mount [27; 28].

TABLE 9.3. Endpoints in a fertility and early embryonic development study (ICH 4.1.1/ Segment 1) from the ICH S5(R2) guideline.

Evaluation of stages A* and B* of Reproductive Process	Standard Parameters	Additional Parameters
Females		
Effects on: Estrus cycle Tubal transport Implantation and development of preimplantation stages of the embryo Assessment of: Maturation of gametes Mating behavior Fertility Preimplantation stages of the embryo Implantation.	Clinical signs and mortalities at least once daily, Body weight and body weight change at least twice weekly Food intake at least once weekly (except during mating) Record vaginal smears daily, at least during the mating period, to determine whether there are effects on mating or precoital time Observations that have proved valuable in other toxicity studies Necropsy (macroscopic examination) of all adults Preserve organs with macroscopic findings for possible histological evaluation; keep corresponding organs of sufficient controls for comparison Preserve ovaries and uteri from all animals for possible histological examination and evaluation on a case-by-case basis Count corpora lutea, implantation sites, live and dead conceptuses	Monitoring of the estrus cycle during premating period Specific clinical observations related to sexual behavior
Males		
Detection of functional effects, that may not be detected by histological examinations of the male reproductive organs: Libido Epididymal sperm maturation Assessment of: Maturation of gametes, mating behavior, and fertility	Clinical signs and mortalities at least once daily, Body weight and body weight change at least twice weekly Food intake at least once weekly (except during mating), Observations that have proved of value in other toxicity studies Recording of positive matings Necropsy (macroscopic examination) of all adults, Preserve organs with macroscopic findings for possible histological evaluation; keep corresponding organs of sufficient controls for comparison Preserve testes and epididymides from all animals for possible histological examination and evaluation on a case-by-case basis Sperm count in epididymides or testes as well as sperm viability	Specific clinical observations related to sexual behavior Abnormal sperm forms

ICH: International Conference on Harmonisation.

* A = Premating to conception (adult male and female reproductive functions, development and maturation of gametes, mating behavior, and fertilization). B = Conception to implantation (adult female reproductive functions, preimplantation development, and implantation).

In a regulatory study, males are treated for at least 4 weeks prior to mating during the mating period and until (at least) sacrifice of the females. Males are kept under treatment until females are sacrificed in order to remate them with another batch of untreated females if there is doubt as to the outcomes of the study (e.g., a suspected decrease in fertility). At sacrifice, a sperm analysis is performed on at least the content of one epididymis. Table 9.3 summarizes details of the parameters to be recorded. Characterization of abnormal forms of spermatozoa is not mandatory; however, when there are signals of a potential effect on fertility (from previous toxicity studies, suspected class effects, and the like), this evaluation is of great value. As for a female fertility study, a specific follow-up evaluation of the mating behavior can be done when necessary.

Segment 2 Study (ICH 4.1.3: Embryofetal Development Study)

In the ICH embryofetal development study, animals are treated during the period of organogenesis, which is usually, from day 6 to day 17 of gestation in rats, from day 6 to day 15 of gestation in mice, and from day 6 to day 18 of gestation in rabbits. Based on experience, it is often necessary, at least for the New Zealand white rabbit, to prolong treatment until day 19 of gestation to ensure that palate formation is complete. Females are euthanized one or two days prior to littering (on day 20 or 21 of gestation for rats, on day 18 of gestation for mice, and on day 29 of gestation for rabbits) and a Cesarean section is performed. Cesarean sections should be performed as close as possible to the time of littering. For example, on day 21 of gestation in rats this is a great help in interpreting the results, as the background "noise," in terms of apparent delays in development (e.g., a high number of control and treated fetuses presenting an unossified fifth metacarpal bone or moderate dilatation of the renal pelvis), is reduced. Therefore, treatment related delays in development are better evidenced. A wide range of parameters are recorded (Table 9.4). For example, number of corpora lutea and implants, number of live and dead fetuses and number of early and late resorptions. Fetuses are examined for external anomalies, including the buccal cavity, then euthanized and examined for visceral and skeletal defects. Visceral examination is performed routinely on fresh specimen for rats and rabbits but less commonly on mouse fetuses, which are usually fixed in Bouin Allen fluid before dissection [29]. As a general rule, and following regulatory guidelines, half of the fetuses are examined for visceral defects and the other half stained with Alizarine Red S [30] for detection of skeletal defects and delays in ossification in rodents while all fetuses undergo both examinations (visceral and skeletal) in rabbits. Use of a double staining technique, which visualizes cartilages and bones, is not mandatory but may present advantages especially when the test compound is suspected of affecting normal bone development. For example, double staining could be used to discriminate between a delay in ossification and abnormal bone structure. Double staining would make visible the underlying cartilaginous structure in the former case and help verifying whether an apparent deformed or even "split" bone is really deformed or split or whether this is only a delay in ossification.

TABLE 9.4. Endpoints in an embryofetal development study (ICH 4.1.3/Segment 2) from the ICH S5(R2) guideline.

Evaluation of Stages C*–D*of the Development Process	Standard Parameters	Additional Parameters
Adverse effects to be assessed: Enhanced toxicity relative to that in nonpregnant females, Embryofetal death, Altered growth Structural changes	During study for dams: Signs and mortalities at least once daily Body weight and body weight change at least twice weekly Food intake at least once weekly Observations that have proved of value in other toxicity studies At Terminal Examination: Necropsy (macroscopic examination) of all adults Preserve organs with macroscopic findings for possible histological evaluation; keep corresponding organs of sufficient controls for comparison Count corpora lutea, numbers of live and dead implantations Individual fetal body weight Fetal abnormalities Gross evaluation of placenta	Toxicokinetics in pregnant females on at least last day of treatment Evaluation of fetal exposure on last day of treatment Evaluation of test compound concentration in amniotic fluid or placenta Histopathological evaluation of selected fetal organs Double staining for skeletal evaluation

* C = Implantation to closure of the hard palate (adult female reproductive functions, embryonic development, major organ formation). D = Closure of the hard palate to the end of pregnancy (adult female reproductive functions, fetal development and growth, organ development, and growth).

Segment 3 study (ICH 4.1.2: Pre- and Postnatal Study Including Maternal Function)

In a pre- and postnatal study, pregnant females are treated from the beginning of organogenesis until the weaning of their litters. The mostly widely used species is the rat and involves treatment from gestation day 6 to postnatal day 21. Females are allowed to litter; the duration of gestation and, when feasible, of parturition are recorded. Pups are counted at birth, or on postnatal day 1, sexed and weighed. Their growth and survival are then followed during the whole lactation period at regular intervals and key development

TABLE 9.5. Endpoints in a pre- and postnatal study including maternal function (ICH 4.1.2/ Segment 3) from the ICH S5(R2) guideline.

Evaluation of Stages C*–F*	Standard Parameters	Additional Parameters
Adverse Effects to Be Assessed: Enhanced toxicity relative to that in nonpregnant females Pre- and postnatal death of offspring Altered growth and development Functional deficits in offspring, including behavior, maturation (puberty), and reproduction (F1)	Maternal Animals: Clinical signs and mortalities at least once daily Body weight at least twice weekly Food intake at least once weekly at least until delivery, Observations that have proved of value in other toxicity studies, Duration of pregnancy and parturition Terminal Examination: Dams and pups Necropsy all adults Preservation and possibly histological evaluation of organs with macroscopic findings Implantations Abnormalities Live offspring at birth Dead offspring at birth Body weight at birth Pre- and postweaning survival and growth/body weight Maturation and fertility Physical development Sensory functions and reflexes Behavior	Toxicokinetics: full profile or verification of maternal exposure during at least lactation) Transfer of test compound to milk Verification of pups' exposure to test compound

* = Implantation to closure of the hard palate (adult female reproductive functions, embryonic development, major organ formation). D = Closure of the hard palate to the end of pregnancy (adult female reproductive functions, fetal development and growth, organ development and growth). E = Birth to weaning (adult female reproductive functions, neonate adaptation to extrauterine life, preweaning development and growth). F = Weaning to sexual maturity (postweaning development and growth, adaptation to independent life, attainment of full sexual function).

time points for the pups recorded (Table 9.5). Examples of these key time points in rats are the time for full implementation of the lactation process (usually postnatal day 4), the beginning of the decline in lactation with pups starting to ingest solid food (usually postnatal day 12 and/or -15) and (time to the weaning of pups (usually postnatal day 21).

The development of progeny can be monitored using either complete litters or "culled" litters before weaning. When culling is performed (to minimize the influence of the litter size on pup development), litters are usually reduced on postnatal day 4, to a fixed number of pups, usually 4 males and 4 females. All the sacrificed pups are autopsied and examined for any gross morphological malformation. Any pup dying during the study, during the pre- and postweaning periods is also examined for malformations. During the lactation period, pre-weaning tests are performed, in order to monitor physical and reflex development of the young animals. Physical development markers, such as tooth eruption, fur growth, pinna unfolding or auditory canal opening are directly linked to the body weight of the pups. In addition, not all development markers need to be monitored. For example, in rats it is unnecessary to evaluate both pinna unfolding and hair growth since they both appear, in general, on postnatal day 5. However, tooth eruption should be monitored, as this appears concurrent with modifications to the feeding behavior of the pups (see above). The day developmental tests are performed, each pup must be weighed to allow for correlation between physical markers of general development and body weight. However, the time needed to the opening of the eyes is without apparent relationship to the body weight of pups. The time to eye opening is an excellent marker for the development of the cornea and, when altered, can be a potential risk of blindness in humans; this is discussed in detail in the review by Zieske [31]. Development of the cornea in the human embryo initiates as early as 5 weeks of pregnancy. The vertebrate cornea begins its development as the ectoderm overlaying the lens. This primitive epithelium (two cell layers thick) then stratifies to three to four cell layers thick, the lens completes its formation and detaches from the ectoderm, and the eyelids form and fuse. The next step is the separation of the lens from the corneal epithelium with waves of neural crest cells migrating into the space between the lens and epithelium to form the corneal endothelium and the stromal keratocytes. This migration of cells appears to be species specific. Following eyelid fusion, the primitive corneal epithelium decreases to two cell layers until the time of eyelid opening (24 weeks in humans). During the period of eyelid closure, the cornea gradually enlarges and matures. These maturation events include cell proliferation in the epithelium, stroma, and endothelium; differentiation of the epithelium; appearance of a tear film and tear film–associated proteins; and swelling and thinning of the stroma. These events are easily observed and described in rodents. Because rodents are born with closed eyelids when a delay in eyelid opening occurs, this might indicate a perturbation in the corneal maturation process and an alteration in the gene expression linked to eye opening. When such an event occurs, in absence of other markers of a general delay in development, we recommend performing an in-depth evaluation of visual function in test animals in a complementary study if necessary.

Evaluating sensory functions is difficult in pups before weaning, as most of the tests are based on active or passive avoidance tasks. The difficulties in learning an avoidance task is related to the expression of the conditioned response and is hindered by high levels of stress produced in the immature animal by the "punishment" (most often an electric shock) and by their inability to find an escape route (lack of spatial orientation) [30]. However, functions already developed at birth can be explored. For example, olfaction is developed during intrauterine life. Recognition of the odor of the amniotic fluid spread on the nipples by the dam during parturition acts as a signal for finding the nipples in the neonate [31]. At 7 days of age, using olfactory stimuli, rats can orient themselves in a small arena to reach a nest-scented area. They can also make their way through a Y maze to reach the anesthetized mother [32]. During this preweaning period, the appearance of reflexes is monitored using the same principles as for the markers of physical development. For example, in rat pups, the surface and air-righting reflex can be recorded on postnatal days (PND) 5 and 17, respectively. Additional tests such as cliff avoidance, measuring the onset of the perception of space, can be also performed, generally on PND 11 in rats.

At weaning, young animals are separated from their mother. A limited number of animals is selected (in general, two per sex and per litter) for physical and neurobehavioral postweaning tests and to produce a second generation. It is advisable at this time, when feasible, to keep the weanling pups from the same litter, or at least by pairs of males and females from the same litter, together for a few days in order to reduce the stress of weaning. These animals are then housed singly and monitored for survival and growth (regular weighing). The animals not selected at weaning are euthanized and examined at least for gross morphological lesions. Puberty is evaluated from the occurrence of balanopreputial separation in males (usually between PNDs 30 and 50 in rats) and vaginal opening in females (which occurs between PNDs 25 and 40 in rats). The exact time these events happen differ depending on the strain of animals used. Historical data for a control population should be established, as for other tests and are specific for a given animal, strain, and test facility. Because the onset of puberty is also related to the general development of the animals, the body weight of each animal must also be recorded at least on the day when puberty is reached.

The days following weaning, general motor activity and behavior are monitored using a functional observation battery. Pups are placed in a small arena and observed for clinical signs, activity, and/or reflexes. Clinical observations include changes in skin, fur, eyes, mucous membranes, occurrence of secretions, and autonomic activity (e.g., lacrimation, piloerection, pupil size, unusual respiratory pattern and/or mouth breathing, and any unusual signs of urination or defecation). The level of spontaneous activity, changes in body position, activity level (decreased or increased exploration of the standard area), and coordination of movement are recorded. Changes in gait (e.g., waddling, ataxia) and posture (e.g., hunched back) and reactivity to handling, placing, or other environmental stimuli, clonic or tonic movements, convulsions, tremors, stereotypes (e.g., excessive grooming, unusual head movements, repetitive circling), bizarre behavior (e.g., biting or excessive licking, self-mutilation, walking backward, vocalization), or aggression are recorded. In addition, animals are manipulated to test their reactivity to handling, their palpebral reflex, pinna reflex, and grip strength, among others. Postweaning neurobehavioral testing is focused on the development of sensory functions, (locomotor) activity, and learning and memory processes. Auditory function, at least in rats, is the easiest sensory function to evaluate; vision and olfaction are more difficult to assess. In rats, at about PND 28, testing the auditory startle response is generally performed. When there is a suspected alteration in audition, a more precise evaluation of this function can be performed using an audiogram, generally in a specific additional study [33]. For vision, simple first-approach tests exist such as recording the pupillary reflex and ophthalmological examination. However, are they good indicators of the absence of any disturbance of visual function, especially in albino rats, the most commonly used strains of rodents for such studies? Many attempts have been made to develop specific tests for evaluating the visual function of rodents such as a modified cliff avoidance test, optokinetic tracking, or other tests of binocular vision. The developing mammalian visual system progresses through "sensitive" or "critical" periods early in life in which mature vision is facilitated through adaptive feedback from the visual environment. This is visual plasticity and, as a key component of visual function, this has been evaluated mainly through "loss-of-function" experiments where eyelids of animals were sutured, for example. Glenn Prusky and his team recently developed [34] methods evaluating the enabling properties of visual experience during development in rats. They used a virtual optokinetic system [35] for measuring visual thresholds of optokinetic tracking, a visual behavior that facilitates the stabilization of retinal images. This methodology allows measurements through each eye separately in untrained and freely moving laboratory animals daily from eye opening [36]. These techniques should have a use limited to secondary and complementary exploration of the visual function when an alteration is suspected.

Olfactory function is probably the most difficult sense to test in young animals to date. In general, this function is not tested routinely, although methods have been developed, such as using olfactometers [37]. In brief, rats deprived of water are trained to discriminate between different odors, using water as a reward for correct odor discrimination. This active avoidance test has limited use in routine studies.

Spontaneous locomotor activity is measured in about 8-week-old rats using an actimeter, preferably with an automated recording system, as this can be used without the presence of a technician in the testing room. Movements of the animal in the front and back of the cage, circular clockwise and counterclockwise, rearing, and stereotypic movements for at least 20 min are recorded. Note that when the animal is placed in the center of the test arena, the first 5 min are needed for habituation to this new environment. Therefore, recording activity during this period should be either omitted or monitored separately.

Learning and memory are evaluated using a maze in most cases. The more complex the maze is, the better the evaluation of both learning and memory is. We recommend Morris and Cincinnati water mazes [38]. In brief, these mazes use the aversion of the rat to water and its natural desire to escape as quickly as possible from a hostile environment. The rat, after verification of its swimming ability in a straight channel, is placed at the entrance of the maze (A site) and has to swim within a complex path made of series of successive T-shaped channels, following a logical sequence of turns either left or right, to reach a platform, and escape (B site). Four trials constitute the learning phase. Approximately 1 week later, the rat is placed in the maze again entering the B site. Therefore, it must reverse the series of turns to escape at the A site. In both phases, the animal is left for a maximum of 5 min in the water whatever the result of the test (success or failure to escape). In both test phases, the following parameters are recorded: result of the test itself (positive or negative), time to escape, number of errors (wrong direction), and number of correct orientations.

Postweaning tests are usually performed twice during the study: once during the postweaning phase but before puberty and a second time at adult age. At about 3 months of age, young F1 adults are mated to check their reproductive capacity, avoiding brother–sister matings, following the process already described above for a fertility study. Females are sacrificed midpregnancy. Positive and negative matings, number of corpora lutea, and implantation sites (viable and dead) are recorded. At the end of the study, all animals are sacrificed and submitted to macroscopical examination at a minimum to detect gross anomalies. In the light of the outcome of the macroscopic examination, a microscopic examination is performed.

JUVENILE TOXICITY STUDIES

The decision to conduct a juvenile toxicity program should initially be based on an in-depth review of available human data in both adults and children and the pharmacology and toxicology data for adult animals. Juvenile toxicity studies should be performed to address any gaps in this data and are not intended to duplicate the studies, or data, already available. The study strategy that is developed must consider the target organs or functions to be evaluated and the timing of the development of these organs/functions in both test animals and humans. Preliminary studies are usually necessary to determine the tolerance of juvenile animals, of the age retained for the main studies, to the test compound and fill any gaps in the TK and/or metabolism data. The design of each study is based on key considerations; some cases are not specific to juvenile animals:

- the intended therapeutic use or indication,
- the duration of (clinical) treatment,
- interspecies differences in sensitivity to and metabolism, of the test compound and
- knowledge of the profile of target organ toxicity of the test compound.

Objectives of Juvenile Toxicity Studies. Regulatory juvenile toxicity studies are designed to detect two distinct types of hazard: those related to the different and specific vulnerability of a developing organism to the general toxic effects of a drug and those related to the direct or indirect effect of that test drug on the development of the organ, function, or whole individual. General toxicity on the immature animal is most often detected at the end of the treatment period; however, a reversibility period is advisable in order to characterize residual toxic effects/lesions that may persist in the adult. Juvenile toxicity studies may also provide information about specific biomarkers that can be used in clinical studies with children.

Selection of Animals. When selecting an animal model, the same criteria are used as those for adult toxicity studies: differences and similarities to humans with respect to pharmacokinetics, pharmacology, and pharmacodynamics. In addition, in terms of organ and functional development, similarities and differences to humans must be considered and any practical constraints linked to the use of immature animals being considered. In addition, the age, or the various age classes, of the patients to be treated

TABLE 9.6. A comparison of postnatal age and developmental stage between humans and various animals [7].

Species	Developmental Stage				
	Preterm	Newborn	Infant	Child	Adolescent
Human		0–28 days	1–23 months	2–12 years	12–16 years
Monkey	*	0–15 days	0.5–6 months	0.5–3 years	3–4 years
Dog	*	0–21 days	3–6 weeks	6–20 weeks	5–7 months
Pig	*	0–15 days	2–4 weeks	4–14 weeks	4–6 months
Rabbit	0–4 days	0–10 days	1.5–5 weeks	5–12 weeks	3–6 months
Rat	0–4 days	0–10 days	1.5–3 weeks	3–6 weeks	7–11 weeks
Mouse	0–4 days	0–10 days	1.5–3 weeks	3–5 weeks	5–7 weeks

* Not defined. In humans, premature viable babies may be less than 6 months of intrauterine age. In monkeys, dogs, and pigs, correspondence with human prematurity has not been consistently established.

must also be considered. This is important for two reasons. First, to ensure that animals of the right age are selected for the study. A comparison between humans and various animals of age and developmental stage is given in Table 9.6. Second, because intra- and interspecies differences in the timing of development milestones, kinetics and toxicity can considerably vary with age. As an aid to selecting the appropriate species for a study, we have found it useful to ask the following questions:

- for each animal model under consideration, what is known about the toxicity, pharmacology, pharmacodynamics, and TKs for the test compound in the adult?
- if the target organs and the functional adverse effects of the test compound in adults are known, at what age do these effects occur?
- when do target organs in adults reach maturity?
- is sufficient information on the comparative development between this species and humans to allow selection of animals of the right age?
- is the route of administration practicable in the age range chosen for the species under consideration?
- can toxicity to the target organs and/or functions of interest be evaluated in the juvenile animal and the adult of the same species?
- are suitable validated methods, experiential equipment, and historical data available?
- are one or two test species needed to fully evaluate the potential adverse effects being investigated?

For example, what test species can be chosen to evaluate the toxicity of a drug developed to treat pulmonary diseases in children aged ≤6 years? In making this choice, the toxicologist is faced with two issues. One is a *case-specific issue,* for example, that children will receive treatment before their lungs are fully developed; another issue is that functional maturity of the lungs does not occur until 6–8 years of age. The second issue is a *general issue*, which relates to the impact of chronic treatment on a growing organism. From studies of the comparative development of the pulmonary alveolus [39], several species appear to be relevant for testing such a drug in juvenile animals. Human alveoli begin to develop during the 36th week of pregnancy, are partially developed at birth, and are fully functional at 6–8 years of age. The first 2 years of life constitute the most critical period of development for the lungs. Therefore, the choice of animal species will be oriented to one for which the corresponding critical period is well characterized and where the administration by the chosen route to the juvenile animal is feasible. The juvenile dog could be used for such a study, because in this species, alveoli are partially developed at birth and become fully functional at the age of 16 weeks; the critical development period lasts for this full period. The rat is another alternative. The alveoli continue their development after birth (day 4 postpartum) and become fully functional at 3 weeks of age; the critical development period occurs over 10 days (days 4–14 postpartum). The rat has the additional advantage that the toxicity of the test compound on the general development of juvenile animals to maturity can be readily evaluated, adulthood being reached only about 3 months after birth. This example also illustrates the fact that the rat and the dog are the species most often used for juvenile toxicity studies. Both species are commonly used in adult toxicity studies; therefore, a wide body of data is available for both species in terms of toxicity, physiology, anatomy, metabolism, reproduction, and development. Moreover, toxicology research laboratories have a wide range of historical data for these species and well-established procedures for housing animals, dosing animals using a variety of routes, and using them in a range of nonclinical studies including DART studies. There are some critical pros and cons to the use of each species. The rat is small, easy to handle, easy to mate, has a short gestational period, and produces large litters. However, it is highly immature and dependent on the dam at birth. The dog is large, has a relatively long gestational period, and produces small litters. It is also poorly developed at birth and highly dependent on its mother for several weeks after birth. Moreover, dogs need a high level of socialization with humans to be good experimental models. Housing must be correctly equipped to avoid cannibalism with a large enough space, nesting area, toys, bones, and the like. The weaning process must be spread over at least a week to be successful. Other species are less commonly used for juvenile toxicity studies. For the rodent, the choice is limited; the mouse, despite its smaller size and greater activity, can be an alternative to the rat. As alternative nonrodent species, the monkey and the pig present interesting advantages. The macaque is a good model with which to explore early postnatal development (up to about 4 years of age), as it is very immature at birth and has a great phylogenetic similarity to humans. The macaque is particularly interesting when exploring the effects of test compounds on behavior and for which there is a well-described battery of tests to assess the development of motivation, color discrimination, time estimate, learning, and memory. However, their use is limited because their "mother–child" relationships are not well understood; the young macaque is highly dependent on its mother for several months after birth. In addition, such studies are extremely expensive to conduct because usually only a very small number of young macaques are available at any given time, thus the study must be spread over a long period using different batches of juvenile animals and because it is manpower intensive.

Given the high degree of similarity between humans and pigs in the development of the gastrointestinal tract, use of the minipig can present significant advantages over the dog. The piglet is easy to train and to handle. Most routes of administration commonly used in nonclinical studies are feasible for the minipig with the exception of intravenous and inhalation routes. Piglets can be bottle fed to reduce interactions with the mother and avoid problems due to suckling difficulties. However, the birth of animals should be closely monitored (there is a high risk of mortality) and the animals must be housed in a facility that has a strictly controlled temperature (there is a risk of hypothermia). In addition, there is still a limited amount of historical toxicology data available for piglets [40]. Rabbits are rarely used for juvenile studies, as general toxicity data are rarely available in this species despite being routinely used in embryo/fetotoxicity studies. In addition, handling litters often results in maternal cannibalism or rejection.

Overall, therefore, in the absence of specific issues, the rat remains the species of choice for testing the impact of xenobiotics on juvenile development. It is a well-understood model, its sexual and physical development (including skeletal development) is well characterized, and a range of specific functions can be investigated in a single study at reasonable cost.

Target Organs and Functions that Should Be Monitored. Based on regulatory guidelines, a study should evaluate the development of at least five key target organs or functions: the central nervous system (CNS), the reproductive system, the immune system, and pulmonary and renal functions. In addition, general growth (body weight and body weight gain, growth speed, growth markers such as tibial length) and sexual maturity should be studied. Other parameters are added, on a case-by-case basis to characterize the potential effects of the test compound better and to identify possible biomarkers of toxicity that could be used in clinical studies. These additional endpoints can be monitored in a single study; however, this would be a highly complex study that might increase the risk of errors. In practice, it is better to conduct a series of studies with a limited number of endpoints that are aligned with the timing of the clinical development studies and that take into account the different timing for organ/system development between experimental animals and humans.

Choice of Dose Levels. As for any toxicology study, three dose levels and a vehicle control group are used in a majority of cases. The choice of dose levels is based on the information already available: the doses already used in general toxicity studies, DART studies and TK data. However, the final choice of doses used should be made in the light of the results of a dose range–finding study. Usually, doses are chosen on the basis on three general principles:

1. Dose levels should be on the lowest part of the dose–response curve derived from toxicology studies in adult animals.

2. The lowest dose should give a systemic exposure close to the therapeutic exposure expected in the target population.
3. One of the doses should have been used previously in general toxicity studies in the same species.

Again, as for any toxicology study, the highest dose should induce some toxicity. However, this toxicity should not be exaggerated; the results would be impossible to interpret when massive agonal signs preceding death may obliterate more subtle markers of the toxic effect such as modification of the clinical chemistry parameters or histopathological lesions that are no longer visible in moribund (or even dead) animals. The rules for limiting a high dose are the same as for toxicological studies in adult animals (see Chapter 7)

Constitution of Dose Groups. In the absence of regulatory guidance on the number of animals required per dose group, the approach used in other toxicology studies should be used for juvenile toxicity studies. Considering that two groups are used for each dose level (one for behavioral testing and assessment of fertility, the other for necropsy at the end of the treatment period), we think that 16 rodents/sex/group is reasonable. The same group numbers should be used in rabbit studies, whereas for other nonrodents, 8 animals/sex/group is acceptable. There is no precise guideline on how to for constitute the dose groups. Therefore, three alternatives should be considered: the use of split litters, the use of whole litters, and cross-fostering litters. Each option has advantages and inconveniences.

In a split-litter design, pups in a given litter are distributed to several dose groups and remain with their mother. There is a good distribution of doses among the lactating females, reducing the influence of the mother on the outcome of the study, and, in general, the number of litters needed to obtain the required size of each group is minimized. On the other hand, the risk of a dosing error is increased and cross-contamination between dosage groups (pups and mother) and of control pups may occur. In the whole-litter design, all pups from a given litter receive the same dose level, the risk of dosing error is reduced, and because there are separate control pups the risk of cross contamination is minimized. However, the influence of maternal behavior and a reduced intergroup genetic variability can introduce bias into the outcome of the study. With a cross-fostering design, pups of the same litter are reared by a foster dam. Again, there is a minimum risk of dosing error and the influence of the mother is abolished. Fostering rarely occurs before PND 4 to avoid the occurrence of hypolactasia or agalactia and to reduce the risk of pups being rejected by the foster mother. Fostering requires a relatively long period of adaptation and strict monitoring of the process during the first days. The complexity of this option increases the technical workload dramatically.

Dosing Animals. In principle, the route of administration should be the anticipated route for the treatment of children. However, depending on the age of the animals to be treated, or on the test species, the use of some routes is not feasible; in this instance, the dosage route used should be the one giving the highest systemic exposure in the

TABLE 9.7. Age at which dosing can start in juvenile animals by various routes of administration.

Species	Oral Gavage	sc	iv	Inhalation	im
			Age at Which Dosing Starts		
Rodent	≥PND 4	≥PND 0	≥PND 10	PND	Not recommended
Rabbit	≥PND 14	≥PND 14	≥PND 14	Not recommended	≥PND 14
Dog	≥PND 7	≥PND 4	≥PND 0	≥PND 1	≥PND 14
Minipig	≥PND 7	≥PND 4	Not recommended	≥PND 1	Not recommended

PND = postnatal day.
Abbreviations: sc = subcutaneous; iv = intravenous; im = intramuscular.

test species and producing minimal interspecies (test species vs humans) differences in absorption and distribution. The age at which animals are first treated is a function of the developmental parameters to be evaluated (see above) and the route of administration that is used (Table 9.7). Intramuscular injection is difficult for rodent pups because the muscular mass of the pups is extremely small, whereas administration by inhalation, using the whole body technique is feasible where the whole litter plus the mother are exposed in the inhalation chamber. Although intravenous administration is difficult for the minipig at any age, juvenile studies have been performed using implanted vascular access ports. Because the oral route of administration is often chosen for pediatric use, it is the route used most often in juvenile toxicity studies. Administration is rapid when compared to other routes; however, there is a high risk of gavage error and/or a high level of mortality due to esophageal perforation and/or asphyxiation due to regurgitation. In addition, there can be interference with feeding if the dosing volume is relatively high. In rodents, this route is difficult from PND 1, possible from PND 4 and relatively easy from PND 6 or PND 7. Puppies can be gavaged from PND 1 if a small dosing volume is used (e.g., ≤5 ml/kg/day). Other, less common, methods of oral administration can also be viewed. The deposition of a small amount of test compound into the mouth of juvenile animals abolishes the risk of gavage error and esophageal perforation; however, this technique is complex and time consuming. There is also a risk of taste aversion and of subdosage due to loss of test compound during application. When the effects of a compound administered by artificial gavage to children should be explored, a gastric catheter is installed in the stomach of rats aged ≥4-days; small aliquots of the test compound can be delivered several times a day (e.g., three times an hour every 2 hours).

Subcutaneous administration can cause problems of local tolerance, and there is a high risk of compound loss because of swelling at the injection site. Intraperitoneal administration, especially in very young animals, requires a high degree of skill to avoid causing lesions of the abdominal viscera and is thus not adapted to the high volume needs of regulatory nonclinical studies. Using the inhalation route in rodents, when both the litter and the mother are exposed, can result in contamination of the milk, and this should be considered when calculating the administered dose. Puppies can be treated with an oral-nasal mask from postnatal day 1 but only for a short time (e.g., 15 min/day).

Duration of the treatment period should be as close as possible to the duration envisaged in children of the target developmental age/period and cover all relevant developmental stages. This may involve a treatment until adulthood or up to the age used in toxicity studies. Latent defects or delayed adverse effects can be readily explored in rodents where the treatment and/or the observations can be prolonged until adulthood. Such an approach is not usually required in nonrodents.

Formulation of the Test Compound. General principles are discussed in Chapter 6. The ideal is to test the final (commercialized) formulation of a drug to be used in children, especially for oral formulations because pediatric oral formulations are quite different from those used in adults (i.e., a syrup instead of a capsule), there is a need to test the innocuity of this novel formulation with all the used excipients. Nevertheless, general considerations for the formulation of test compounds are similar to those for adults; there are some noteworthy differences, however. Liquid formulations can cause problems in a juvenile toxicity study. A large volume of administration, which is sometimes necessary to reach the target dose level, can adversely affect pup feeding due to filling of the stomach and can lead to nutritional deficiency. These deficiencies can either mask a treatment effect or result in false positives (e.g., a decrease in body weight gain) or accentuate true positive effects. In contrast, if too small a volume of administration is used, there is potentially a higher level of imprecision in the dose administered. These problems can be overcome if variable, progressively increasing volumes, depending on the age and the weight of the pup, are used. As for adult studies, for parenteral administration, the viscosity and pH of the formulation should be carefully controlled to avoid local reactions at the injection sites, pain due to a too-slow resorption of the injected volume (subcutaneous or intramuscular routes), or lesions of the vessels. Careful consideration should be given to the excipients, which are used to ensure that there are no differences in response between adults and juvenile animals.

Study Conduct. In general, breeders supply lactating rodents with litters from about 1 day postpartum. Because a very large number of animals are required to give birth at the same time, using animals of this age is an advantage, as it is less expensive than using time-mated females produced at the test facility. It is not considered ethical to transport neonatal dogs, minipigs, rabbits, or monkeys; thus, it is necessary either to obtain pregnant females or to mate animals at the experimenter's facility. As for rodents, it is important to ensure that a sufficient number of pups are born within a limited period. For all animals, as soon as possible after birth, pups must be individually identified. In general, tattooing is used: the paws of rodents and the ears of nonrodents. Older animals can be implanted subcutaneously with a transponder chip.

As in any toxicology study, pups are examined at least once daily. Rodents are weighed every 2 or 3 days and nonrodents at least once a week. Unnecessary handling of pups, or prolonged separation from the mother, can cause problems: an increase in mortality, reduced body weight gain, and modification of the mother's behavior. Separation from the mother for longer than 1 hour/day can lead to changes in the behavior of pups and an increased risk of cannibalism by the mother and/or a modification of feeding patterns. The impact of alterations to milk quantity and quality will be greater in species that suckle often than for species that suckle only once or twice a day (e.g., rabbits).

Preweaning Evaluations. The growth and development of rodent pups is assessed by monitoring developmental milestones and reflex testing daily using similar techniques to those routinely used in developmental toxicity studies (see above for pre- and postnatal studies); specific measures, such as measurement of external tibia length, are determined every 2 or 3 days. For rabbits, developmental monitoring is similar to that of the rat. In dogs and minipigs, growth measures, such as standing shoulder height and external tibia length, are recorded at least twice a week. The animals are examined daily to assess landmark events, such as tooth eruption and eye opening; auditory, papillary, labial reflex, and timing of the acquisition of locomotion (crawling, standing, walking, running) are evaluated at different ages, depending on the species. Blood sampling is performed for TKs and to measure clinical pathology parameters. In rodent studies, blood is taken from additional animals added to each dosage group and the volume of blood that can be sampled is very limited until PND 12 or 14. Blood sampling is performed under light anesthesia. Rat pups can be sampled sublingually from PND 4 or by cardiac puncture from birth. Dogs are sampled at the jugular vein. Minipigs can be sampled at the cranial vena cava and even without anesthesia from birth [41]. Rabbits can be sampled at the ear artery from about 2 weeks of age. Although, reference data for clinical pathology parameters for rats and dogs at various ages are available in the literature [42], the ideal is to use reference values generated in house. Cardiovascular parameters (heart rate, blood pressure, and ECG) can be recorded in piglets and puppies as well as in rat pups from the age of about 1 week. Piglets and dogs are restrained in a hammock for the ECG and heart rate recording. However, interpretation of the ECG data remains difficult until weaning due to the high interanimal variations in waveforms.

Postweaning Evaluations. Weaning occurs at 3 weeks in rodents, 7 weeks in dogs, and 5 weeks in pigs and rabbits. Single housing of animals immediately after weaning is not recommended whatever the species, and even more so for nonrodents. Delaying this change in habitat decreases the risk of behavioral changes due to a sudden change in the environment and avoids effects that may adversely affect postweaning investigations. Because social contacts are necessary to allow normal neurobehavioral development, we recommend group housing; groups should be composed of a single sex; animals should be of similar age and can be drawn from the same or different litters. If animals are being treated with test compound prior to weaning then after weaning, the same treatment regime is continued; however, consideration should be given to adjusting the dosing regime to allow for age-dependent differences in TKs or metabolism. The routine examinations, described for the preweaning phase, are continued after weaning, although the frequency of body weights and growth measurements can be reduced to twice weekly in view of the slower rate of growth. Specific postweaning examinations are similar to those performed in an adult toxicity study (see Chapter 7) along with the assessment of sexual maturity (vaginal opening in females and balanopreputial separation in males) and reproductive performance. When neurobehavioral testing is required, assessments are performed twice with animals that have reached sexual maturity: once during the treatment period and once after the end of the treatment period. In rodents, these tests generally include an evaluation of motor activity, cognitive functions (learning and memory) in complex mazes, and auditory function (startle reflex with habituation and prepulse inhibition).

The experimental assessment of fertility is different in nonrodents and rodents. Nonrodents are rarely mated at sexual maturity to verify their fertility; a histological examination of their reproductive organs at the end of the study is usually used to evaluate their reproductive capacity. Rodents, on the other hand, are mated at about 3 months of age. One male and one female from the same treatment group (no siblings) are housed in the same cage until copulation occurs (as evidenced by the presence of sperm in a vaginal smear). A Caesarean section is performed midpregnancy, and corpora lutea and implantation sites (viable and dead) are counted. Additional, nonroutine endpoints are incorporated into the study to evaluate the development of specific organs/functions on a case-by-case basis, including sperm analysis, hormone determinations, X-ray imaging or bone densitometry at termination, and immune function evaluation for the detection of immune depression (note that there are no validated tests available currently to evaluate adverse effects that result in immune stimulation, which may make a child more vulnerable to autoimmune disease or hypersensitivity [43]).

At the end of the study, each subgroup (end of treatment period or maturity) is sacrificed, and necropsied; a histopathological examination of a range of organs similar to those collected in a subchronic toxicology study (see Chapter 7) is conducted. A more specific histological examination can be performed on the CNS and reproductive organs if needed.

DATA INTERPRETATION AND RISK EVALUATION

In this section, we discuss the interpretation of data from DART studies that are commonly encountered and that, when they are too vague, can lead to questions from regulatory agencies as to the relevance of such findings to human beings and the evaluation of risk for the population being treated.

Influence of Maternal Toxicity

Poor health status in a female fertility study can induce modifications of the estrus cycle and of libido, cause refusal to mate, decrease fecundity and fertility, and increase preimplantation losses. This in turn can lead to an unusual dose–response curve and misinterpretation of results. For example, in a female rat fertility study with an inhaled steroid tested by the oral route, animals were treated from 14 days prior to mating to gestation day 6. The high dose was selected as the maximum tolerated dose in this strain of rats; it induced severe female toxicity, essentially because of the pharmacological effects of the treatment on hormonal balance. Only 25% of the high-dose females mated; there was a decrease in mean fetal weight at the low- and middose levels when compared to the control group but not at the high dose. However, this apparent absence of effect at the maximum tolerated dose is irrelevant, as only females showing no or minimal maternal toxicity produced viable litters.

In embryofetal studies (Segment 2 studies), it is a mistake to establish direct links between fetal adverse effects and maternal toxicity or, conversely to conclude there is maternal toxicity based on adverse fetal effects. For example, an antibiotic given by gavage to female rats during organogenesis induced a 15% reduction (statistically significant) of weight gain in pregnant females during the treatment period at mid- and high-dose levels when compared to controls. In Cesarean sections, fetal body weights were significantly smaller at both doses. At the high-dose level, there was an increased number of fetuses presenting general delays in ossification. A statistically significant increase in the number of short ribs was also noted at both mid- and high dose. Initially, all fetal effects were considered to be a consequence of maternal toxicity. However, if decreased fetal body weights and delays in ossification can reasonably be considered as linked to the maternal toxicity of the test compound (at least in part), this is not the case for the rib shortening. First, shortening of the ribs is not a delay in ossification but an anomaly of development, and second, even if it were not statistically significant, the number of affected fetus and litters increased at the low-dose level (i.e. in the absence of any maternally toxic effect). Another example is provided by a study in which aspirin was given subcutaneously to female rats during organogenesis at a high dose of 400 mg/kg or to mice at a high dose of 600 mg/kg. There were statistically significant reduced body weight gains during the treatment period and until the end of pregnancy when compared to controls without modifications of food consumption and in the absence of other signs of maternal toxicity. However, when comparing the corrected female body weights at a Cesarean section (i.e., the terminal body weights of the females minus the weight of the gravid uterine horns), this difference was considerably attenuated in both species. Plotting individual female body weights against litter weights showed a clear relationship between the decrease in maternal body weight gain and fetal weight. Therefore, the apparent effect on females was only a reflection of a direct effect of aspirin on the fetal weight; there was a fetal effect in absence of maternal toxicity. In a pre- and postnatal study (segment 3), maternal toxicity may negatively impact the littering process and the postpartum nursing leading to early postnatal deaths and weakness of the surviving pups that cannot correctly suckle their mothers. The absence of nipples stimulation will modify the implementation of lactation (quantity and quality of milk) and modify the survival and growth and development of pups.

Apparent Inconsistent Findings between Studies

A compound known to present weak general toxicity in adult rodents at acceptable systemic exposure levels was tested in mice for its embryo fetal effects (Segment 2 study). In a dose range–finding study (using only 6 females per dose level), there was a high number of fully resorbed litters at the mid- and high-dose levels and an increased number of postimplantation losses at the low dose. The low dose from the range-finding study was retained as the high dose for the definitive study (using 25 females per group) to confirm this embryotoxic effect in absence of maternal toxicity. Again, there was an apparent effect at the high dose and possibly at middose. However, when excluding the data for the (2/25) females in each group showing a complete resorption of their litters, the difference from controls were no longer significant. The number of totally resorbed litters was within the range of historical data for the strain in this test site. Therefore, the high dose, initially considered as potentially embryotoxic on a limited number of data, was found to be the NOAEL in the definitive study. When such a phenomenon occurs, we recommended reporting both studies to regulatory authorities and providing a detailed explanation of the apparent discrepancies rather than changing the conclusions of the first study *a posteriori*.

Malformation or Variation?

The simplest way to differentiate between a malformation and a variation is by referring to an updated internal classification established at the test site where the study was performed. Although there is an international consensus regarding the terminology to be used for naming various fetal anomalies [44], the distinction between malformations and variations is left by the authors to the discretion of each laboratory. An international panel of experts considered that categorization of finding to be a diagnostic procedure, and therefore it remains an individual decision. To build its own glossary, a laboratory should start from the general definitions of malformation and variation [45]. Malformation refers to permanent structural change that is likely to affect the survival or health of the fetus adversely and for a given species. Variation refers to a change that is often reversible, occurs within the normal population under investigation, and is unlikely to affect survival or health adversely (this might include a delay in growth or morphogenesis that otherwise followed a normal pattern of development). During a workshop on terminology in developmental toxicology [46], a series of very useful recommendations were made to classify fetal findings adequately:

- interpreting an anomaly as a variation or a malformation should be universal. regardless of the type of substance tested (drug, biocide, pesticide, industrial chemical, or residue in food). The definitions given above often do not apply to fetal findings that are classified in a "gray zone"
- severity should be clearly described for each gray zone anomaly to classify it as a malformation or a variation
- historical data of the control population for each species and strain for a given supplier and test site should be considered (frequency of occurrence)
- reference to historical data for classification should be from contemporaneous studies (one often considers a maximal period of 3 to 5 years preceding the study as contemporary, depending on the known level of variability of the strain)
- observation of permanent structural and functional changes should be considered as a warning to humans, even if the finding has apparently no serious consequence on health and survival of the species when it appeared.

Some findings can be classified in a third category called "not malformation" or "unclassified" when functional change is not the result of a direct abnormal process but when the adverse effect is higher than a variation. To facilitate the understanding of an internal glossary, we strongly recommend that findings (especially malformations) should be illustrated using drawings or photographs whether the anomaly is found in a single or multiple species, whether it occurs in isolation or as part of a syndrome, or whether this anomaly occurs in humans. This data should be compared with data of other test sites that used the same species and strains.

Weak Incidence of Findings

This is frequently observed in embryofetal toxicity studies (Segment 2) and possibly occurs in the absence of a dose relationship for the finding being considered. For instance, four isolated cases of craniofacial malformations are observed in a rat study (one cleft palate at mid- and high doses, one cyclopia combined with micrognathia, microphthalmia, and astomia at the mid-dose, and a microphthalmia at the high dose). At the same maternal exposure levels in rabbits, there was one case of "open eyes" at the low dose. In such a configuration, should these craniofacial malformations be attributed to the compound and additional studies performed to clarify the issue? A review of the historical control data the test site for rats showed that a cleft palate was not found in the control population in the 5 years preceding the study. However, in historical data generated for the same strain, during the same period but in a different test site from the same company, cleft palate was found in the control population at a similar incidence than in the study under evaluation. Both sites received their animals from the same supplier and had similar animal housing conditions and identical operating procedures. Regarding the finding in the rabbit study, the anomaly had been recorded in the previous 3 years in the control population at a similar incidence to anomalies found in the study under analysis. After a detailed review of the literature regarding potential dysmorphogenetic effects of the class of the test compound and pharmacodynamics of the test compound, these malformations were not considered compound related, and there was no need for an additional study seen in a first instance. It was decided that based on the results of the fertility study (where animals are allowed to litter and their progeny examined for external malformations) and of the results of the pre- and postnatal study, the decision of doing a complementary study might be considered (presence of malformations or related adverse findings in the fertility and re- and postnatal study). Based on this example, we recommend the following approach when encountering such an issue. First evaluate the possible variations in the strain used: in its own test site, in other sites with similar experimental conditions, at the breeder's facility, and in different laboratories. Regularly update (and use quality control) historical data. Then use a derisking strategy: use the integrated analysis (see below) to solve the issue (differentiate between spontaneous and drug induce anomaly) and consider the implementation of additional study. However, avoid repeating the same study; a "clean" study never erases the results of a previous one. Perform an explanatory study focused on the issue to be solved.

Integrated Analysis for Data Interpretation

DART studies are designed to cover the complete continuum of the reproductive cycle. Similarly, interpretation of the data generated by these studies should not be done in "isolation," that is study per study, but holistically, integrating the data from all studies together. Only a holistic approach optimizes evaluation of the potential risk, as each DART study identifies a specific set of hazards to reproduction and development:

- An integrated analysis is based on a determination of the quality of the package of studies, the choice of test species, the exposure levels, the comparison of exposure levels between species, study design and the robustness of the tests.
- Results are analyzed endpoint by endpoint and then in combination.
- Animal data are compared with human data when available for the same compound (clinical studies in male and female) or for the same or similar class of active substance (exposure, threshold of toxicity, probability of use during pregnancy, and/or lactation).
- The benefit/risk ratio and level of concern (null, weak, strong) can be defined.
- The product label (warnings, contraindications, precautions) can be determined.

However, there are several factors that make such an analysis difficult; depending on the endpoints and the evaluated parameters, the power of each study may vary. In some studies, there is no way to determine a dose–response curve, all the doses not providing an effect. When there is an adverse effect, it does not occur in all animals and it is not always possible to define a subgroup based on the level of sensitivity. These intersubgroup differences in response are often observed between the main group and the satellite animals for evaluating TK at the same dose level, for instance. Low-dose effects are not always considered, even on a classical dose response curve—the statistical significance is often considered erroneously, whereas the biological significance is not. There are various ways to perform this risk evaluation through an integrated analysis, listed as follows:

- The *reference dose* approach based on the use of the NOAELs, LOAELs, and safety margins. This is one of the most commonly used ways to evaluate the risk using drugs.
- The *benchmark dose* approach based on the shape of the dose–response curve and the safety margins
- The *Gailor/Sikker* approach based on the variability of the control population and the dose–response curve
- The *probit and logit* approach based on the determination of thresholds of toxicity.
- The *mechanistic* approach based on understanding the toxic phenomenons.

In evaluating the risk in reproductive and developmental toxicology, two very similar and nice models were developed by the FDA in 2001 [47] and by the EMA in 2005 [48]. Both are based on a systematic approach using successive decision trees and lead to a decision regarding the level of risk and the precautions or contraindications that should be taken and mentioned in the label ("categorization" of the drug) with the drug under review:

Step 1: are the studies available, are they relevant. and is there at least one signal of an adverse effect?

Step 2: when there is no reported signal, were the models and the dose levels adequately chosen, is there a class alert?

Step 3: when there is a positive signal (reproductive or developmental signal), take it through a series of screens to determine the level of concern. Consider the strength of the signal, the pharmacodynamics of the test compound, the metabolism data (in animals vs humans), the TK profile (in reproductive and developmental toxicity studies and toxicity studies in general), and the class alerts.

CONCLUSIONS

As for general toxicology studies (Chapter 7), information on the potential adverse effects of test compounds on reproductive function and development is needed to process a compound. This is particularly important for clinical trials involving a broad population, including women of childbearing potential or children or for long-term trials. These data are also a regulatory requirement in support of a marketing application. DART and juvenile toxicity studies should be tailored to the therapeutic use of the test compound, the type of test, and the age of the patients. The conduct of studies must be adapted to the overall development plan for the test compound and be closely integrated with the clinical study plan. Last, but not least, interpreting data from DART studies is progressive and constantly evolving, which occurs throughout the development cycle of the test compound and which must integrate information from other toxicology studies. This systematic approach is essential to ensure that conditions for safe use (i.e., the protection of reproductive capacity) of novel drugs are reached in women of childbearing potential, pregnant women, children from birth to adolescence, and adult males or females generally.

REFERENCES

1. *Encyclopædia Britannica*, 2009. Life cycle. http://www.britannica.com/EBchecked/topic/340084/life-cycle

2. Colborn T, vom Saal FS, and Soto AM, 1993. Developmental effects of endocrine-disrupting chemicals in wildlife and humans. *Environ Health Perspect* **101**:378–384

3. Guo YL, Lambert GH, and Hsu CC, 1995. Growth abnormalities in the population exposed in utero and early postnatally to polychlorinated biphenyls and dibenzofurans. *Environ Health Perspect* **103**:117–122

4. Szabo DT, Bigsby R, Chapin RE et al., 1999. Evaluating the effects of endocrine disruptors on endocrine function during development. *Environ Health Perspect* **107**:613–8

5. Castro DJ, Löhr CV, Fischer KA, Pereira CB, and Williams DE., 2008. Lymphoma and lung cancer in offspring born to pregnant mice dosed with dibenzo[a,l]pyrene: The importance of in utero vs. lactational exposure. *Toxicol Appl Pharmacol 233*:454–458

6. Eriksson P, Lundkvist U, and Fredriksson A, 1991. Neonatal exposure to 3,3′,4,4′-tetrachlorobiphenyl: hanges in spontaneous behaviour and cholinergic muscarinic receptors in the adult mouse. *Toxicology 69*:27–34

7. Recabarren SE, Rojas-García PP, Recabarren MP et al., 2008. Prenatal testosterone excess reduces sperm count and motility. *Endocrinology 149*:6444–6448

8. Richardson VM, Ross DG, Diliberto JJ et al., 2009. Effects of perinatal PBDE exposure on hepatic phase I, phase II, phase III, and deiodinase 1 gene expression involved in thyroid hormone metabolism in male rat pups. *Toxicol Sci 107*:27–39

9. Lilienthal H, Hack A, Roth-Härer A et al., 2006. Effects of developmental exposure to 2,2,4,4,5-pentabromodiphenyl ether (PBDE-99) on sex steroids, sexual development, and sexually dimorphic behavior in rats. *Environ Health Perspect 114*:194–201

10. Talsness CE, Shakibaei M, Kuriyama S et al., 2005. Ultrastructural changes observed in rat ovaries following in utero and lactational exposure to low doses of a polybrominated flame retardant. *Toxicol Lett 157*:189–202

11. Eriksson P, Viberg H, Jakobsson E et al., 2002. A brominated flame retardant, 2,2′,4,4′,5-pentabromodiphenyl ether: uptake, retention, and induction of neurobehavioral alterations in mice during a critical phase of neonatal brain development. *Toxicol Sci 67*:98–103

12. Viberg H, Johansson N, Fredriksson A et al., 2006. Neonatal exposure to higher brominated diphenyl ethers, hepta-, octa-, or nonabromodiphenyl ether, impairs spontaneous behavior and learning and memory functions of adult mice. *Toxicol Sci 92*:211–218

13. Herbst AL, Ulfelder H and Poskanzer DC, 1971. Adenocarcinoma of the vagina. *Association of maternal stilbestrol therapy with tumor appearance in young women. N Engl J Med 284*:878–881

14. Hatch EE, Palmer JR, Titus-Ernstoff L et al., 1998. Cancer risk in women exposed to diethyl-stilbestrol in utero. *JAMA 280*:630–634

15. Klip, H, J. Verloop et al., 2002. Hypospadias in sons of women exposed to diethylstilbestrol in utero: A cohort study. *The Lancet 359*:1081–1082

16. Brouwers, MM, Feitz WF et al., 2006). Hypospadias: A transgenerational effect of diethyl-stilbestrol? *Hum Reprod 21*:666–669

17. Wilson JG, 1959. Experimental studies on congenital malformations. *J Chron Dis 10*:111–130.

18. International Conference on Hybridization, 2005. S5(R2) guideline. Detection of toxicity to reproduction for medicinal products & toxicity to male fertility. http://www.ich.org/LOB/media/MEDIA498.pdf

19. U.S. Food and Drug Administration, 2006. Guidance for industry: nonclinical safety evaluation of pediatric drug products. http://www.fda.gov/cder/guidance/5671fnl.html

20. European Medicines Agency, 2005a. Draft guideline on the need for non-clinical testing in juvenile animals on human pharmaceuticals for paediatric indications. http://www.ema.europa.eu/pdfs/human/swp/16921505en08.pdf

21. Barrow P, 1990. *Technical Procedures in Reproduction Toxicology. Laboratory Animals Handbooks 11*. London: Royal Society of Medicine.

22. Baldrick P., 2004. Developing drugs for pediatric use: a role for juvenile animal studies? *Regul Toxicol Pharmacol 39*:381–389

23. Hurtt ME, 2004. Workshop Summary Juvenile animal studies: Testing strategies and design. *Birth Defects Res B: Dev Reprod Toxicol 71*:281–288

24. ICH, 2000. E11 guideline: Clinical investigation of medicinal products in the pediatric population. http://www.ich.org/LOB/media/MEDIA487.pdf

25. Stahlmann R, Chahoud I, Meister R, et al., 1988. Gentamicin plasma concentrations in pregnant and nonpregnant rats and fetuses after single and multiple injections. *Arch Toxicol 62*:232–235

26. McElhatton PR, Sullivan FM and Toseland PA, 1997. The metabolism of primidone in nonpregnant and 14-day pregnant mice. *Xenobiotica 7*:611–615

27. Mercier O, Perraud J, Stadler J, and Kessedjian MJ, 1985. A standardized method to test the copulatory behaviour of male rats: A basis of evaluation of drug effects. *Teratology 32*:28A

28. Mercier O, Perraud J, and Stadler J, 1987. A method for the routine observation of sexual behaviour in rats. *Lab Animals 21*:125–130

29. Wilson, JG, 1965. Methods for administering agents and detecting malformations in experimental animals. In: J.G. Wilson and J. Warkany, editors, *Teratology, Principles and Techniques*. Chicago and London: The University of Chicago Press. Pp. 262–277

30. Dawson, AB, 1926. A note of the staining of the skeleton of cleared specimens with alizarin red S. Stain Technol *1*:123–124

31. Zieske JD, 2004. Corneal development associated with eyelid opening. *Int J Dev Biol 48*:903–911

32. Calamandrei G, 2004. Ethological and methodological considerations in the use of newborn rodents in biomedical research. *Ann Ist Super Sanità 40*:195–200

33. Pedersen PE, Stewart WB, Greer CA, Shepherd GM, 1983. Evidence for olfactory function in utero. *Science 221*:478–480

34. Amsel A, Burdette DR, and Letz R, 1976. Appetitive learning, patterned alternation, and extinction in 10-d-old rats with non-lactating suckling as reward. *Nature 262*:816–818

35. Bourdois PS, Junghani J, Perraud J, and Reinert H, 1975. Transplacental effects of drugs on hearing, vision and behaviour. Poster 87. 14th Meeting of the Society of Toxicology, Williamsburg.

36. Prusky GT, Silver BD Tschetter WW et al., 2008. Experience-dependent plasticity from eye opening enables lasting, visual cortex dependent enhancement of motion vision. J Neurosci *28*: 9817–9827

37. Prusky GT, Alam NM, Beekman S, and Douglas RM, 2004. Rapid quantification of adult and developing mouse spatial vision using a virtual optomotor system. *Invest Ophthalmol Vis Sci 45*:4611–4616

38. Douglas RM, Alam NM, Silver BD et al., 2005. Independent visual threshold measurements in the two eyes of freely moving rats and mice using a virtual-reality optokinetic system. *Vis Neurosci 22*:677–684

39. Sokolic L, Laing DG, and McGregor IS, 2007. Asymmetric suppression of components in binary aldehyde mixtures: behavioral studies in the laboratory rat. *Chem Senses 32*:191–199

40. Vorhees CV, Reed TM, Acuff-Smith KD et al., 1995. Long-term learning deficits and changes in unlearned behaviors following in utero exposure to multiple daily doses of cocaine during different exposure periods and maternal plasma cocaine concentrations. *Neurotoxicol Teratol 17*:253–264

41. Zoetis T and Hurtt M, 2003. Species comparison of lung development. *Birth Defects Res Part B: Dev Reprod Toxicol* **68**:121–124

42. Chevalier G, Forster R, and Bouchez C, 2009. Evaluation of the feasibility of juvenile toxicity study in the Göttingen Minipig. *Toxicol Lett* **189**:S144

43. Diehl KH, Hull R, Morton D, Pfister R et al., 2001. A good practice guide to the administration of substances and removal of blood, including routes and volumes, *J Appl Toxicol* **21**:15–23

44. Beck MJ, Padgett EL, Bowman CJ et al., 2006. Nonclinical juvenile toxicity testing. In: RD Hood, editor. *Developmental and Reproductive Toxicology: A Practical Approach*, 2nd ed. Boca Raton, FL: CRC Press. pp. 263–328

45. Barrow P, 2007. Toxicology testing for products intended for pediatric populations. In: WK Sietsema and R Schwen, editors. *Nonclinical drug safety assessment: practical considerations for successful registration*. Washington DC: FDA News. pp. 411–440

46. Makris SL, Solomon HM, Clark et al., 2009. Terminology of developmental abnormalities in common laboratory mammals (version 2). *Birth Defects Res B* **86**:227–327

47. Chahoud, I. Buschmann J, Clark R et al., 1999. Classification terms in developmental toxicology: need for harmonisation. *Reprod Toxicol* **13**:77–82

48. Solecki R, Bergmann B, Bürgin H et al., 2003. Conference [roceedings: Harmonization of rat fetal external and visceral terminology and classification. Report of the Fourth Workshop on the Terminology in Developmental Toxicology, Berlin, 18–20 April 2002. *Reprod Toxicol* **17**:625–637

49. U.S. Food and Drug Administration, 2001. Draft reviewer guidance integration of study results to assess concerns about human reproductive and developmental toxicities. http://www.fda.gov/downloads/Drugs/GuidanceComplianceRegulatoryInformation/Guidances/UCM079240.pdf

50. European Medicines Agency, 2008. EMEA/CHMP/203927/2005. Guideline on risk assessment of medicinal products on human reproduction and lactation: from data to labeling. http://www.ema.europa.eu/pdfs/human/swp/20392705enfin.pdf

10

DATA ANALYSIS, REPORT WRITING, AND REGULATORY DOCUMENTATION

Monique Y. Wells

INTRODUCTION

The drug development process is at once simple and complex. It is simple because regulatory guidelines indicate what studies need to be conducted, how they should be conducted, and at what time they should be conducted during the development process. The guidelines tell us which documents need to be filed and at what time. They also tell us which criteria must be fulfilled for acceptance of preclinical dossiers in support of final regulatory approval of compounds.

The complexity arises because, as is commonly said, "The devil is in the details." Even with the road map of *in vivo* toxicity studies to be conducted and the time line for conducting them, any number of things may happen to derail the plan. Animal availability may be limited, requiring considerable delay in beginning a study. During the initial phase of development (e.g., during pilot studies), the chemical properties of the compound may engender unexpected waste during administration, raising questions about the adequacy of dosing (in the absence of toxicokinetic (TK) data), and requiring the production of additional amounts of drug or reformulation of the test compound before the next study can begin. Unexpected toxicity may occur, requiring that a study be repeated at different (lower) doses. The study may be conducted as planned, but results may be equivocal, requiring that the study be repeated. Poor interpretation and/or

Pharmaceutical Toxicology in Practice: A Guide for Non-Clinical Development, Edited by Alberto Lodola and Jeanne Stadler
© 2011 John Wiley & Sons, Inc.

poor reporting of data may be discovered late in the process of creating a dossier, leading to the reopening of finalized studies for review and amendment.

Of all the aforementioned scenarios, poor interpretation and reporting can almost always be avoided by having an ironclad commitment to quality, beginning with the creation of the study plan (protocol) and ending with the final review of the study report. This requires practical knowledge of how studies should be planned and conducted, and scientific knowledge of how the chemistry of the compound may affect its formulation, influence its TK profile, and alter the normal physiology and histology of the species being tested. The sponsor retains complete control for studies conducted "in house," and should reasonably expect the staff to possess the knowledge base required. However, for studies conducted at contract research organizations (CROs), the sponsor may or may not have staff that is capable of effectively assessing the practical and scientific expertise of the laboratories that it selects. When this is not the case (e.g., when the sponsor is a start-up biotech company with no toxicology department or a small pharmaceutical company with limited staff in toxicology), the sponsor should be especially vigilant with regard to the oversight of its CROs. To accomplish this, the sponsor is well advised to engage the services of one or more consultants with the requisite expertise to select its CROs and to monitor, or even subcontract certain parts of, its studies (see Chapter 4).

Because of the logistical complications and the difficulties in maintaining quality that arise when multiple parties are involved in generating and interpreting data for a given study (some of which are addressed under Data Analysis and Interpretation below), the Organisation for Economic Co-operation and Development (OECD) created a specific guideline for this situation. Entitled "The Application of the OECD Principles of GLP to the Organization and Management of Multi-Site Studies," it addresses the "planning, performance, monitoring, recording, reporting and archiving" of multisite studies [1].

Excellence in data analysis and interpretation presumes excellence in the quality of the data that have been collected and recorded. Technicians who generate qualitative data must be well trained and should have a thorough understanding of the biology of the animal species with which they work. Data generated by instrumentation (e.g., electrocardiography and clinical pathology data) must be reliable, with the methodologies selected for the generation of these data having undergone validation and extensive periodic quality control. The scientists who interpret the data, from the study director to the specialists in ophthalmology and pathology, must be well versed in the conventions applicable to their fields as they relate to the regulatory toxicology environment. Following the principles of Good Laboratory Practice should help to ensure that quality data are available for analysis and interpretation; the details of these principles as they apply to each part of the regulatory toxicity study are beyond the scope of this publication.

DATA ANALYSIS AND INTERPRETATION

To conduct any study with quality, the first requirement is to understand its purpose. The purposes of the nonclinical toxicity study are to:

1. identify any organs that may be affected by exposure to the compound,
2. identify any correlations among clinical signs, in-life measurements, and evaluations (e.g., body weight, food consumption, clinical pathology, electrocardiology, and ophthalmology), organ weights, necropsy findings, and histopathology.
3. determine whether these effects are adaptive, adverse, or noncompound-related or not.
4. identify the dose(s) at which no compound-related effects occur.

Information obtained from preclinical studies will be used to determine the dose levels for first-in-man and subsequent clinical studies, as presented in the U.S. Food and Drug Administration (FDA) guidance document, *Estimating the Safe Starting Dose in Clinical Trials for Therapeutics in Adult Healthy Volunteers* [2] and the International Conference on Harmonisation (ICH) guidance document M3(R2), *Guidance on Nonclinical Safety Studies for the Conduct of Human Clinical Trials and Marketing Authorization for Pharmaceuticals* [3]. These data will also be used to identify parameters to be monitored for toxicity during clinical trials. The data generated from each preclinical study should be analyzed and reported with these goals in mind. *Presenting Toxicology Results* is an excellent reference work for this topic [4]; additional details can be found therein.

Several types of data are generated during preclinical toxicity studies:

*   Descriptive: including clinical signs, ophthalmology findings, and histopathology findings
*   Numerical: including means and standard deviations for measurements such as body weight, food consumption, clinical pathology and TK parameters (these data are frequently subjected to statistical analysis); incidence of mortality, clinical signs and histopathology findings (incidence data [mortality, preneoplastic lesions, neoplastic lesions] are subjected to statistical analysis in carcinogenicity studies); severity of clinical signs and histopathology findings
*   Frequency: number of days that clinical signs occurred (derived from evaluating table containing descriptive data)

Data commonly collected from a mammalian repeat–dose toxicity study are summarized in Table 10.1. Prior to writing a study report, rigorous analysis and thoughtful interpretation of all study data should be performed. The study director is responsible for gathering all the data generated during the study as well as the interpretations made by the scientists who contribute data to the study (e.g., ophthalmologist, biochemist, pathologist) to create a coherent report of the toxicologically meaningful effects observed. For all scientists involved, the most difficult part of identifying these effects is avoiding the enticing, yet inappropriate and sometimes dangerous, "crutch" of depending too heavily on statistical significance and historical reference ranges to interpret data.

One of the most common and major pitfalls in interpreting and presenting data in toxicity studies is overreliance on statistical significance of numerical data (see above) as evidence of toxicological relevance. The dictionary has multiple definitions of the

TABLE 10.1. Data commonly collected in mammalian repeat-dose toxicology studies.

Study Phase	Data
In-life	• Mortality
	• Clinical signs
	• Body weight
	• Food consumption
	• Electrocardiography
	• Ophthalmology
Laboratory investigations	• Hematology (with or without bone marrow smears)
	• Clinical chemistry
	• Urinalysis
	• Toxicokinetics
Postmortem	• Gross (macroscopic) observations
	• Organ weights
	• Histopathologic (microscopic) observations

word "significant." For the purposes of data interpretation in the regulatory toxicology setting, the definition to retain for this word is "probably caused by something other than mere chance" [5]. This does not necessarily mean that the statistically significant event is "important" (another definition that one can find for the word "significant").

For all data to which statistical analysis is applied, a healthy skepticism of the flags that frequently result is required. Statistically significant values may fall within the normal reference range of the parameter evaluated, reflect trends that are not considered adverse (e.g., increased serum alanine aminotransferase levels of <2-fold [6]; normal maturation of gonads in pubescent animals), or occur for analytes that have question-able significance for risk assessment in humans (e.g., cholesterol and triglycerides in rats [7]. Therefore, statistical significance does not automatically confer biological or toxicological relevance on a result. Whenever statistical flags occur, evaluation of in-dividual animal data is warranted to ascertain whether the significant event is in fact toxicologically relevant or not.

More importantly, the absence of statistical significance does not negate the bio-logical or toxicological relevance of a result. For example, if high-dose rats had non-statistically significant decreases in body weight and food consumption at the end of a study compared to controls due to the inability to eat properly because of compound-related tooth fractures, it would not make sense to conclude that these changes were not biologically relevant. As another example, one would not logically consider a 10% decrease in mean red blood cell count that is not statistically significant an incidental finding when the mean hemoglobin and hematocrit for the same group are decreased by 10%–12% and are statistically significant. Similarly, an increase in absolute kidney weight that is not statistically significant may well be toxicologically relevant when the accompanying relative kidney weight is increased and statistically significant. Again, evaluation of individual animal data is advisable under such circumstances to arrive at a robust interpretation of the results that is capable of withstanding intense regulatory scrutiny.

Too much reliance on historical control data is also problematic. Concurrent control data generally represent the best data set that one can use to determine whether a change observed in animals administered a xenobiotic is toxicologically relevant or not. (An exception to this rule is the *in vivo* micronucleus study, where historical control data are used as part of the acceptance and evaluation criteria for the study (see Chapter 6). However, historical control data do have their place—if they are used correctly. First, the use of these data should be restricted to strain-, age-, and sex-matched controls. Data should ideally have been obtained from studies performed at the same laboratory and under the same environmental conditions within the last 5 years of the date of the current study. When applicable, the method of sample collection and handling for the historical controls should be the same as that used for the current study. For example, small organs such as the pituitary and adrenal glands may sometimes be preserved in fixative prior to being weighed. Data from such specimens should not be combined with organ weights from fresh tissues.

For parameters that are rarely measured in traditional toxicity studies, such as hormone levels, blood gases, and serum immunoglobulins, published literature may be the only source of reference ranges available. Because there is often no information on the methods used to collect these data, ranges from literature should be used even more sparingly and cautiously than historical control data generated in the laboratory that conducted the study.

When there is doubt as to whether or not a compound-related change is toxicologically relevant, a look at the historical control data may help to make this determination. If the value for the suspected change falls within the historical control range, this is evidence to support the conclusion that the change is not biologically relevant (other supporting reasons would include lack of a dose response and a low incidence of the finding). In contrast, if there is evidence to sustain the conclusion that a change that falls within the historical control range is toxicologically relevant, then this conclusion should be maintained. It is inappropriate to dismiss such effects just because the values fall within the reference range of the laboratory. If, after consultation of all available information, including historical control data, no conclusion can be reached, then the report writer should indicate that the toxicological significance of the finding is uncertain.

The results of carcinogenicity studies often provide an opportunity to put the aforementioned advice into practice. There have been many occasions when a neoplasm that commonly occurs on a spontaneous basis appears to be compound-related; this is statistically significant. In such cases, consultation of a robust historical control database plus other pertinent data, such as incidences of the tumor cited in the literature, can be very helpful in ascertaining whether the contested result is truly toxicologically relevant under the conditions of the study conducted or not.

For example, consider the case of the assessment of carcinogenic potential of Exelon^{TM}, an acetylcholinesterase inhibitor used for treating Alzheimer's disease. In a 2-year carcinogenicity study performed with mice, a statistically significant increase in mammary adenocarcinoma was observed at the highest dose level administered to females in the study [8]. This neoplasm was found to be increased compared to the combined, but not the individual, control groups. In an evaluation of the historical control database for studies conducted by the sponsor at two different CROs, it was determined

TABLE 10.2. Degree of percent intimal thickening in balloon-injured vessels after different doses of the somatostatin analog HBF101.

Dose of HBF101 (μg/kg/day)	Aorta	Brachiocephalic artery	Left subclavian artery
		% Post-injury Intimal Thickening	
0	21.5 ± 6.0	24.8 ± 2.7	30.3 ± 6.0
2.5	$10.1 \pm 3.2^*$	$11.5 \pm 4.0^*$	$14.7 \pm 3.6^*$
25	$14.1 \pm 1.1^*$	$13.6 \pm 2.8^*$	$23.6 \pm 3.2^*$
250	$12.6 \pm 5.9^*$	$16.3 \pm 7.7^*$	$22.9 \pm 5.4^*$

$^*p < 0.05$, *Student's t test*

that the incidence observed in the study was within the reference ranges from those institutions. Furthermore, the incidence of mammary hyperplasia and adenoma was not increased, there was no clear indication of earlier time-to-tumor onset for mammary adenocarcinoma, and there was no similar effect observed in the rat carcinogenicity study. Therefore, the lesion was not attributed to compound administration.

One should be aware that toxicologically significant findings might not necessarily occur in a classic, ascending dose-related pattern. U-shaped or inverted U-shaped dose response curves can result from compound administration. This is called a nonmonotonic dose response, and it occurs when the action of the test item is stimulatory at low doses and inhibitory at high doses [9]. This type of response is often observed for hormones and other endocrine-active compounds [10].

For example, consider the following measurements for serum growth hormone levels (ng/mL; mean $\pm$ SEM) after administration of an endocrine-active chemical to female rats:

- Control: 107.1 ± 10.1
- Low dose: 155.6 ± 132.5
- Mid dose: 193.8 ± 58.7
- High dose: 8.0 ± 3.0

Mean values increase in a dose-related pattern at the low and mid doses compared to concurrent control mean, but the high dose mean is much lower than that of the concurrent control. Because the compound of interest is a hormone, one should suspect that this dose-response curve is "real." Of course, verification that no technical problems occurred in the evaluation of the specimens is required. However, once this has been ruled out, and in the absence of other contradictory evidence, the data set should be considered representative of a compound-related effect.

Table 10.2 shows a fictionalized example of histopathology data that indicate a nonmonotonic dose response, presented in tabular form. In the true experiment, investigators tested the hypothesis that injection of the somatostatin analog angiopeptin would reduce the degree of intimal hyperplasia induced by injuring the endothelium of three large blood vessels (the aorta, the common iliac artery, and the external iliac artery) with a balloon catheter in rabbits. The investigators found that although all three doses were effective, the lowest dose of the compound tested -2 μg/kg/day, was the most effective one administered for each of the three arteries selected for evaluation [11].

It is common practice to analyze data in comparison to concurrent study control values. As stated above, this data set is generally the best one to use to determine whether a compound-related change is toxicologically relevant or not. For large-animal studies (e.g., dog, nonhuman primate, rabbit, and minipig), however, it is more meaningful to compare clinical pathology values from a given group to *pretest* values. In this situation, each group serves as its own control. Because evaluating data on an individual animal basis is also more important in large-animal studies, each animal also serves as its own control. This approach is particularly valuable for studies that last up to 3 months but is less useful for longer studies due to the physiological changes that occur due to aging.

When pretest data are to be used in a study, it is important to compare pretreatment values for the animals destined for compound administration to those of the animals destined to be study controls. This permits the identification of biologically relevant differences among the groups prior to the beginning of the study and allows for the replacement of animals with outlying values if necessary. If the number of animals per group is small (≤ 3 per group), and if no differences are identified among pretest animals, their values may be combined to form one large pool of pretest data.

When multiple sacrifice dates are scheduled for a toxicity study, comparison of results between or among sacrifice dates is a critical part of data analysis and interpretation. This is the opportunity for the study director and the other scientists involved with the study to assess whether or not an abnormal clinical sign, in-life measurement, or histopathologic lesion occurs transiently, has a delayed onset, or becomes progressively worse with compound administration. If a recovery sacrifice is scheduled, then the opportunity exists to evaluate whether the abnormal finding persists, regresses, or disappears completely when dosing is stopped. This exercise represents the correlation of a particular finding with itself across time. Such correlations should be discussed in the appropriate section of the report.

The evaluation and discussion of correlations among different effects is also important, whether one or multiple sacrifice dates are planned for a study. Understanding how clinical signs, in-life measurements such as electrocardiology and clinical pathology parameters, and terminal findings such as organ weights and histopathologic lesions relate to each other can provide clues for interpreting data of studies where effects may be less obvious. This task is often difficult when studies are performed at a CRO or at multiple sites (TK analysis and histopathology are often subcontracted) because study personnel frequently do not have access to all the data for the study at the time that they are required to make an assessment of their own data. For example, it is disturbingly common for the consulting or CRO study pathologist to evaluate the histopathology of a study without having complete information on clinical pathology or in-life observations. The sponsor may not appreciate the negative impact of failing to make such information available or may simply not wish to do so. In such situations, the optimal practice would be to ask all the scientists involved in the creation of the report to read the sections to which they had no prior access and make comments and changes to the draft report prior to the release of the report to the sponsor.

Information on the effects of dose and time on exposure to the test compound and its metabolites allow for the most informed interpretation of data. However, toxicity data must often be interpreted and reported in the absence of these TK data, due to their unavailability when the draft report was generated. For preliminary evaluation, exposure levels may be presumed based on TK data from studies conducted in the same species and sex at the same or similar dose levels by the same route of administration, if dosing occurred for a similar length of time (see Chapter 6). Subsequently, there is a need to reevaluate the interpretation of study results once the actual TK data from that particular study are available.

Pathology data can be the most challenging data to interpret and report for a study because of the dynamic nature of the physiologic processes controlling the parameters measured for clinical pathology and the inherent inexactitude of the slide evaluation process for histopathology. Interpreting these data should always be left to a professional with appropriate education, training, credentials and, most importantly, awareness of the specific nature and requirements of the field of toxicologic pathology. (An example that illustrates the importance of this last criterion is discussed later in this section.) Ideally, the histopathologist should have access to, and the competence to integrate, all available information about the compound being tested, from its known activities (information from the literature and from previous toxicity studies), the experimental design of the study being evaluated, pharmacokinetic or TK data, and all observations and measurements made during the in-life phase of the study. In addition, histopathologists need the organ weight and necropsy data to optimize their ability to evaluate and interpret microscopic lesions.

Because CROs may not employ clinical pathologists, interpreting the clinical pathology data is often the responsibility of the study director. It is not uncommon for the study director to lack sufficient understanding of the pathogenesis of various disease processes to make the appropriate connections between in-life, clinical pathology, and histopathology data. Under these circumstances, conclusions drawn about study data may be incomplete, misleading, or even erroneous. The study director is well advised to have his or her interpretations reviewed by a scientist with expertise in clinical pathology prior to finalizing this portion of the study report.

For example, consider the following scenario in a short-term study evaluating dog oral toxicity where there were three animals per sex per group:

Tubular degeneration and necrosis of the kidneys were observed in three out of three males and one in three females at the high dose of 400 mg/kg/day, in no animals at 200 mg/kg/day, and in one female at 100 mg/kg/day. The study report indicated that the change at 100 mg/kg/day was not likely to be compound related because it was unilateral and minimally severe and because it was likely due to decreased renal perfusion secondary to the marked salivation that the animal displayed during the study. It further stated that the slight increases in inorganic phosphorus and potassium observed in the affected animal were indicative of decreased renal perfusion. Table 10.3 presents clinical chemistry data corresponding to this case. This interpretation was erroneous, given that marked salivation is not commonly observed to affect potassium levels in

TABLE 10.3. Selected clinical chemistry parameters for female animals from a dog oral toxicity study.

Group and Animal number	Potassium mmol/L		Phosphorus mmol/L		Urea mmol/L		Creatinine μmol/L	
	Predose	Week 5	Predose	Week 5	Predose	Week 5	Predose	Week 5
Control Animal 1	4.24	4.41	1.89	1.77	4.8	4.8	77	72
Control Animal 2	4.21	4.62	1.98	1.85	5.4	4.6	72	67
Control Animal 3	3.93	4.43	2.10	1.92	5.9	4.9	79	66
100 mg/kg/day Animal 1*	4.05	5.46	1.92	2.37	5.1	5.9	73	76
100 mg/kg/day Animal 2	4.47	4.31	1.97	2.10	5.3	6.1	75	78
100 mg/kg/day Animal 3	3.97	4.73	1.91	2.20	7.3	6.0	80	85

Tubular degeneration/necrosis was observed histologically in this animal.

laboratory animals, and has been noted to cause a *decrease* in potassium levels in some species [12]. More importantly, the primary parameter that should change with decreased renal perfusion is urea (with or without creatinine) [13]. There were no changes in urea or creatinine in the affected animal compared to other animals in its group or control animals. No indication was given regarding to what the inorganic phosphorus and potassium were compared to make the assessment that they were slightly increased. Furthermore, the study report indicated that clinical chemistry parameters for all individuals were "within physiological range," which by definition should have included the potassium and phosphorus levels of the affected animal. In short, the arguments presented did not adequately support the presumption that decreased renal perfusion was present. The renal lesion observed in the female at 100 mg/kg/day may have occurred by chance, but the line of reasoning presented to support this conclusion was ill informed and weak.

    In another example, increased mean leukocyte counts (due to increased neutrophils) and fibrinogen levels compared to concurrent control values were observed in an oral toxicity study in rats where compound-related necrosis and associated acute inflammatory lesions of the gastrointestinal tract occurred (see Table 10.4 for hematology data corresponding to this case). Both fibrinogen levels and neutrophil counts are expected to increase with acute inflammation; however, the study director dismissed the increased fibrinogen levels as incidental because they were "slight" and noted the increased neutrophil counts but did not correlate them with the inflammation associated with the necrosis. It is likely that the study director did not make these correlations because he looked only at mean incidence tables and did not consider each individual animal as a biological entity when he assessed the clinical pathology and anatomic pathology data. Though one generally has confidence in the meaningfulness of mean values for data in rodent studies, it is always useful to look at individual animal data as well to completely understand what is happening in these studies. In this case, the larger standard deviations

TABLE 10.4. Selected mean ($\pm$ standard deviation) hematology parameters from a rat oral toxicity study.

	Compound X (mg/kg/day)							
	0		50		150		450	
Sex	M	F	M	F	M	F	M	F
Leukocytes (G/L)	10.28	7.87	11.33	8.66	10.93	8.35	12.32	10.96*
	(2.38)	(2.08)	(3.11)	(2.10)	(2.79)	(2.91)	(3.78)	(3.71)
Neutrophils (G/L)	1.16	1.45	1.02	1.19	1.35	1.57	1.40	2.48*
	(0.24)	(1.45)	(0.25)	(0.48)	(0.26)	(0.76)	(0.40)	(1.98)
Fibrinogen (g/L)	3.24	2.75	3.28	2.78	3.39	3.87*	3.30	3.93**
	(0.20)	(0.28)	(0.27)	(0.31)	(0.27)	(1.46)	(0.20)	(1.28)

$* p < 0.05; ** p < 0.01$

presented for the statistically significant mean high dose values served as an indication that the reason(s) for the variation in the individual values merited investigation. There is a greater chance that the connection between these data would not have been missed if a clinical or an anatomic pathologist had had access to these data and had been allowed to make clinical pathology and anatomic pathology correlations in his or her part of the study report.

In a third example, a small (maximum 11%) decrease in red blood cell count, hemoglobin, and hematocrit compared to concurrent control values was observed in males only at the high dose level in a 2-week oral toxicity study in rats (see Table 10.5 for hematology data corresponding to this case). This change was considered not to be

TABLE 10.5. Selected mean ($\pm$ standard deviation) hematology parameters from a rat oral toxicity study.

	Males		
Dose (mg/kg/day)	RBC (T/L)	Percent reticulocytes	Absolute reticulocytes (T/L)[1]
0	7.71	3.4	0.26
	(0.24)	(0.00)	(0.00)
1	7.53 [NC][2]	3.3 [NC]	0.25 [NC]
	(0.42)	(0.03)	(0.00)
5	7.32 [NC]	3.9 (+15)	0.28 [NC]
	(0.31)	(0.02)	(0.00)
30	6.84 [−11]	8.0	0.55 [+2.1 fold]
	(0.33)	[+2.3-fold]	(0.00)
		(0.05)	

[1] *Absolute reticulocytes = (RBC x percent reticulocytes)/100*
[2] *NC = change < 10% of mean control value*

toxicologically relevant due to its low magnitude. However, this finding should have been considered relevant, given the following facts:

1. Serum urea was increased in high-dose males, meaning that the extent of the real decrease in red blood cell values was likely masked due to dehydration [14].
2. Increased erythropoiesis (grades 3–4 out of 5) was present in the spleen in all high-dose males
3. A modest increase in mean absolute and percent reticulocytes was observed in affected animals, with five of six high-dose males having absolute reticulocyte values (the more pertinent parameter to evaluate for meaningful interpretation of possible effects) higher than the highest concurrent control value.

It is not likely that an experienced toxicologist/pathologist would have missed these correlations.

PEER REVIEW

Peer review is the tool that is used to ensure the accuracy and consistency of data and their interpretation. Some companies use this process, which should be performed only by qualified personnel with experience in toxicology, to evaluate all sections of the study report.

In most cases, peer review is restricted to pathology data—to verify that the nomenclature used for diagnoses is current and meaningful, and to ensure that the interpretation of findings as toxicologically relevant and adverse is reasonable. It is more often performed for anatomic pathology data than for clinical pathology data. Peer review of these data by competent personnel is invaluable for avoiding the inclusion of errors and omissions in study reports such as those described in the previous section. The results of studies that have undergone formal peer review are more readily accepted by regulatory authorities than those that have not been reviewed.

To provide the most comprehensive and informed review, the peer review pathologist should have access to information about the compound being tested as well as the results of the study being reviewed. This assists the reviewer in assessing whether or not the interpretation of the findings in the report is reasonable in the context of the study.

The following are three examples of how peer review of histopathology data can be useful.

Example 1

A histopathologist was asked to evaluate a rat study where there were no changes in mean alanine aminotransferase (ALAT) or aspartate aminotransferase (ASAT), decreased mean bilirubin due to low values in a few individual animals (which had concomitant increases in ALAT and ASAT), and no change in mean relative liver weights in the high-dose group compared to concurrent control values. Animals with decreased bilirubin also had slightly increased relative liver weights compared to the highest concurrent control value. The pathologist diagnosed hepatocellular hypertrophy in several animals at this dose level, but not in those with decreased bilirubin and increased liver enzymes and relative liver weights. Evidence of hepatocellular hypertrophy is generally detectable once liver weights are increased by ~20% over control values [15]. Hepatocellular hypertrophy is considered to be histopathological evidence of enzyme induction, which is a possible cause of decreased serum bilirubin levels [16]. A pathologist who is aware of the strong correlation between increased relative liver weight and hepatocellular hypertrophy, and who found evidence of hypertrophy in the absence of increased relative liver weight, would reasonably be expected to comment on this remarkable finding. In addition, the pathologist would be expected to comment on the lack of correlation between histopathology findings and the decreased bilirubin, increased enzymes, and increased relative liver weights observed in a few animals. No such comments were found in the study report, leading a knowledgeable reviewer to question whether the diagnosis of hepatocellular hypertrophy had been made correctly and to ask whether a peer review had been performed. In fact, a peer review had not been scheduled for the study. Because of the reviewer's observations, a peer review was finally undertaken.

Example 2

In a more dramatic—but not uncommon—situation, a CRO hired a study pathologist who had been trained as a diagnostic veterinary pathologist (one who is trained in the pathology of domestic animals and who works in a clinical setting) to evaluate rodent studies. Neither the CRO's management nor the pathologist was aware that today's toxicologic pathologist uses a standardized system of nomenclature and diagnostic criteria when evaluating regulatory toxicity studies and that peer review is a standard exercise performed for evaluating quality control of the study pathologist's work. The study pathologist evaluated all studies, including carcinogenicity studies, using nontraditional nomenclature and inappropriate diagnostic criteria. The CRO only discovered this by chance when a sponsor requested that a peer review be performed on a study that was critical to a regulatory filing. The study in question was so error-laden that it required reevaluation. The burden placed on the sponsor because of the time lost in filing the regulatory submission and the additional expense of having the work repeated was colossal.

Example 3

A study pathologist faced the challenge of diagnosing a complicated lesion that had multiple components. Because this particular lesion had not been seen before, the pathologist deliberately diagnosed the components of the lesion separately in an attempt to be certain not to miss aspects of the change that might be compound-related. This resulted in a lengthy diagnosis list that was difficult to interpret. The peer reviewer for the study also had not seen such a lesion but was able to approach the study from a fresh perspective. The study and peer review pathologists examined the different components of the lesion separately and together. After extensive discussion, they finally agreed that it would be best to combine certain elements of the diagnosis list while leaving others distinct so that the best analysis of the potential pathogenesis of the lesion could be made.

REPORT PREPARATION

The writer of the study report should always remember that the reader's ease in comprehending the report is one of the most important hallmarks of report quality. This is particularly important when the writer must create reports that are partially composed of subreports for various data sets (e.g., ophthalmology, toxicokinetics, and pathology) that are written by multiple specialists. Therefore, we consider various philosophies for reporting toxicity data in this section. These concern both form (organization, reporting format) and substance (presentation of data and their interpretation). The following discussion focuses on the information to be presented in the results, discussion, and summary sections of the toxicology report.

FORMAT OF THE REPORT

The principal part of a complete toxicology report contains the following: title page, Summary, Introduction, Materials and Methods, Results, Discussion, and Conclusion. A reference section should be included if necessary. These sections will be followed by data tables, figures, and appendices. Tables generally present mean data, whereas appendices generally present individual animal data. Appendices may also include complete reports for subcontracted parts of the study (e.g., TKs, histopathology), analytical data concerning the test compound, and study plan and amendments.

Study results can be presented in two basic formats. Using a traditional format, results from all parts of the study are presented first, followed by a comprehensive discussion of the results in a separate, designated section. The Results section is conventionally divided into subsections so that data for clinical signs, ophthalmology, and clinical pathology, for example, are communicated separately. Historically, the writer of the study report who uses this format has presented and discussed *all* results, regardless of their toxicological relevance. This engenders a report that is much longer than necessary, which may provoke frustration and negative bias in the reviewer of the report (see Substance of the Report below). Therefore, it is advisable for toxicology report writers to use the Results section to present only the findings judged to be toxicologically relevant and to dismiss any irrelevant findings in a short paragraph in that section. The Discussion section can then be reserved for presenting arguments supporting the conclusion that certain findings reported in the Results section are toxicologically relevant.

Alternatively, one can combine the Results and Discussion of toxicologically relevant findings in one section—Results and Discussion. Using this format, a discussion of each toxicologically relevant result is presented after the result is communicated. This style is particularly suited for small studies or studies with few findings. If this form of reporting is selected, it is best to present the Discussion as indented text in a different typeface so that the reader can easily discern the difference between the result and the discussion.

The following is an example of the Results and Discussion format for a histopathology finding in an imaginary oral toxicity study with a compound called Gen2AntibacT.

Histopathology

"Compound-related changes induced by the oral (gavage) administration of Gen2AntibacT were limited to vacuolar degeneration of the kidneys at all dose levels in males and at 2500 mg/kg/day only in females.

Vacuolar degeneration of the distal tubular epithelium (tubular degeneration) was observed in 1 in 10 males at 250 mg/kg/day, 2 in 10 males at 750 mg/kg/day, and 2 in 5 males and 1 in 5 females at 2500 mg/kg/day for Gen2AntibacT, compared to an incidence of 0 in10 in control males and 0 in10 in control females. No changes in kidney weight were observed in the affected 250 mg/kg/day males compared to control values. In 750 mg/kg/day males, relative kidney weights were increased by 49%–51% over control values. No comparison of kidney weights with control values was possible for 2500 mg/kg/day animals because of premature death." All other lesions observed in this study were considered spontaneous in nature and are commonly observed in rats of this strain and age.

> Vacuolar degeneration of distal tubules occurred with the dietary administration of 0.75% Gen1AntibacT (equivalent to 648 mg/kg in males and 564 mg/kg in females) over a 90-day period. Ten out of 10 (10/10) males and 9 out of 10 females were affected (reference). The results of the current study indicate that the second generation of AntibacT produces similar lesions at a comparable dose level (750 mg/kg/day) when administered by oral gavage.

Whichever style is selected, the primary factor in making the selection should be the facilitation of the reader's comfort in reading the report.

The format used for study reports should be consistent throughout the preclinical dossier for the compound as much as possible. This will greatly assist the person or team reviewing the dossier to find pertinent information quickly, thereby reducing frustration and the potential for creating unfavorable bias toward the regulatory submission. In cases where studies are performed by more than one CRO, the sponsor is well advised to provide a report template to each CRO so that all reports will have the same form.

Data for each sacrifice date should be presented separately when a study has been designed with multiple sacrifice dates (e.g., interim sacrifice, final sacrifice, and recovery sacrifice). This can be done in one of two ways: either the traditional subheadings for the results section are further subdivided by sacrifice date, or the sacrifice dates are the major headings and the observations and measurements for each sacrifice date serve as subheadings (see Table 10.6). For reproductive toxicity studies, the Results section is best divided into subsections that present the data specific to each phase, for each sex (when applicable, as in fertility studies), and for each generation for the study conducted. Table 10.7 shows an example of part of the outline of a report from a combination reproductive function and male fertility study.

TABLE 10.6. Possible subheadings for the results section of a general toxicology report.

Format of subheading for reports	
"Traditional"	Modified
1. Mortality	1. Interim Sacrifice
1. A. Interim sacrifice	1. A. Mortality
1. B. Terminal sacrifice	1. B. Clinical signs
1. C. Recovery sacrifice	1. C. Body weight
	1. D. Food consumption
	1. E. Laboratory investigations
	1. E. i. Hematology
	1. E. ii. Clinical chemistry
	1. E. iii. Urinalysis
	1. F. Pathology
	1. F. i. Organ weights
	1. F. ii. Necropsy findings
	1. F. iii. Histopathology findings
2. Clinical Signs	2. Terminal Sacrifice
2. A. Interim sacrifice	2. A. Mortality
2. B. Terminal sacrifice	2. B. Clinical signs
2. C. Recovery sacrifice	2. C. Body weight

SUBSTANCE OF THE REPORT

At one extreme, all data, no matter how trivial, are described in detail in the study report. This is presumably done for the sake of completeness, so that no one can accuse the writer of the report of concealing information. Data may be reported with no apparent concern for toxicological relevance so that incidental findings may be presented before adverse or adaptive ones. There may be no discussion of the data, no attempt to put them into perspective for the reader. Even if data are discussed, there is frequently no attempt made to correlate findings across the study.

At the other end of the spectrum, and by far more preferable than the aforementioned scenario, data are presented to inform the reader of the most important findings first. These are the indications of toxicity. Adaptive findings are presented next, followed by findings of uncertain significance. Incidental findings are presented last; these are not communicated individually but are addressed in one or two summarizing sentences. The writer is well advised to strive for brevity in the report but not at the expense of conveying all pertinent information.

Finally, the no-effect level (NOEL) and/or no-adverse effect level (NOAEL) for the findings in the study are identified. Because the distinction between these levels is important, it is imperative that study results be discussed so that the reader may know which findings are adverse and why. As discussed under Data Analysis and Interpretation

TABLE 10.7. Possible subheadings for the results section of a reproductive toxicology report.

Generation of animals	Data Sequence
1. F_0 Generation	1. A. General condition and mortality
	1. B. Male bodyweight
	1. C. Food consumption
	1. D. Mating performance and fertility
	1. E. Bodyweight of females during gestation
	1. F. Developmental toxicity phase
	1. F. i. Necropsy of females
	1. F. ii. Litter responses
	1. F. iii. Fetal observations
2. F_0–Postnatal Phase (females allowed to litter)	2. A. Gestation length, parturition and gestation index
	2. B. Bodyweight during lactation
	2. C. General condition of offspring
	2. D. Litter size and viability indices
	2. E. Offspring bodyweight
	2. F. Sex ratio
	2. G. Physical development
	2. H. Auditory and visual function
	2. G. Activity monitoring
	2. H. Learning activity
3. F_0–Terminal Studies	3. A. F_1 offspring
	3. B. F_0 females
	3. C. F_0 males
4. F_1 Generation	

earlier, the NOAEL is the critical element for the selection of the doses to be used for the first clinical trial of the drug product.

RESULTS SECTION

A short summary sentence or paragraph of toxicologically relevant findings should open each subsection of the results section of the study report. This allows the reader to learn immediately what is important for the data set(s) concerned. Opening sentences or paragraphs conceived this way may also be used to create the text of the results section of the summary of the study. (For a model of such an opening sentence, see the example of the Results and Discussion format for presenting data given previously.)

All data in all parts of the Results section should be presented in terms of the sexes affected and the dose(s) at which they were affected. The incidence of the change per sex and per dose is valuable information that should be included when pertinent. Quantitative data should be presented prior to qualitative data. Quantitative data should be presented numerically in the text, either as percent change or -fold change compared to concurrent control or pretest values. This provides the reader with an objective assessment of the changes observed. Absolute numerical data may be presented if percentages or -fold changes cannot be provided, but this occurs only rarely. When a value is statistically significant, this should be mentioned in the same sentence in which the value is presented. The specification of the p-value is optional. Complex data should be presented in tabular and text form whenever possible. This allows the writer to provide numerical information in the table while limiting the text to conceptual information, which lightens the reader's burden of comprehension. Data from satellite groups (e.g., toxicokinetic groups) should be presented separately from data obtained from principal groups.

Data and other information from animals found dead or killed for humane reasons should be presented in a section entitled "Mortality." It is important to include the study day of death or euthanasia and the reasons for terminating animals prior to their scheduled sacrifice date in this section. Pertinent clinical signs, body weight, food consumption, and clinical pathology data for the affected animals should also be reported. Cause of death should be determined by gross and/or histopathology (or more rarely, by clinical pathology results alone) and reported whenever possible. If no definitive cause of death can be identified, this should be stated in the text.

For clinical signs, clinical pathology and anatomic pathology data, the writer is well advised to avoid the use of diagnostic terminology. It is better to describe an animal as "unresponsive" as opposed to "comatose" (which implies that a neurological evaluation has been performed), and to indicate a "decrease in red blood cell mass" instead of reporting an "anemia" (which implies clinical impairment of the blood's oxygen-carrying capacity). It is also better to say that there was a "nodule" or a "mass" observed at necropsy as opposed to a "tumor" (which implies the presence of a neoplasm). Diagnostic terms are frequently used inappropriately and may unnecessarily alarm the regulatory reviewer or the clinician conducting a clinical trial.

Diagnostic terms are medical terms, but not all medical terms are diagnostic terms. Sometimes using a descriptive medical term is warranted when clinical signs are recorded. When such a term is used, it should be defined clearly—preferably in the same sentence in which it is used for the first time. Examples include "nystagmus" (rapid, involuntary movement of the eye) and "opisthotonos" (abnormal posture in which the head and tail are bent upward and the abdomen is bowed downward because of severe muscle spasm). Alternatively, the writer may include a glossary of terms in the report.

Individuals who write reports for reproductive and developmental toxicity studies should prefer the terms "embryofetal toxicity" or "developmental toxicity" to "teratogenicity" and should be careful about the terms used to define specific congenital abnormalities in the fetus (malformations vs variations). The incidence of findings in the offspring of dams should be evaluated and presented with reference to both the litter and the individual fetus. The writer should describe the relationship between maternal toxicity and developmental toxicity to the greatest extent possible.

Similar parameters should be presented together within a given section. This is particularly important for clinical pathology parameters. It would be nonsensical to present information on red blood cell parameters (red blood cell count, hemoglobin, and hematocrit), followed by information on white blood cell parameters and hemostasis and subsequently present data on red blood cell indices (mean corpuscular hemoglobin, mean corpuscular volume, mean corpuscular hemoglobin concentration). Similarly, one would not separate a discussion of increased liver enzymes and increased bilirubin by inserting a paragraph on electrolyte changes between the two.

Data may be presented by sex (best used to emphasize gender effects):

> ALAT and ASAT in 25 mg/kg/day male rats were increased 3-fold and 4-fold, respectively, at the end of the study. Bilirubin was also increased 2-fold in these animals. In female rats, ALAT and ASAT were increased 3-fold at 5 mg/kg/day and 4.5-fold at 25 mg/kg/day, whereas no change in bilirubin was observed at any dose level.

or alternatively, by parameter:

> ALAT and ASAT were increased in male rats at 25 mg/kg/day only (+3-fold and +4-fold, respectively) and in female rats at 5 mg/kg/day (+3-fold for both parameters) and at 25 mg/kg/day (+4.5-fold for both parameters). Bilirubin was increased +2-fold in male rats at 25 mg/kg/day, but no change in this parameter was observed in female rats at any dose level.

For studies that are devoted to specific endpoints, such as TK and carcinogenicity studies, the Results section should concentrate on the data that are relevant to those endpoints. The writer should not focus on reporting in-life findings in a TK study or nonneoplastic findings in a carcinogenicity study unless these findings impact the interpretation of the results of the study negatively or are unexpected based on the results of previous studies. For *in vivo* micronucleus studies, the writer should always state whether evidence of systemic exposure of the test system to the compound (e.g., TK data, clinical signs or other indications of toxicity) was observed or not.

TK results may be presented at various locations in the study report. However, it has been recommended that TK results be presented at the beginning of the results section because the degree of systemic exposure achieved in the study strongly influences the occurrence of toxic and adaptive effects in the species tested [4]. When TK data are generated at a site other than the laboratory that conducted the study, they are commonly presented in an appendix to the study report or in a report separate from that of the principal study. Regardless of where the data are presented, the results and interpretation of these data should be included in the text of the main report.

Optimally, TK results should be presented in narrative and tabulated form with the tables providing the numerical details of the evaluation performed. It is essential to include the following in the TK section:

- degree of exposure (Cmax and AUC) at each dose
- proportionality of exposure related to dose
- any evidence of metabolism of the compound
- any evidence of accumulation of the compound with repeat dosing
- any gender differences

Concentrations should be indicated using the same units found in the principal report. Results should always be interpreted after the formulation analysis of the compound are reviewedto ensure that the compound administered was stable and present at the concentrations desired.

For carcinogenicity studies, the writer should emphasize the reporting of compound-related neoplastic and preneoplastic or hyperplastic lesions. Mortality should be addressed first to inform the reader of the number of animals surviving until the end of the study (indicating the adequacy of the power to be expected from the statistical analysis of the neoplasm data) and to indicate whether compound-related neoplasms contributed to the early death or sacrifice of animals or not. Subsequently, the writer should communicate the number of palpable or otherwise grossly observable masses found and their relationship to histopathology findings, the number of animals that developed neoplasms, the number of primary neoplasms found, the number of malignancies found, the number of systemic neoplasms found, the frequency of neoplastic incidence in affected organs, and time-to-tumor onset per group. Any decreases in tumor incidence should be reported. Statistical significance should be indicated where applicable.

The FDA provides guidance on the design, analysis, and interpretation of rodent carcinogenicity studies in its Guidance for Industry series available on its Web site [17], including information on the number of surviving animals considered acceptable to validate the design of a study with negative results, as well as graphic indications of how to present survival and tumor data.

The number of benign tumors, malignant tumors, the combined number of malignant and benign tumors, and the total number of proliferative lesions (hyperplastic, benign, and malignant) should be indicated for neoplasms found in each organ. For neoplasms that have been shown to develop along a morphologic continuum from hyperplasia to neoplasia, this is particularly important. Examples of such proliferative lesions in rodents include bronchioloalveolar adenoma and carcinoma [18, 19], interstitial cell adenoma of the testis [20, 21], acinar cell adenoma and carcinoma of the pancreas [22], and islet cell adenoma and carcinoma [23].

It is important to mention the absence of effects in the results section for all types of studies, whether this occurs at one or all dose levels. Statements indicating that no effects occurred allow the reader to be certain that the writer of the report has not forgotten to report information on parameters measured or clinical signs observed. When findings are not considered compound-related, it is better to state this in the Results section as opposed to the Discussion section. The writer should always present the reason(s) that the effects were judged not to be compound-related.

Examples of sentences that present negative results are:

The remaining clinical signs observed in this study are frequently seen in Wistar rats of similar age at our laboratory.

and

Other variations in organ weights, even those that were statistically significant, were considered incidental and not related to compound administration because of the absence of a dose-response pattern and the presence of outlying values that altered certain control mean values.

DISCUSSION SECTION

Whether presented in a separate section or incorporated into a Results and Discussion section, the discussion of the report should address the following:

1. toxicologically relevant effects observed, including identification of target organs
2. existence of correlations among the effects observed (in developmental toxicity studies including whether or not maternal and fetal toxicity are related, when feasible)
3. how these effects compare with those observed in other studies conducted with the test compound or other compounds of the same class, when possible
4. how these effects compare with toxicologically relevant effects of compounds from different classes, when possible
5. whether or not the effects represent exaggerated, on-target pharmacology or off-target pharmacology ("true" toxicity)
6. whether or not the changes are reversible
7. whether or not there are compound-related effects that are toxicologically irrelevant to humans (of no biological significance, species-specific, etc.)
8. whether or not there are any vehicle-related or methodology-related (e.g., dosing by gavage or continuous infusion) effects
9. whether or not there is a NOEL or a NOAEL for each of the toxicologically relevant changes observed

These points should be addressed in the Discussion section of all study reports, whether they are produced by the sponsor or by a CRO. If the sponsor does not require its CRO to discuss these points in its study reports, then the sponsor should be prepared to address these issues in the regulatory dossier that it files with the appropriate authorities at the time that it seeks approval for clinical trials. Physicians conducting clinical trials will need to understand these issues thoroughly to manage effectively any risks associated with the administration of the new drug product to human patients.

As in the Results section, similar parameters should be discussed together. After reading the Discussion section of a report, the reviewer of the report should understand why the writer believes that each compound-related finding is relevant to the toxicological profile of the chemical that has been tested.

For TK studies, it is useful to note any differences in methodology, dose, and formulation between the toxicity study and the protocol to be used for compound administration in humans. Correlations with signs of toxicity should be discussed when possible.

When discussing findings in relation to observations made in other regulatory or experimental studies, lesion pathogenesis, or irrelevance of findings to human health, references should be provided. Conjecture should absolutely be avoided—speculative statements may lead to unnecessary questions from regulatory authorities that are difficult to impossible to answer. Care should be taken not to discuss the toxicological relevance of data for which the Materials and Methods section indicates that sampling or other technical problems caused the evaluation of parameters to be confounded, inadequate, or impossible.

SUMMARY SECTION

The Summary section of the toxicology report is the most critical section of all. This section may be copied verbatim from the study report and placed in the common technical document (CTD), investigational medicinal product dossier (IMPD), investigational new drug (IND), and new drug application (NDA) filings, the investigator's brochure (IB), expert reports, and other documents that are to be submitted to regulatory authorities. It may also be submitted to databases that are made available to the public or placed in product safety summaries. As such, it becomes the only representative of the study report and must be both accurate and succinct. A first-rate summary will give a reviewer confidence that it is not necessary to read the entire study report to obtain pertinent information.

The Summary should contain all the elements of a complete report. There should be an introduction that provides information on the objective of the study, a Materials and Methods section that provides a brief overview of the study design, the animals used for the study (strain, number of animals per group, total animal number), doses administered, and route by which doses were administered. Any nonstandard procedures or parameters evaluated should also be mentioned in the principal Materials and Methods section. For studies for which dose selection depended on the conduct of range-finding studies, the rationale for dose selection should be indicated. Toxicologically relevant results should then be presented, beginning with changes observed at the highest dose administered or at the lowest dose administered. The report writer should be consistent in the order chosen to report effects by dose (from highest to lowest dose or visa versa) so that the reader is not confused. The affected dose levels should be specified instead of using the terms "high," "mid," and "low" to describe the dose groups. Results should be presented in numerical terms (percentages; ratios of affected animals/number of animals per group) whenever possible.

Results of uncertain relevance should also be described in the Summary. Statements regarding negative results should be used judiciously. It may be useful to include a statement summarizing negative results for a particular group of data, but, more importantly, negative results should be mentioned if (1) they are unexpected or (2) they highlight the absence of a certain change at a dose level that is lower or higher than other doses for which that change was observed.

Example of a summary statement of negative results:

There were no compound-related hematology or clinical chemistry findings in this study.

Example of a statement of unexpected negative results:

Despite the development of tremors in rats treated at similar doses in other studies with the test compound, no tremors were observed in rats treated at 300 mg/kg/day in this study.

Example of a statement highlighting negative results at a specific dose level:

Although maternal toxicity was observed at 1, 10, and 50 mg/kg/day, adverse effects on pregnancy rate, number of implantations, and litter size were only observed at 50 mg/kg/day.

Results that were not discussed as relevant changes in the report should not be presented in the Summary. The Summary section will also contain a discussion and a conclusion. Questions to be addressed in the Discussion portion of the summary are the same as those addressed in the Discussion section of the study report. The conclusion, which is generally a "cut and paste" of the Conclusion section of the study report, will indicate the principal effects and target organs identified and specify the NOEL or NOAEL for the study, if identified. The maximum tolerated dose should be specified for range-finding or other studies that will be used to determine the dose levels for future studies.

All toxicologically relevant findings should be indicated in the Summary. Any toxicity that is observed in the clinic that has not been reported in the IB is considered an unexpected adverse event that must be reported to the FDA. A sponsor should never be faced with the need to file such a report for a finding that was observed preclinically but not appropriately recorded in the report or its summary.

USING REFERENCES AND PUBLICLY ACCESSIBLE DATABASES

Pharmaceutical development often involves the assessment of compounds that are part of an already marketed class of chemicals. More and more frequently, it involves combining two or more preexisting drugs into a new compound. Under these circumstances, data from relevant, previously conducted, toxicity studies may be available in the scientific literature or as part of the database of governmental or other not-for-profit organizations. Such information can be useful in designing studies (particularly with regard to dose selection), as well as determining the level at which adverse effects can be expected and tolerated. Alternatively, this information can be used as evidence that the new compound has caused an unexpected adverse effect that may not be tolerable for the envisioned application of the drug. Journal articles may provide mechanistic data that can be helpful in extrapolating effects observed in animals to potential or recognized effects in humans.

Myriad scientific journals publish safety data on pharmaceuticals and other chemicals. Clinical data may be found in publications such as the *New England Journal of Medicine*, *Journal of Clinical Research*, and *Clinical Trials*, to name a few. Journals that publish preclinical data include *Toxicological Sciences*, *Toxicologic Pathology*, and *Fundamental and Applied Toxicology*.

The Internet is an invaluable resource for obtaining safety information on pharmaceuticals and other xenobiotics. PubMed® is an abstract service that references MEDLINE® and other life science journals to provide over 17 million citations. PubMed is provided by the U.S. National Library of Medicine (NLM). Some links to full text articles are available. Other sources of information are discussed as follows.

FDA DRUG APPROVAL PACKAGES

The U.S. Food and Drug Administration (FDA) posts drug approval packages for marketed products on its Web site [24]. These documents contain Pharm/Tox reviews that summarize the data obtained in preclinical studies. Sometimes the Pharm/Tox review is presented in an independent document on the site; sometimes, the toxicology data are presented in a document called *Pharmacology Review*. Drug approval packages are covered by the Freedom of Information (FOI) Act and may be used by scientists and others; however, information found in original IND and NDA filings is confidential and permission to access and use data from such documents must be granted by the filing institution. It is possible to request documentation on compounds that are not represented on the Web site by writing to the FDA.

NATIONAL TECHNICAL INFORMATION SERVICE, U.S. DEPARTMENT OF COMMERCE

The National Technical Information Service (NTIS) has served as a centralized resource for U.S. government-funded scientific, technical, engineering, and business-related information (STEI products) created by or for U.S. federal agencies for more than 60 years. There are now close to three million documents [25]. NTIS considers all STEI products to be information produced and released by the sponsoring federal agency, which is solely responsible for the quality and objectivity of the products. Therefore, documents obtained through NTIS do not represent the views of the NTIS. However, NTIS does decide whether a given document is useful enough to be added to its collection or not. NTIS does not conduct or fund scientific research, does not create or fund original STEI products, and does not use third-party STEI to develop new or improved STEI products [26]. Documents accessible through this organization include journal articles as well as technical reports from the National Institute of Environmental Health Sciences (NIEHS) and the National Toxicology Program (NTP). Users must pay a fee to access the information on the NTIS Web site.

The NTP is another major source of documentation. Its mission is to evaluate agents of public health concern in the United States. NTP, working with other U.S. governmental agencies, provides scientific data, interpretations, and guidance concerning the appropriate uses of data to regulatory agencies and other groups involved with health-related research. Through its interactive relationship with regulatory agencies, NTP plays an indirect, but important, role in shaping public health policy [27]. Technical reports for NTP toxicity studies and articles from the journal *Environmental Health Perspectives* can be found on the NTP Web site. Although the focus of this organization is on environmental chemicals, some data on pharmaceuticals used as AIDS therapeutics (e.g., antibiotics, AZT) can be found there. Information is available free of charge.

NTP no longer registers reports and documents with NTIS because reports are now available on its Web site in downloadable and printable PDF format. Some older documents that are not available in downloadable format from the NTP Web site may still be ordered from NTIS by providing the chemical name, CAS (Chemical Abstracts Service) number, and NTIS number to identify the document [28].

THE TOXICOLOGY AND ENVIRONMENTAL HEALTH INFORMATION PROGRAM (TEHIP)

This organization evolved from the Toxicology Information Program (TIP) that was established by the NLM in 1967 to create automated toxicity databanks and provide toxicology information and data services. TEHIP's mandate includes environmental health as well as toxicology. It is part of the Specialized Information Services division of the NLM [29]. TEHIP databases are accessible free of charge.

TEHIP maintains the Toxicology Data Network (TOXNET®), which includes several databases that contain toxicology information. Three of these—the Hazardous Substances Data Bank, TOXLINE®, and the Chemical Carcinogenesis Research Information System—are discussed as follows:

HAZARDOUS SUBSTANCES DATA BANK

The Hazardous Substances Data Bank (HSDB®) summarizes safety data from a number of sources, including scientific texts and journals. For each entry, the notation "peer reviewed" is made if the content for that particular source is critically reviewed prior to publication. Information on known human health effects, including evidence of carcinogenicity; data from animal toxicity studies (including NTP studies); absorption, distribution, metabolism, and excretion (ADME); half-life; chemical interactions; existing drug warnings; pharmacology; mechanisms of action; and idiosyncratic reactions can be found in these documents. Physicochemical properties and characteristics of known preparations/formulations are also provided.

HSDB is peer reviewed by a committee of experts in toxicology, chemistry, pharmacology, industrial hygiene, medicine, and other pertinent scientific disciplines. The committee meets several times a year to review and discuss the scientific information in new and updated chemical records [30].

TOXLINE

TOXLINE® is a bibliographical database that contains information on the biochemical, pharmacological, physiological, and toxicological effects of drugs and other chemicals. TOXLINE contains over three million bibliographic citations, most with abstracts and/or indexing terms and CAS registry numbers. Sources of information include biomedical and toxicology abstract services such as PubMed and MEDLINE, developmental and reproductive toxicology literature (DART®), and databases for technical reports such as the one found at NTIS [31].

CHEMICAL CARCINOGENESIS RESEARCH INFORMATION SYSTEM

The Chemical Carcinogenesis Research Information System (CCRIS®) is sponsored by the National Cancer Institute. Its databank contains information on studies performed on carcinogens, mutagens, tumor promoters, cocarcinogens, metabolites, and carcinogen inhibitors. Information is scientifically evaluated and fully referenced, with test results being reviewed by scientific experts. Over 9000 chemicals are currently represented on the site [32].

Following are two examples using information in the public domain to interpret the results of pharmaceutical toxicity studies:

Example 1: Octreotide and Intimal Hyperplasia

In the case of octreotide, a somatostatin analog that has been on the market for several years for the treatment of acromegaly, neuroendocrine gastrointestinal tumors and other neoplastic, endocrine and gastrointestinal diseases [33–35], a multitude of publications exist that describe the inhibitory effect of this compound on intimal hyperplasia of coronary and other arteries [36, 37]. In a 13-week rat study performed by subcutaneous injection, octreotide was observed to enhance the incidence of intimal hyperplasia in arteries and veins of the dermis and subcutis compared to that observed in vehicle controls [38]. Because the available literature indicated that the opposite effect was to be expected in vessels, the intimal hyperplasia observed in the skin was interpreted as an adverse finding.

Example 2: Isoniazid and CNS Vacuolization

Isoniazid, rifampicin, and pyrazinamide are well known antibiotics that are used in a cocktail for the treatment of tuberculosis. Gatifloxicin is a broad-spectrum antibiotic used to treat respiratory, skin, and urinary tract infections. Safety data for these drugs are available in the Hazardous Substance Databank, NIEHS technical reports and pharmacology/toxicology reviews for the Center of Drug Evaluation and Research (FDA). In a 13-week oral (gavage) rat study that tested various combinations of these drugs for potential toxicity, vacuolation of the cerebellar roof nuclei and several areas of the cerebrum was identified in a dose-related pattern. After a review of the literature and the aforementioned sources of information, the cerebellar lesion was determined to be due to the isoniazid component of the formulations [39]. Journal articles and textbooks described in detail the morphologic features and locations of vacuoles observed with the administration of isoniazid, whereas none of the references for the other antibiotics described vacuolation of nervous tissue as a compound-related lesion.

NTP TECHNICAL REPORTS

NTP Technical Reports are excellent examples of literature available in the public domain that scientists can use to support their arguments in the discussion of the toxicologic potential of compounds that they investigate. In reading any NTP summary, one will see that NTP investigators also use literature available in the public domain extensively. In fact, they perform an extensive literature search for both animal and human toxicity and write a comprehensive summary of the literature available to date before they present and discuss the results of studies that they have conducted. Their literature summaries include information on general toxicity, reproductive and developmental toxicity, carcinogenicity, and genetic toxicity. The reference list for an NTP summary of a given chemical entity can function as a partial literature search for information on that chemical.

IMPACT OF UNCLEAR REPORTING ON REGULATORY SUBMISSIONS

Regulators are trained to spot inconsistencies and discrepancies in dossiers; therefore, all documents that are destined for review by regulatory authorities should be created with this in mind. Examples of regulatory submissions include the following:

- IND: investigational new drug application. Sponsors must file an IND with the FDA to obtain permission to test the therapeutic or diagnostic potential of a new drug product in humans [40].
- IB: investigator's brochure. This document provides the physician conducting a clinical trial with a new drug product the information required to understand the rationale behind the clinical protocol, including the doses to be administered, the method(s) and frequency of administration, and safety monitoring procedures [41].
- IMPD: investigational medical product dossier. This dossier forms the basis of approval for clinical trials in the European Union [42].
- CTD: common technical document. This document provides for a "harmonised structure and format for new product applications." It includes sections on organization of the application, and the quality, safety, and efficacy of the drug product [43].

Guidelines for the compilation and submission of these dossiers are provided in the aforementioned references.

As stated in the reporting section, the summary portion of the study report is what is generally used as the representative text for that study in regulatory documents. When poorly written (albeit consistent) summaries or summaries that have been written in different styles are placed into a single regulatory document, it is often difficult for a reviewer to follow which changes are considered to be related to compound administration within or across species and whether said changes are considered adverse or not. When studies for a preclinical dossier have been performed at multiple locations, the sponsor of the regulatory dossier is advised to review and edit all study summaries thoroughly as required to harmonize the order and style in which information is presented. For each summary, it should be clear to the reader which effects are considered compound-related, at what doses they were found, and whether or not the effects are considered adverse.

Summaries for small-animal studies should be presented before summaries for large-animal studies. If the summary of a study refers to information that will be presented later in the regulatory document, the exact location of the information should be indicated. The pertinent sentence in the summary should be phrased so as not to imply that the reader has already encountered said information. For example, a CTD included a study summary for a 13-week intravenous toxicity study that contained the sentence "The changes encountered in this study were similar to those observed in the subcutaneous study." However, no summary for any subcutaneous study had been previously presented in the document and there was no indication as to where the reviewer could find this summary. The reviewer was forced to return to the table of contents to look for the page number of the subcutaneous study, only to find that there were summaries for four subcutaneous studies in two species in the dossier.

In the same 13-week intravenous toxicity study summary, alkaline phosphatase increases were said to be "possibly related to 'the' bone changes," information about which was only to be encountered for the first time four paragraphs later. This phrase would have been better formulated as follows: " . . . alkaline phosphatase increases were possibly related to the increased trabecular bone formation in the femur identified microscopically (see page X for details)."

Under no circumstances should a summary mention data that have not been presented in the dossier.

Information in tabulated summaries should be cross checked with information presented in written summaries, as discrepancies will almost certainly generate unnecessary questions from the authorities. Particular care should be taken to avoid the classification of numerical changes as increased in the text of the written summary when the tabulated summary indicates that the change represents a decrease, or visa versa. Such mistakes are easily made—and are perhaps even spotted more easily by reviewers. This lack of attention to detail is a red flag for regulators, who will likely begin to look for other types of errors because of finding this sort of avoidable blunder.

Additionally, the sponsor should verify that effects identified as indicative of toxicity in one study have been similarly identified as such in other studies. If a valid reason for the difference in classification among studies exists, it should be presented. For example, in the reproductive toxicity section of a preclinical safety dossier, decreased body weight gain and food consumption were classified as maternotoxic effects in two study summaries and as exaggerated pharmacologic effects in two other summaries. No reason for this distinction was presented. This led the reviewer to go back to the general toxicity part of the dossier to search for any studies in which these findings were mentioned and to see how they were classified, if at all.

Biologically irrelevant data should never make their way into a document that is to be submitted to a regulatory authority. They make dossiers unnecessarily longer to read and may lead the authority to raise questions that require an official response. This, in addition to adding significant time to the review process, increases the risk of discovering additional errors and omissions in data presentation or in data interpretation within the submitted dossier. A thorough evaluation of each study report as described in the section on data analysis above should minimize, if not eliminate, this problem.

Regulatory submissions will necessarily contain a discussion section for preclinical results. The discussion section for individual study reports may be used for these documents, including any references that may be required to explain the reasoning used to arrive at the conclusions that are presented in the dossier. These sections should also be carefully reviewed for consistency of style and form and appropriately edited to maximize the coherence of the regulatory submission.

The conclusion section of each study summary ("the summary of the summary") presented in a regulatory submission should be clearly labeled as such. This will allow the reviewer to understand that he or she has reached the end of the information supplied for the study in question.

REFERENCES

1. Organisation for Economic Co-operation and Development, 2002. The application of the OECD principles of GLP to the organisation and management of multi-site studies. 17 pp. http://www.olis.oecd.org/olis/2002doc.nsf/LinkTo/NT00000B8A/$FILE/JT00128856.PDF

2. U.S. Food and Drug Administration, 2002. Estimating the safe starting dose in clinical trials for therapeutics in adult healthy volunteers. 26 pp. http://www.fda.gov/ cber/gdlns/dose.pdf

3. U.S. Food and Drug Administration, 2010. Guidance for Industry. M3(R2) Nonclinical Safety Studies for the Conduct of Human Clinical Trials and Marketing Authorization for Pharmaceuticals. http://www.fda.gov/downloads/Drugs/GuidanceCompliance-RegulatoryInformation/Guidances/ucm073246.pdf

4. Nohynek G.J, editor, 1996. *Presenting Toxicity Results: How to Evaluate Data and Write Reports*. G Copping, and MY Wells, contributing editors. London, Bristol: Taylor & Francis. 139 pp.

5. Gove PB, editor-in-chief, 1981. *Webster's Third New International Dictionary Unabridged*. Springfield, MA: Merriam-Webster Inc.

6. Boone L, Meyer D, Cusick P, Ennulat D et al., 2005. Selection and interpretation of clinical pathology indicators of hepatic injury in preclinical studies. *Vet Clin Pathol 34*:182–188

7. Wagner JD, Greaves KA, Schwenke DC, and Bauer JE, 1999. Lipids and lipoproteins. In: WF Loeb and FW Quimby, editors. *The Clinical Chemistry of Laboratory Animals*. Philadelphia: Taylor & Francis. pp. 181–228.

8. Center for Drug Evaluation and Research Application. Pharmacology Review(s). Exelon[TM] (rivastigmine tartrate) NDA No. 20–823. Part 2. http://www.fda.gov/cder/foi/nda/2000/20823_Exelon_pharmr_P2.pdf

9. Calabrese EJ and Baldwin LA, 2001. The frequency of U-shaped dose responses in the toxicological literature. *Toxicol Sci 62*:330–338

10. Welshons WV, Thayer KA, Judy BM, Taylor JA et al., 2003. Large effects from small exposures I. Mechanisms for endocrine-disrupting chemicals with estrogenic activity. *Environ Health Perspect 111*:994–1006

11. Foegh ML, Asostra S, Conte J, Howell M et al., 1994. Early inhibition of myointimal proliferation by angiopeptin after balloon catheter injury in the rabbit. *J Vasc Surg* **19**:1084–1091

12. Stockham SL and Scott MA, 2002. Monovalent Electrolytes and Osmolality. In: SL Stockham and MA Scott, editors. *Fundamentals of Veterinary Clinical Pathology*. Ames: Iowa State Press. pp. 337–380

13. Hall RL and Everds NE, 2008. Principles of clinical pathology for toxicology studies. In: AW Hayes, editor. *Principles and Methods of Toxicology*, 5th ed. Boca Raton, FL: CRC Press. pp. 1318–1358.

14. Brockus CW and Andreasen CB, 2003. *Erythrocytes*. In: KS Latimer, EA Mahaffey, and KW Prasse, editors. *Duncan and Prasse's Veterinary Laboratory Medicine. Clinical Pathology*. Ames: Blackwell Publishing. pp. 3–45

15. Amacher, DE, 1998. The relationship among microsomal enzyme induction, liver weight and histological change in rat toxicology studies. *Food Chem Toxicol* **36**:831–839

16. Gough, H, Goggin T, Crowley M, and Callaghan N, 1989. Serum bilirubin levels with antiepileptic drugs. *Epilepsia* **30**:597–602

17. U.S. Food and Drug Administration, 2001. *Statistical Aspects of the Design, Analysis, and Interpretation of Chronic Rodent Carcinogenicity Studies of Pharmaceuticals*. 44 pp. http://www.fda.gov/Cder/guidance/815dft.pdf

18. Boorman GA and Eustis SL, 1990. Lung. In: GA Boorman, SL Eustis, MR Elwell, CA Montgomery, and WF MacKenzie, editors. *Pathology of the Fischer Rat*. San Diego: Academic Press. pp. 339–368

19. Dixon D, Herbert RA, Sills RC, and Boorman GA, 1999. Lungs, pleura, and mediastinum. In: RR Maronpot, editor. *Pathology of the Mouse*. Vienna, IL: Cache River Press. pp. 293–332

20. Boorman GA, Chapin RE, and Mitsumori K, 1990. Testis and epididymis. In: GA Boorman, SL Eustis, MR Elwell, CA Montgomery, and WF MacKenzie, editors. *Pathology of the Fischer Rat*. San Diego: Academic Press. pp. 405–418

21. Radovsky A, Mitsumori K, and Chapin RE, 1999. Male reproductive tract. In: RR Maronpot, editor. *Pathology of the Mouse*. Vienna, IL: Cache River Press. pp. 381–408

22. Eustis S L, Boorman GA, and Hayashi Y, 1990. Exocrine pancreas. In: GA Boorman, SL Eustis, MR Elwell, CA Montgomery, and WF MacKenzie, editors. *Pathology of the Fischer Rat*. San Diego: Academic Press. pp. 95–108

23. Riley MGI, Boorman GA, and Hayashi Y, 1990. Endocrine Pancreas. In: GA Boorman, SL Eustis, MR Elwell, CA Montgomery, and WF MacKenzie, editors. *Pathology of the Fischer Rat*. San Diego: Academic Press. pp. 545–556

24. U.S. Food and Drug Administration, 2008. Drugs@FDA. http://www.accessdata.fda.gov/scripts/cder/drugsatfda/

25. National Technical Information Service, 2008a. About NTIS. http://www.ntis.gov/about/index.aspx#npolicy

26. National Technical Information Service, 2008b. Information quality standards. http://www.ntis.gov/help/quality.aspx

27. National Toxicology Program, 2008a. Mission statement. http://ntp.niehs.nih.gov/?objectid=72015D13-BDB7-CEBA-FCC75AAEAA3A08E6

28. National Toxicology Program, 2008b. NTIS ordering information. http://ntp.niehs.nih.gov/index.cfm?objectid=072FAE73-B72E-D758-A017E83B5A213140

29. National Library of Medicine, 2008a. Toxicology and Environmental Health Information Program. http://www.nlm.nih.gov/pubs/factsheets/tehipfs.html

30. National Library of Medicine, 2008b. Toxnet—Hazardous Substances Database. http://toxnet.nlm.nih.gov/cgi-bin/sis/htmlgen?DescSRP.htm

31. National Library of Medicine, 2008c. TOXLINE®. http://www.nlm.nih.gov/pubs/factsheets/toxlinfs.html

32. National Library of Medicine, 2008d. Chemical Carcinogenesis Research Information System. http://www.nlm.nih.gov/pubs/factsheets/ccrisfs.html

33. Dasgupta P, 2004. Somatostatin analogues: Multiple roles in cellular proliferation, neoplasia, and angiogenesis. *Pharmacol Ther 102*:61–85

34. Eriksson B and Öberg K, 1999. Summing up 15 years of somatostatin analog therapy in neuroendocrine tumors: future outlook. *Ann Oncol 10*:31–38

35. de Herder WW and Lamberts SWJ, 2003. Somatostatin analog therapy in treatment of gastrointestinal disorders and tumors. *Endocrine 20*:285–290

36. Aavik E, Luoto,N-M, Petrov L, Aavik, S et al., 2002. Elimination of vascular fibrointimal hyperplasia by somatostatin receptor 1,4-selective agonist. *FASEB J 16*:724–726

37. Yumi K, Fagin J.A, Yamashita M, Fishbein MC et al., 1997. Direct effects of somatostatin analog octreotide on insulin-like growth factor-I in the arterial wall. *Lab Invest 76*:329–338

38. Wells MY, Voute H, Lonchampt M.-O, Fisch C et al., 2009. Intimal hyperplasia in rats after subcutaneous injection of a somatostatin analog. *Toxicol Pathol 37*: 235–243

39. Wells MY and Krinke GJ, 2008. Cerebral vacuolation induced in rats by the administration of LUP-3FDC, an anti-tuberculosis cocktail. *Exp Toxicol Pathol 59*:365–372

40. Center for Drug Evaluation and Research, 2009. Investigational new drug (IND) application process. http://www.fda.gov/cder/Regulatory/applications/ind_page_1.htm#Introduction

41. International Conference on Harmonization, 1996. Guideline for Good Clinical Practice. E6 (R1) 53 pp. http://www.ich.org/LOB/media/MEDIA482.pdf

42. European Commission, 2005. Detailed guidance for the request for authorisation of a clinical trial on a medicinal product for human use to the competent authorities, notification of substantial amendments and declaration of the end of the trial. 55 pp. http://ec.europa.eu/enterprise/pharmaceuticals/pharmacos/docs/doc2005/10_05/ca_14-2005.pdf

43. International Conference on Harmonization, 2000. M4. The Common Technical Document. http://www.ich.org/cache/compo/276-254-1.html

11

RISK MANAGEMENT

Alberto Lodola

INTRODUCTION

In Chapters 5–9, we discussed nonclinical studies that are used to identify the adverse effects of test compounds. This is the *hazard identification* phase of drug development. The outcome of this series of studies is a comprehensive set of data from which the *potential risks to humans* are identified. Ideally, we all want a drug with the desired pharmacological effect and no risk of adverse effects, but as we know, all drug therapy carries a degree of risk. Although no pharmaceutical company wants to waste scarce resources on developing a drug that is not safe for clinical use, there is also a need not to discard potentially effective new drugs because of a lack of understanding of the potential risk to humans. Therefore, as the development program unfolds, the relevance to humans of the adverse events identified in animals is assessed. The *hazard assessment* phase aims to answer the question: which of the adverse findings in animals is of relevance to humans and what degree of risk do they represent? The third, and final, step in the process is the *risk management* phase; the U.S. Food and Drug Administration (FDA) defines risk management [1] as an iterative process:

- assessing a product's benefit–risk balance,
- developing and implementing tools to minimize its risks while preserving its benefits,

Pharmaceutical Toxicology in Practice: A Guide for Non-Clinical Development, Edited by Alberto Lodola and Jeanne Stadler
© 2011 John Wiley & Sons, Inc.

- evaluating tool effectiveness and reassessing the benefit-risk balance, and
- making adjustments, as appropriate, to the risk minimization tools to improve the benefit–risk balance further.

The European Medicines Agency (EMEA) defines a risk management system as a "set of pharmacovigilance activities and interventions designed to identify, characterize, prevent, or minimize risks relating to medicinal products, and the assessment of the effectiveness of those interventions" [2]. Risk management should be applied throughout a drug's lifetime and must be modified in the light of technical/scientific advances, legislative changes, and the perceived impact on public health of the drug. Hazard identification and assessment phases usually involve drug development experts within a pharmaceutical company, clinical investigators, and regulatory authorities. However, as soon as it is practical, the needs of the patient must also be integrated into the risk management process. The response of individuals to the potential adverse effects of a drug is different and is conditioned, in part, by their understanding of the issue/s in hand. In a general sense, therefore, risk management involves dealing with scientific issues but also the information needs and cultural background of all the constituents involved in the process. In this chapter, we discuss how these goals can be met.

RISK

Understanding the factors that shape the common perception of risk is essential when elaborating a risk management strategy. Risk can be defined in a number of ways depending on the field of activity to which it is applied; see the Merriam-Webster dictionary, for example [3]. For nonclinical drug development, because we are concerned with the impact of the risks identified on humans, we define risk as "the possibility that harm or injury will result to patients as the consequence of exposure to a drug."

The common perception, and acceptance, of risk is highly complex and conditioned by several factors [4]:

- the nature of the hazard and its probability of occurrence,
- a subjective assessment of its importance (which varies from person to person),
- the degree of understanding (risks which are not understood are the most unacceptable) and
- whether the risk activity is imposed or not (there is greater acceptance of a risk undertaken voluntarily than an imposed risk).

There is also a significant paradox in risk perception [5]. People appear to apply greater significance to small risks that are difficult to understand and that are outside their control (e.g., the potential carcinogenicity of trace amounts of chemicals in food and water), while at the same time ignoring large risks over which they have control (the obvious example is smoking). Moreover, there is an expectation that "scientific knowledge is absolute and unchanging"—clearly something that scientists know to be unrealistic. All these factors point to the need to clearly define the nature, and potential impact, of the risk under consideration and, as we discuss below, underline the importance of an effective communications strategy in any risk management process. An absolute standard cannot be applied to the acceptable risk associated with a novel pharmaceutical product; there is no single risk–benefit benchmark. For a drug intended to treat an advanced aggressive cancer for which there is no effective treatment, the acceptable risk will be much greater than for a novel drug intended for the treatment of a non–life-threatening condition (e.g., migraine). It should also be borne in mind that the risk assessment (and risk management) of a drug may change during the lifetime of a drug, due to availability of novel drugs with a better risk–benefit ratio or an increased understanding of the nature of the risk. Risk management is, therefore, not a static exercise but a dynamic process that evolves as experience with a drug increases.

THE RISK MANAGEMENT PROCESS

Guidance documents are available from the FDA: Premarketing Risk Assessment [1], Development and Use of Risk Minimization Action Plans [6], and Good Pharmacovigilance Practices and Pharmacoepidemiologic Assessment [7]. The EMEA has also produced guidance on risk management, for Marketing Authorisation Holders (MAH) and Marketing Authorisation Applicants (MAA). In general, a risk management plan (RMP), which is composed of a "a safety specification and a pharmacovigilance plan" [8] and "an evaluation of the need for risk minimization activities" should be submitted with the application for a new marketing authorization:

- for any product containing a new active substance,
- for a biological drug or a generic/hybrid drug where a safety concern has been identified,
- when the MAA/MAH identify a safety issue at any stage in the life cycle of a drug, and
- in some circumstances, for products that are not in the above categories that are seeking a new authorization via the centralized procedure

The ICH E2E guideline [9] is also of interest, as it deals with the planning of pharmacovigilance activities, particularly during the early postmarketing period of a new drug. Overall, although these guidelines provide a good general background to the concept of risk management, they are focused on clinical data. Our concern is how to apply the risk management process to nonclinical data, with a view to supporting drug development decisions and the risk–benefit analysis for new drugs. In preparing to develop a nonclinical risk management strategy, we have found that a team approach is best in most cases, given the complex nature of the problem/s to be resolved and usually the need to develop and implement a strategy in a relatively short time. The team should be as small as possible to facilitate discussion and decision making while at the same time contain members that bring all the necessary expertise to deal with the problems at hand. A suitable team would be composed of the Study Director (SD), subject matter experts (e.g., pathologist, toxicokinetics specialist), and a management representative other members should be co-opted ad hoc as needed, including external experts (i.e., consultants) who are recognized opinion leaders in their field or who have direct experience of the issue/s in question. As discussed previously (see Chapters 3 and 4) the SD is the central point of accountability for a study and, as such, must be involved in risk management to ensure continuity within the project. Leadership of the team should go the person who is best placed to drive the issue to resolution; this is not necessarily a subject matter expert but someone with sufficient experience and expertise to keep the team focused on the task in hand. The involvement of a management representative on the team is not essential, but it can be of great benefit. Follow up studies are often part of risk management strategies and therefore require a commitment of resources. The management representative can ensure that team members clearly understand the trade-offs involved in making this decision in the context of the companies drug development pipeline. Moreover, experienced managers may have already dealt with similar issues and can thus guide strategy development. In developing a risk management strategy, it is essential to do the following:

- ensure that although it is comprehensive, the risk management process is simple and focused,
- assemble all available nonclinical and clinical data that define the hazard,
- conduct a comprehensive review of the open scientific literature,
- review data for marketed drugs with similar chemical structures and/or pharmacological activity and
- regularly review and modify the strategy in the light of additional nonclinical and clinical data

Based on these needs, a series of iterative steps can be described to guide the risk management process and are summarized in Fig 11.1. It should be noted that although we discuss this process in terms of nonclinical findings, this is broadly applicable to the analysis and resolution of any drug development issue.

Step 1: Identify Risk

All treatment-related (nonclinical) findings that are regarded as having a potential risk to humans should be identified (see Chapters 5–9) and taken forward to Step 2.

Step 2: Analyze Risk

Once a preliminary assessment has been made, findings of interest can be analyzed separately or grouped according to a preliminary hypothesis. For example, cardiac lesions in rats and dogs often results from a treatment with drugs that induce hypotension and reflex tachycardia [10]. Treatment-related findings that are known to have no relevance

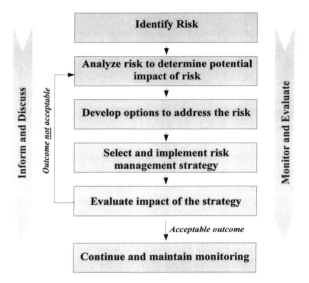

Figure 11.1. Overview of the Risk Management process

to humans can be discarded (e.g., effects of the Harderian gland in the rat. The external adnexa of the eyes of rodents (and other species with a third eyelid) include the Harderian gland, which is located within the orbit behind the eye, almost encircling the optic nerve. It is found in humans in vestigial form during embryonic development and occasionally as a developmental abnormality [11]. Given these facts, it is highly improbable that abnormal findings to the Harderian gland in nonclinical studies signal a potential hazard to humans). Continuing this analysis, findings with the greatest potential (adverse) impact and the greatest probability of occurring in humans are dealt with first, and risks with lower probability of occurrence and/or lower impact are dealt with later. In practice, this idealized approach is very difficult to follow, as deciding how to prioritize between risks with a high probability of occurrence but low impact vs a risk with high impact but low probability is challenging. Resources and time permitting, from a pragmatic viewpoint, it is best to address all adverse findings at the same time.

Step 3: Develop Options

For toxicities, identified in Step 2, a risk management strategy must be developed that does the following:

- allows a decision to be made about the future of the test compound, that is should development continued or, not and/or
- identifies conditions for safe use of the compound, that is how to maximize the risk–benefit ratio, and/or
- supports safe clinical development of the test compound.

If the nonclinical findings fall into a group of pathologies that are well characterized and whose relevance to human safety are understood, this may step may simply involve the development of a communication strategy. If the toxicity in question is poorly understood, additional supportive/mechanistic studies may be needed. The scientific literature provides a wealth of background information and mechanistic hypotheses to explain the pathogenesis of toxicities. The FDA makes freely available the data used in support of marketing applications for all drugs approved in the USA [12] on its Web site. Although commercially sensitive information has been deleted from the dossiers, they describe the nonclinical (and clinical) data from regulatory and investigative studies that were included in the submission document for many marketed drugs. Similarly, following the granting of a marketing authorization by the European Commission, the EMEA makes the European Public Assessment Report (EPAR) available [13]. EPARs reflect the scientific conclusion reached by the Committee for Medicinal Products for Human Use (CHMP) at the end of the centralized evaluation process for new drug submissions. Although there is no detailed presentation of nonclinical data, the overview and discussion of findings is highly informative. Access to this type of information can provide insight into adverse events related to the pharmacology or chemical class of a test compound, the types of mechanistic studies that have been used by others to investigate the pathogenesis of lesions, and insight into how to risk manage findings.

Step 4: Implement Strategy

The actions identified in Step 3 are put into action and usually involve one or more of the following:

- preparing review documents to identify, explain, and put data into context
- seeking expert advice from external experts (recognized opinion leaders)
- consulting with the regulatory authorities
- conducting a series of studies to better characterize the finding in question

Step 5: Evaluate Outcome

When the risk management strategy has been implemented, the outcome of the action taken must be monitored and its impact on the degree of risk to the patient reassessed. At this stage, with the additional data that has been developed, there should be sufficient information to answer one or more of the following questions:

- DO the nonclinical findings predict potential effects in humans?
- If the nonclinical findings were to occur in humans, would they pose an unacceptable risk?
- If the nonclinical findings were to occur in humans, can we attenuate or, ideally eliminate their impact?
- If the nonclinical findings were to occur in humans, can we define conditions for safe usage?

If, after the first iteration of the risk management cycle, it is not possible to answer all, or indeed any, of these key questions, a new round of analysis (Step 2) should be started and additional options developed (Step 3).

Step 6: Monitor Outcome

Once a suitable risk management strategy has been implemented, there must be continued monitoring of the data. New, nonclinical, and clinical data are constantly produced, which can alter understanding of the hazard (i.e., toxicity) profile of the test compound. Additionally, there can be changes to the formulation and/or the manufacturing process for the test compound that can affect the nonclinical and/or clinical toxicity profile and, consequently, the risk–benefit ratio of the test compound. Therefore, this monitoring phase usually accompanies a drug throughout its life.

EFFECTIVE COMMUNICATION

The risk management process must be supported by a robust communication strategy that should take account of three groups with distinct, but overlapping, needs: the company, the regulatory authorities, and the public.

The Company

The nonclinical scientist is usually part of a drug development team that has overall responsibility for advancing the test compound; team members often have varied expertise and/or experience of drug development. As a result, there will be varying degrees of understanding of nonclinical studies, data and, more importantly, the significance of nonclinical findings. To the nonspecialist, or the novice, the range of lesions produced in nonclinical studies can be daunting and result in calls for abandoning what may be a novel, effective, and safe drug. It is essential, therefore, that when presenting nonclinical data within the company nonclinical findings are reviewed describing the potential risk of each finding, if and how the risk can be monitored in clinical studies, and the impact on the development potential of the test compound. To do this, nonclinical findings should be presented in detail (type, incidence, severity), their pathogenesis described, and the potential risk to humans listed wherever possible. This process should be undertaken at key stages in the drug development process, for example, when preparing for Phase 1 clinical studies, when data from pivotal (regulatory) nonclinical studies are available, or if a new finding emerges in a study. In addition, ad hoc discussion should be initiated in a timely manner any time significant new findings of concern are identified.

Regulatory Authorities

Nonclinical data are presented to regulatory authorities at intervals. This occurs when specific advice is sought, or in advance of key development milestones (e.g., with the FDA there are pre-IND meetings, end of Phase 2 meetings, and so on) building up to the

TABLE 11.1. Summary of key findings from the Kaiser Public Opinion Spotlight [15].

Issue/Question	Response	
Adults taking prescription medication	54%	
Perception that prescription drugs have generally made the lives of people better	"Agree"	73%
How much do you agree that pharmaceutical companies provide reliable information about the side effects and safety of pharmaceuticals?	"A lot"	21%
Overall confidence in prescription drug safety	"Very"	27%
Do pharmaceutical companies do enough to test and monitor the safety of their drugs?	"Agree"	55%

final submission for marketing authorization. These meetings provide an opportunity to present nonclinical findings to the authorities, to discuss their potential risk to humans, and to gather the authority's perspective of the potential risk and the risk management strategy that has been deployed. Although there will be nonclinical specialists in the regulatory team involved in these discussions that will usually have broad experience and expertise, it should not be assumed that they are experts in the issue under consideration. Therefore, great care must be taken in describing the issue/s, potential risk/s, and risk management strategy. Once clinical development is initiated, the Investigator's Brochure (IB) [14] brings together all the data from a given drug development program and is used in support clinical studies. The IB is a valuable tool for communicating key issues (e.g., nonclinical, clinical, pharmaceutical, manufacturing) to regulatory authorities, clinicians, and volunteers/patients. The organization of safety information in a well-prepared IB allows investigators to identify potential risks, their severity, potential relevance to humans, and how to manage those risks. Although it is not primarily intended as a communication tool within the pharmaceutical company, development issues are presented within a risk management context in a well-prepared IB so that preparing the IB provides an additional opportunity to develop and communicate a risk management strategy.

General Public

An insight into how the public views the pharmaceutical industry can be gained from an opinion poll conducted in the United States [15]. We have summarized the findings in Table 11.1. Based on these data, it would appear that there is room for improvement in communicating the risk–benefits of drugs to patients: at least to U.S. patients and most probably patients in other countries. An effective communication strategy must help reassure patients that their medication is "safe and effective," but this is not an easy undertaking. An understanding of the often complex issue/s involved, and hence rational risk–benefit decision, is based on the analysis and interpretation of a large body of complex, sometimes contradictory, data. A critical, and sometimes overlooked part of a risk management strategy, is to ensure that the description/discussion of these complex

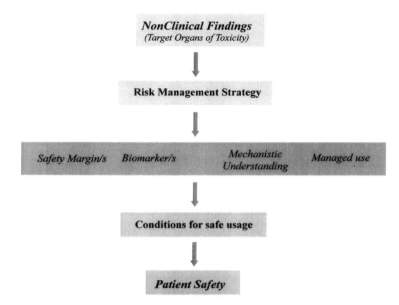

Figure 11.2. Commonly used risk management strategies

issues is simplified and made accessible to patients and the wider public in general. The preparation of a clear, concise description in layman's terms of nonclinical issues, their significance, and how they are being managed and monitored should form a part of all risk management strategies. In our view, this should be a specific exercise and build on, but not replace, the nonclinical summaries prepared for clinical trials consent forms and the package inserts.

COMMONLY USED RISK MANAGEMENT STRATEGIES

No single strategy can be used to manage potentially adverse nonclinical findings; however, there are several commonly used approaches (Fig. 11.2). Typically, nonclinical studies produce findings ranging from those for which there is a significant understanding to those for which there is limited understanding. The following risk management approaches can be used individually, but more usually multiple approaches are used and, when necessary, the toxicologist must develop new approaches.

Use of a Safety Margin

This risk management option can be applied to all nonclinical findings whether their pathogenesis is known or not and whether their significance to humans is known or not. Thus, the highest dose at which the adverse finding does not occur in nonclinical studies, allometrically scaled for humans (e.g., see [16]) is compared to the therapeutic dose of the drug so that a safety margin is determined. Better still, this safety margin is calculated based on systemic exposure to the drug, that is, the C_{max} or AUC at these doses. This clearly leads to the question: what is an acceptable safety margin? There is no right answer to this question. Although the safety margin should be as large as possible, an acceptable value depends on a number of factors:

- knowledge of risks for other drugs of the same pharmacological class
- knowledge of risks of structural analogues
- the therapeutic indication, and
- the availability of effective, alternative drugs to treat the target indication.

Taking these factors into account, it follows that an acceptable safety margin for a drug/compound under development for the treatment of a life-threatening condition for which there is no effective therapy will be smaller than that for a non–life-threatening condition for which there is effective treatment. In this instance, even the absence of a safety margin may be acceptable. If marketed drug/s are available to treat the target indication, then the safety margin for a novel drug must be compared with that for the marketed drug/s. If the novel drug does not have significant advantages in terms of efficacy, as compared with the marketed drug/s, then it is probably unrealistic to expect that a lower safety margin will be acceptable for the novel drug. In general, two things must be borne in mind when deciding on the size of the safety margin:

- first and foremost, the safety of patients must be ensured, and
- there must be a robust, rational, data-based explanation supporting the selected value.

Nevertheless, even drugs with small safety margins can provide effective safe treatment for patients. For example, consider the use of drugs that have a narrow therapeutic index or ratio (NTI) [17]. In brief, a drug is considered to have an NTI if any of the following conditions apply:

- there is less than a twofold difference in median lethal dose and median effective dose values
- there is less than twofold difference in minimum toxic concentrations and minimum effective concentrations in the blood
- safe and effective use of the drug products require careful titration and patient monitoring

Examples of some commonly used drugs with NTIs are given in Table 11.2. Because small changes in systemic concentration of NTIs can produce significant changes in pharmacodynamic response, the range between too little of the NTI drug, which may result in ineffective treatment, or too much of the NTI drug, which can have toxic effects, is very narrow [18]. For example, with digoxin, two to two-and-a-half times the normal (therapeutic) dose is fatal to a significant proportion of the patient population. Another

TABLE 11.2. Examples of drugs with a narrow therapeutic index [18].

Drug Name
Aminophylline
Carbamazepine
Clindamycin
Clonidine
Digoxin
Disopyramide
Dyphylline
Guanethidine
Isoetharine mesylate
Isoproterenol levoxyine
Lithium carbonate
Metaporterenol
Minoxidil
Oxytriphylline
Phenytoin
Prazosin
Primidone
Procainamide
Quinidine gluconate
Theophylline
Valproic acid
Warfarin sodium

example is provided by the use of warfarin [19–22]. Fortunately, a simple laboratory test allows this problem to be risk managed. Measuring the prolongation of the prothrombin time (PT) is the primary method used to measure warfarin's anticoagulant effect. Thus, the optimal dose of warfarin administered can be individualized by monitoring the patient's international normalized PT ratio. Additionally, other factors that may affect the response to therapy must also be accounted for in developing a risk management strategy for NTIs: the age of the patient, the pharmacodynamics of the drug, comorbid conditions, interaction with comedication, dietary intake of vitamin K, and compliance with the specific drug regimen. Because of their NTIs, these drugs require careful risk management; patients need individualized dosing regimens and close monitoring to achieve and maintain acceptable safety and therapeutic benefit. These complex factors are sometimes difficult to control and, as a result, serious consideration must be given to the viability of developing a test compound once it is recognized to have an NTI.

Use of Biomarkers

Any change (ionic, metabolic, genomic, proteomic, or metabonomic) which occurs coincident with or reflects the biological effect (benign or pathogenic) of interest can

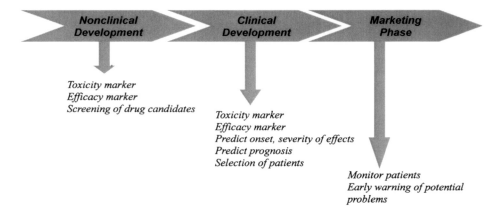

*Nonclinical
Development*

*Clinical
Development*

*Marketing
Phase*

*Toxicity marker
Efficacy marker
Screening of drug candidates*

*Toxicity marker
Efficacy marker
Predict onset, severity of effects
Predict prognosis
Selection of patients*

*Monitor patients
Early warning of potential
problems*

Figure 11.3. Role of biomarkers in drug development and risk management

potentially be used as a biomarker. Once they are proven and shown to be valid and reliable, biomarkers have considerable utility in the whole drug development process in addition to risk management (Fig. 11.3) and can be used to:

- monitor toxicity *and* efficacy,
- allow early identification and attrition of drug candidates with unacceptable risk/benefit ratios,
- provide a bridge between nonclinical and clinical studies, and
- allow the monitoring of subjects/patients in clinical trial and clinical practice.

Ideally, safety biomarkers should be sensitive indicators (although not necessarily predictors) of tissue damage and apply to both nonclinical and clinical testing. Monitoring of biomarkers can be *invasive* or *noninvasive*. Invasive biomarkers rely on obtaining blood, or other tissue samples, for laboratory analysis and or histopathological evaluation [23]. A well-known example of this, which has been used clinically for many years and routinely in nonclinical studies, is using liver enzyme activities as markers of hepatic cell damage [24]. Examples of some commonly used biomarkers are given in Table 11.3. More recently, significant advances in biomarker technology has resulted in the emergence of novel biomarkers based on alterations in gene expression and various "omic" changes [34–39]. Noninvasive approaches rely on the measurement of parameters that do not require tissue sampling. For example, a marked hypotension in nonclinical studies is apparent from measuring blood pressure. Another example is provided by using the QT interval to risk manage the potential of drugs to induce Torsade de Pointes (TdP). Over the years, a large number of drugs have been shown to increase the QT interval in patients (see Table 11.4). Some of these drugs (the antiarrhythmics) would be predicted to increase the QT interval based on their pharmacological actions; however, most would not. Moreover, not only has the link between increased QT interval and TdP

TABLE 11.3. Examples of commonly used biomarkers of toxicity.

	Heart/Muscle	Brain	Kidney	Prostate (Cancer)	Liver	Reference
Creatine kinase	√	√				25–28
Myglobin	√					29
Troponin	√					25, 29
Lactate dehydrogenase	√				√	30
Kallilikrein 2				√		31
Prostate-specific antigen				√		31
PCA3*				√		32
Albumin	√		√			28
α-GST			√			33
NAG			√			33

*PCA3: Prostate cancer antigen 3 gene; α-GST: α-glutathione-S-transferase; NAG: N-acetyl-β-d-glucosaminidase.

TABLE 11.4. Examples of drugs that prolong QT interval (modified from [43]).

	Drug	
	QT Prolongation	
Therapeutic Indication	Well Documented	Some Case Reports
Antiarrhythmics		
	Amiodarone	Dopamine
	Dofetilide	Nicardipine
	Ibutilide	Norepinephrine
	Procainamide	
	Sotalol	
Antipsychotics		
	Thioridazine	Clozapine
	Pimozide	Chlorpromazine
	Zipradazine	
Tricyclic Antidepressants		
	Amitriptyline	
	Amoxapine	
	Clomipramine	
	Doxepine	
Antibiotics		
	Erythromycin	Cotrimoxazole
		Gatifloxacin
		Moxifloxacin
		Clarithromycin
Antimalarials		
	Halofantrine	Chloroquine
	Pentamidine	Mefloquine
		Quinine

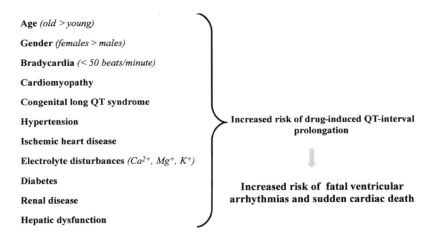

Figure 11.4. Some risk factors for drug induced QT interval prolongation and Torsade de Pointes

has yet to be proven conclusively, but there are also other risk factors that affect the prolongation of drug-induced QT interval and the TdP potential (Fig. 11.4). Nevertheless, this provides an excellent example of a simple rapid (noninvasive) biomarker with which to risk manage potentially drug stopping toxicity. Increasingly new imaging technologies allow noninvasive examination of internal systems [40].

When developing biomarkers a distinction should be made between the qualification of a biomarker and the validation of a biomarker. Qualification provides proof of the relationship between a biomarker and a physiological, pathological, or pharmacological change. Validation provides proof of the accuracy, precision, and reliability of an assay to measure the biomarker. No formal, that is, regulatory, validation of a biomarker is needed for its use by a pharmaceutical company during drug development. In this instance, the biomarker in question need only be tested to a degree that provides the development team with sufficient confidence to use it in (company) decision making. If the same biomarker is to be used in clinical studies, it must be sufficiently validated so that regulatory authorities accept its use. If novel biomarker data are central to the drug submission dossier, a rigorous validation of the proposed biomarker is needed; this has been discussed by the FDA [41]. There is also an International Conference on Harmonization guideline, which by defining a genomic biomarker, pharmacogenomics, pharmacogenetics, and genomic data and sample coding categories is useful in developing standardized validation procedure for new biomarkers [42].

Mechanistic-Based Approaches

In some instances, the nonclinical finding/s of concern may form part of a group of well-characterized pathologies whose relevance to humans is understood, or at least for

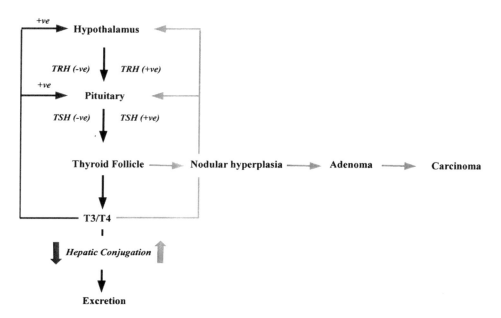

Figure 11.5. Postulated pathogenesis of thyroid hyperplasia and tumor developments in rats The hypothalamus stimulates the pituitary through thyrotropin-releasing hormone (TRH) to produce thyroid-stimulating hormone (TSH), which stimulates the thyroid gland to produce thyroid hormone (Thyroxine (T3) and triiodothyronine (T4)). There is feedback of T4/T3 on the hypothalamus and pituitary to reduce production of TRH and TSH. Thyroid hormone is conjugation by the liver and excreted into the bile. As a result of increased hepatic T3/T4 catabolism activity, there is a feedback stimulation of the thyroid and pituitary with increase in TRH and TSH production. Prolonged stimulation of the thyroid gland initiates a series of changes resulting in carcinoma formation.

which there is significant clinical experience. Two examples of nonclinical findings for which there is a comprehensive body of literature are summarized below.

Increased Incidence of Thyroid Hyperplasia and/or Tumors in Rats Treated with Enzyme Inducers

The long-term treatment of rats with compounds that inhibit thyroid hormone synthesis results in an increased incidence of thyroid tumors. The production of these tumors can be reduced if rats are treated with triiodothyronine (T3) and or thyroxin (T4) or if they are hypophysectomized. There is an increased incidence of thyroid hyperplasia and tumor development [44] in rats treated with phenobarbital (PB). There is a significant body of evidence showing that these changes result from increased thyroid hormone degradation and excretion, due to PB-mediated increases in hepatic levels of the enzyme that catabolizes T3/T4, resulting in stimulation of the thyroid gland by thyroid stimulating hormone (TSH) resulting in thyroid hyperplasia and tumor development (Fig. 11.5). Many drugs (and potential drugs) are hepatic enzyme inducers and produce thyroid hyperplasia and in chronic studies hyperplasia and thyroid tumors thyroid hyperplasia in subchronic studies and PB has been used clinically for many years without evidence of a treatment-related increase in thyroid pathologies. In developing a mechanistic hypothesis to explain the finding/s of concern, the way is open to use the open scientific literature to better assess the potential risk to humans, and/or equal if not greater importance, compare PB with similar effects produced by marketed drugs. The relevance of the proposed mechanism to humans can also be assessed; metabolic processes in the test species (e.g., metabolic pathways, rates of metabolism, susceptibility to inducers) may not be similar to those in humans. One final advantage is that from the mechanistic hypothesis potential biomarkers for the effect of concern can be identified; in the example above circulating levels of T3, T4, and TSH plus hepatic levels of T3/T4 metabolizing enzymes. Using these biomarkers, it could be determined whether conditions suitable for developing the lesion in humans exist.

Hepatotoxicity Due to the Metabolism of the Test Compound/Drug to a Reactive Metabolite

Acetaminophen is one of the worlds most commonly used drugs. It is a nonsteroidal anti-inflammatory (NSAID) drug used to treat pain and fever induced by inflammation. The accidental overdose of acetaminophen is one of the leading causes of hepatic failure in the United States. Under conditions of safe usage, the principal pathway for hepatic acetaminophen metabolism is when acetaminophen is conjugated with glucuronide or sulphate. A smaller proportion of the drug is oxidized by hepatic CYP2E1 to N-acetyl-p-benzoquinone-imine (NAPQI), a highly reactive metabolite, which is conjugated with glutathione. These nontoxic conjugates are excreted [45]. If the ingested dose of the drug is so great that the rate of NAPQI conjugation cannot keep pace with the rate of NAPQI production and/or cellular reserves of glutathione are depleted, NAPQI interacts with cellular proteins and nucleic acids, initiating a cascade of cellular changes that result in cell damage and hepatotoxicity (Fig. 11.6). The production of reactive metabolites is not unique to acetaminophen. Once the mechanism of toxicity is understood, steps can be taken to monitor the effect in humans that would allow quantitation of the potential risk and conditions of safe usage to be established. As with acetaminophen, if the mechanism of toxicity is understood, it may even be possible to develop an antidote to the toxicity [46].

There are many excellent texts describing the pathogenesis of lesions induced by xenobiotics in a range of organs [47–49]; this is required reading for all nonclinical drug developers and provides background information that is essential to the risk management of nonclinical toxicities for novel drugs. In many instances, there is often no mechanistic rational to explain the pathogenesis of a lesion. In these cases, it may be necessary (advisable in our view) to conduct supplemental (mechanistic) studies to gain some understanding of the potential mechanism/s involved. In adopting this approach, it is essential that realistic expectations/goals are set. It is most unlikely that a detailed

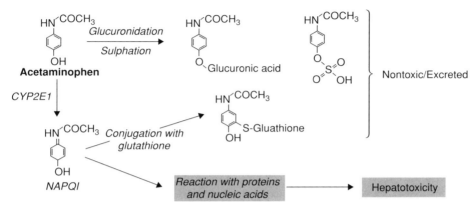

Figure 11.6. Pathogenesis of acetaminophen induced hepatotoxicity
Acetaminophen is either conjugated with glucuronide or sulphate in the live or oxidized by CYP2E1, to N-acetyl-p-benzoquinone-imine (NAPQI) and conjugated with glutathione. These non-toxic conjugates are excreted. If the ingested dose of the drug is so great that the rate of NAPQI conjugation cannot keep pace with the rate of NAPQI production and, or cellular reserves of glutathione are depleted then NAPQI can interact with cellular proteins and nucleic acids, initiating a cascade of cellular changes which result in cell damage and hepatotoxicity

mechanistic rational that explains the pathogenesis of treatment induced lesion will result. Most likely, these studies will provide data that will better describe the lesion in all instances and, for well-thought-out strategies, allow a simple mechanistic scheme to be developed to support or refute a mechanistic hypothesis.

Management of Drug Use

In some cases, the type, incidence, and/or severity of adverse events are such that unrestricted use of a new drug would result in an unacceptable risk/benefit ratio. In this instance, use of a novel drug may need to be restricted to the clinic where patients can be closely monitored throughout their treatment. This approach to risk management implies that there are suitable biomarkers available to monitor the onset of adverse events and that conditions have been determined for stopping/reversing these events.

Instances will arise in which the nonclinical effects are so severe that, a strict management program for drug use must be established. This approach is best illustrated by thalidomide. In the late 1950s, thalidomide was marketed as a sleeping aid, sedative, morning-sickness remedy and antinausea medication, and was prescribed to pregnant women. Thalidomide caused severe birth defects and was removed from the market in the 1960s. Since then, using thalidomide to treat various disorders has been investigated: multiple myeloma (blood cancer), multiple sclerosis, pyoderma gangrenosum, ulcerative bowel disease or Crohn's disease, cutaneous and systemic lupus erythematosus, Behcet's syndrome, aphthous ulcers, Kaposi's sarcoma, myelofibrosis with myeloid metaplasia, kidney, brain, and breast cancers, and complex regional pain syndrome. In many cases, there is no effective treatment available for the conditions that have responded to thalidomide therapy. As a result, using thalidomide in special cases was allowed in the United Kingdom starting in 1968, and in the United States to treat erythema nodosum leprosum since 1998. Renewed use of thalidomide is subject to strict controls. The package insert for Thalomid has an eye-catching warning panel, which is reproduced below:

WARNING

SEVERE, LIFE-THREATENING HUMAN BIRTH DEFECTS. IF THALIDOMIDE IS TAKEN DURING PREGNANCY, IT CAN CAUSE SEVERE BIRTH DEFECTS OR DEATH TO AN UNBORN BABY. THALIDOMIDE SHOULD NEVER BE USED BY WOMEN WHO ARE PREGNANT OR WHO COULD BECOME PREGNANT WHILE TAKING THE DRUG. EVEN A SINGLE DOSE [1 CAPSULE (REGARDLESS OF STRENGTH)] TAKEN BY A PREGNANT WOMAN DURING HER PREGNANCY CAN CAUSE SEVERE BIRTH DEFECTS.

BECAUSE OF THIS TOXICITY AND IN AN EFFORT TO MAKE THE CHANCE OF FETAL EXPOSURE TO THALOMID® (thalidomide) AS NEGLIGIBLE AS POSSIBLE, THALOMID® (thalidomide) IS APPROVED FOR MARKETING ONLY UNDER A SPECIAL RESTRICTED DISTRIBUTION PROGRAM APPROVED BY THE FOOD AND DRUG ADMINISTRATION. THIS PROGRAM IS CALLED THE "SYSTEM FOR THALIDOMIDE EDUCATION AND PRESCRIBING SAFETY (S. T.E.P.S.®)".

UNDER THIS RESTRICTED DISTRIBUTION PROGRAM, ONLY PRESCRIBERS AND PHARMACISTS REGISTERED WITH THE PROGRAM ARE ALLOWED TO PRESCRIBE AND DISPENSE THE PRODUCT. IN ADDITION, PATIENTS MUST BE ADVISED OF, AGREE TO, AND COMPLY WITH THE REQUIREMENTS OF THE S. T.E.P.S. PROGRAM IN ORDER TO RECEIVE PRODUCT.

PLEASE SEE THE FOLLOWING BOXED WARNINGS CONTAINING SPECIAL INFORMATION FOR PRESCRIBERS, FEMALE PATIENTS, AND MALE PATIENTS ABOUT THIS RESTRICTED DISTRIBUTION PROGRAM

In addition, the manufacturer of Thalomid has established the so called S.T.E.P.S. program [50] in collaboration with the FDA, healthcare providers, and patients. S.T.E.P.S. educates patients and doctors and provides a restrictive distribution program for Thalomid. In this instance, the benefits of thalidomide therapy were salvaged in the face of serious adverse events by a risk management strategy based on clear communication of the adverse events, education on the conditions for safe usage of the drug, and a highly restricted and controlled access to the drug.

One rapidly evolving area of managed drug use is that of pharmacogenomics/pharmacogenetics. It has been known for many years that different patients react differently to the same drug because of differences in the age of patients, different body size, diet, gastrointestinal absorption, compliance with therapy, and characteristics of the drug target. However, it has also become increasingly clear that there is also a heritable component to variable drug response; study of this phenomenon has resulted in an increased understanding of *pharmacogenetics* (the use of genetic information to help in the therapeutic treatment of a disease) and *pharmacogenomics* (the study of how a person's genetic makeup determines response to a drug). Because of pharmacogenetic research, the concept of individualized therapy that could result in improved efficacy and reduced toxicity has become a possibility [51]. Indeed, the role of pharmacogenomics in drug development has become increasingly important in drug discovery [52]. Warfarin and tamoxifen are two examples of risk management (and prediction of clinical outcome) that appropriately select patients to maximize the risk/benefit ratio.

Warfarin is converted by CYP2C9 to S-7-hydroxywarfarin, which is inactive [22]. A genetic polymorphism of CYP2C9 contributes to the variability among patients for the required maintenance dose of warfarin [22]. In patients stabilized on low-dose warfarin therapy there is an increased frequency of CYP2C9 allelic variants (such as *CYP2C9*2* and *CYP2C9*3)*. Genetic deficiency of CYP2C9 results in an increased likelihood of major bleeding events compared to the general population [53–58]. Screening patients for CYP2C9 allelic variants could help identity those patients with high sensitivity to warfarin.

There is also genetic and drug induced variation in cellular *CYP2D6* activity that results in interindividual variability in response to drug therapy. *CYP2D6* is involved in the metabolism of up to 25% of all drugs and more than 48 different drug substrates for this enzyme have been identified, including: β-blockers, antidepressants, antiarrhythmics, and antipsychotics [59]. The *CYP2D6* gene is polymorphic, with about 63 different major alleles known at present. Many of these polymorphs are associated with altered or abolished function of the final gene product; thus *CYP2D6* phenotypes associated with these different alleles include poor (PM), intermediate (IM), extensive (EM), and ultrarapid (UM) metabolizers. Moreover, variant allele distribution differs between different ethnic groups [59]. Tamoxifen is a standard endocrine therapy in preventing and treating estrogen receptor (ER)-positive breast cancer. From a retrospective analysis of a tamoxifen trial in postmenopausal women with surgically resected ER-positive breast cancer, it was found that genetic variability in *CYP2D6* might affect the treatment outcomes of patients receiving tamoxifen [60]. These data supported the hypothesis that a *CYP2D6*-mediated formation of antiestrogens may lead to differences not only in response but also in side effects. The major metabolites of tamoxifen include *N*-desmethyltamoxifen (NDM), 4-hydroxytamoxifen (4-OH-Tam), tamoxifen-*N*-oxide, α-hydroxytamoxifen, and *N*-didesmethyltamoxifen [61–65]. NDM, which accounts for approximately 92% of primary tamoxifen oxidation and is then converted to α-hydroxy *N*-desmethyl-, *N*-didesmethyl-, and 4-hydroxy-*N*-desmethyl-tamoxifen (endoxifen) [62, 66, 67]. This conversion is exclusively catalyzed by *CYP2D6*, whereas all other routes of *N*-desmethyl biotransformation are catalyzed predominantly by *CYP3A*24*. With respect to the anticancer activity of tamoxifen metabolites, 4-OH-Tam possesses a much higher affinity for ERs and is 30- to 100-fold more potent than tamoxifen in suppressing estrogen-dependent cell proliferation [68, 69] and possibly the active metabolite of tamoxifen. Endoxifen has identical properties and potency as 4-OH-Tam, but it is present in concentrations up to 10-fold higher than 4-OH-Tam [70]

Goetz et al. [71] analyzed patient data to determine whether potent (fluoxetine and paroxetine) or weak/moderate (sertraline, cimetidine, amiodarone, doxepin, ticlopidine, and haloperidol) *CYP2D6* inhibitors coprescribed with tamoxifen affect the outcome of treatment. Goetz et al. [71] categorized patients as follows:

> *extensive metabolizers*: patients without a *CYP2D6*4* allele who were not prescribed a *CYP2D6* inhibitor
>
> *decreased metabolizers*: patients with one or two *4 alleles, or patients to whom a *CYP2D6* inhibitor was coadministered with tamoxifen (regardless of genotype).

Based on *CYP2D6* genotype and the effects of *CYP2D6* inhibitors on endoxifen plasma concentrations [66, 70] patients with decreased metabolism were further divided into the following:

> *Intermediate metabolizers* (patients heterozygous for the *4 allele (*4/Wt) without coprescription of a *CYP2D6* inhibitor, or no *4 alleles (Wt/Wt) but with coadministration of a weak/moderate inhibitor
>
> *poor metabolizers* (patients homozygous for the *4 allele (*4/*4), or *4/Wt and coadministration of any *CYP2D6* inhibitor, or Wt/Wt and coadministration of a potent inhibitor

Goetz et al. [71] found that there was a stepwise decrement in breast cancer outcome based on the extent of impairment of *CYP2D6* metabolism. Whereas women classified as intermediate metabolizers tended to exhibit worse relapse-free survival (RFS), patients classified as poor metabolizers had the worst outcome with significantly worse RFS [71].

CONCLUSION

Given at a sufficiently high dose, all drugs will produce adverse effects. The *potential* of novel drugs to induce adverse effects in humans is initially assessed in nonclinical studies. A process of risk management must the be initiated to determine the *probability* that the effect will occur in humans, the impact on the risk–benefit ratio, and what steps can be taken to identify conditions for *safe usage and/or to monitor the effect* in clinical trials and for the final marketed drug. Of equal—if not greater—importance is the impact of the risk management exercise on the development strategy for the test compound. In the worst case, the adverse event may be such that conditions for safe usage cannot be defined and development of the test compound is stopped. In many cases, conditions for safe use will be found and/or clinical monitoring will be possible and development of the test compound continued. Because risk management is *an iterative process*, the importance/impact of findings may change in the light of data from toxicity studies of increasingly longer duration or if new nonclinical findings emerge. Once the test compound enters clinical trials, the risk management process must integrate the data from these studies. Sometimes the risk cannot be managed and the drug involved must be withdrawn from the market, but not all may be lost. Consider Baycol. The history of the approval and withdrawal of the Bayer drug Baycol has been reviewed by Angelmar [72]. Baycol (cerivastatin) was launched in the UK in 1997, closely followed by launches in the United States, France, Italy, Spain, and Japan. The drug is a statin and inhibits the activity of HMG CoA reductase, the rate-limiting enzyme in cholesterol synthesis. Because of this inhibition, there is a transient decrease in cellular cholesterol concentration, which activates a cellular signaling cascade, culminating in the activation of sterol regulatory element binding protein (SREBP), a transcription factor that up-regulates expression of the gene encoding the LDL receptor. Increased LDL receptor expression causes increased uptake of plasma LDL and, consequently, decreases plasma LDL–cholesterol concentration [73]. Three key issues emerged with Baycol use:

Rhabdomyolysis

Statin treatment has been associated with rhabdomyolysis, a condition that results in muscle cell degeneration and that can lead to potentially fatal kidney and other organ damage. The precise mechanism of statin-associated muscle toxicity is unclear, but it may involve genetically mediated muscle enzyme defects, drug interactions, intracellular depletion of metabolic intermediates, and intrinsic properties of the statins per se [74]. Although all statins present a risk of rhabdomyolysis, there have been significantly more cases associated with Baycol than other approved statins (e.g., Mevacor, Pravacor, Zocor, Lescol, or Lipitor).

Increased Risk of Myopathy with Combination Treatment

Muscle problems were more likely to occur [75] when treatment with Baycol was combined with gemfibrozil. Baycol/gemfinrozil combination therapy increased the risk of myopathy about 25-fold compared to monotherapy. Other statins showed no increase in risk when combined with gemfibrozil.

A Dose Effect

There was a relationship between the dose of Baycol used and the risk of rhabdomyoly-sis. For example, in the United States, of the 31 people who died from rhabdomyolysis associated with Baycol treatment, 12 were also taking gemfibrozil. Most of the remaining 19 patients who died had started Baycol treatment at 0.8 mg; the recommended starting dose was 0.4 mg. In response to these findings, the 0.8 mg dosage strength was initially withdrawn from the market. However, by 2001, over 480 reported cases of rhabdomy-olysis, including over 52 deaths, was associated with Baycol treatment. Because of this, in early August 2001, Bayer withdrew Baycol from all markets except Japan (in Japan gemfibrozil was not approved at that time so combination therapy was not practiced). However, Baycol was also withdrawn from the Japanese market later the same month due to forthcoming approval of gemfibrozil in Japan. In all, over 100 deaths were linked to the use of Baycol.

There was a significant impact from this tragedy on the risk management of statins. A mechanistic basis for explaining their toxicity and conditions for the safe usage of these drugs was established by integrating data from nonclinical, clinical, and mechanistic studies. Tailored monitoring of patients was developed to prevent a similar outcome with other statins. Finally, this provided a stimulus for developing more predictive nonclinical models for statins; for example, a guinea pig model was developed that can distinguish statins with unacceptable myotoxicity profiles from statins with acceptable safety profile that are likely to have an acceptable therapeutic safety margin [76]. This is an excellent example of how an integrated risk management strategy has enabled a class of drugs, which provide great benefit to patients, to remain on the market while underlining the need for constant vigilance: all drugs have adverse effects; risk management helps to define conditions that maximize the risk–benefit ratio.

REFERENCES

1. U.S. Food and Drug Administration, 2005. Guidance for industry. Premarketing risk assessment. http://www.fda.gov/downloads/Drugs/GuidanceComplianceRegulatoryInformation/Guidances/ucm072002.pdf

2. European Medicines Agency, 2005. EMEA/CHMP/96268/2005. Guideline on risk management systems for medicinal products for human use. http://www.ema.europa.eu/pdfs/human/euleg/9626805en.pdf

3. Merriam-Webster's Online Dictionary, 2008. http://www.merriam-webster.com/dictionary/risk

4. Runciman B, Merry A, and Walton M, 2007. *Safety and Ethics in Healthcare: A Guide to Getting it Right.* Surrey, UK: Ashgate. pp. 31

5. Marks S, 2005. Weighing benefits and risks in pharmaceutical use: A consumer's guide. http://www.acsh.org/publications/pubID.1183/pub_detail.asp

6. U.S. Food and Drug Administration, 2005. Guidance for industry. development and use of risk minimization action plans. http://www.fda.gov/downloads/RegulatoryInformation/Guidances/UCM126830.pdf

7. U.S. Food and Drug Administration, 2005. Guidance for Industry. Good pharmacovigilance practices and pharmacoepidemiologic assessment. http://www.fda.gov/downloads/RegulatoryInformation/Guidances/UCM126834.pdf

8. European Medicines Agency, 2005. Guideline on risk management systems for medicinal products for human use. EMEA/CHMP/96268/2005. http://www.emea.europa.eu/pdfs/human/euleg/9626805en.pdf

9. International Conference on Harmonization, 2004. Guideline E2E. Pharmacovigilance planning. Current Step 4 version. http://www.ich.org/LOB/media/MEDIA1195.pdf

10. Balazs T and Herman EH, 1976. Toxic cardiomyopathies. *Ann Clin Lab Sci*, 6:467–476

11. Chieffi G, Baccari GC, Di Matteo L et al., 1996. Cell biology of the Harderian gland. *Int Rev Cytol* 168:1–80

12. U.S. Food and Drug Administration, 2010. http://www.accessdata.fda.gov/scripts/cder/drugsatfda/

13. European Medicines Agency, 2010. EPARs for authorised medicinal products for human use. http://www.ema.europa.eu/htms/human/epar/eparintro.htm

14. International Conference on Harmonization, 1996. Guideline for good clinical practice E6(R1). http://www.ich.org/LOB/media/MEDIA482.pdf

15. Kaiser, 2008. Kaiser Public Opinion Spotlight. Views on prescription drugs and the pharmaceutical industry. http://www.kff.org/spotlight/rxdrugs/upload/Rx_Drugs.pdf

16. U.S. Food and Drug Administration, 2005. Guidance for industry. Estimating the maximum safe starting dose in initial clinical trials for therapeutics in adult healthy volunteers. http://www.fda.gov/downloads/Drugs/GuidanceComplianceRegulatoryInformation/Guidances/ucm078932.pdf

17. U.S. Food and Drug Administration, 2003. Guidance for industry on bioavailability and bioequivalence studies for orally administered drug products. http://www.fda.gov/downloads/Drugs/GuidanceComplianceRegulatoryInformation/Guidances/ucm070124.pdfregards)

18. Burns M, 1999. Management of narrow therapeutic index drugs. *J Thromb Thrombolysis* **7**:137–143

19. Kirchheiner J and Brockmoller J, 2005. Clinical consequences of cytochrome P450 2C9 polymorphisms. *Clin Pharmacol Ther* **77**:1–16

20. Takahashi H and Echizen H, 2003. Pharmacogenetics of CYP2C9 and interindividual variability in anticoagulant response to warfarin. *Pharmacogenomics J* **3**:202–214

21. Takahashi H and Echizen H, 2001. Pharmacogenetics of warfarin elimination and its clinical implications. *Clin Pharmacokinet* **40**:587–603

22. Aithal GP, Day CP, Kesteven PJ, and Daly AK, 1999. Association of polymorphisms in the cytochrome P450 CYP2C9 with warfarin dose requirement and risk of bleeding complications. *Lancet* **353**:717–719.

23. Salaspuro M, 1987. Use of enzymes for the diagnosis of alcohol-related organ damage. *Enzyme* **37**:87–107

24. Clarke H, Egan DA, Hefferman M, Doyle S et al., 1997. Alpha-glutathione S-transferase (alpha-GST) release, an early indicator of carbon tetrachloride hepatotoxicity in the rat. *Hum Exp Toxicol* **16**:154–157

25. Rosalki SB, Roberts R, Katus HA, Giannitsis E et al., 2004. Cardiac biomarkers for detection of myocardial infarction: Perspectives from past to present. *Clin Chem* **50**:2205–2213

26. Lott JA and Stang JM, 1980. Serum enzymes and isoenzymes in the diagnosis and differential diagnosis of myocardial ischemia and necrosis. *Clin Chem* **26**:1241–1250

27. Gordon W, Lipman B, Gewolb IH, Green JA et al., 1985. Creatine kinase brain isoenzyme: Relationship of cerebrospinal fluid concentration to the neurologic condition of newborns and cellular localization in the human brain. *Pediatrics* **76**:15–21

28. Heerspink L, Hiddo J, Brinkman JW, Bakker JL et al., 2006. Update on microalbuminuria as a biomarker in renal and cardiovascular disease. *Curr Opin Nephrol Hypertens* **15**:631–636

29. Wallace KB, Hausner E, Herman E, Holt GD et al., 2004. Serum troponins as biomarkers of drug-induced cardiac toxicity. *Toxicol Pathol* **32**:106–121

30. Huijgen HJ, Sanders GT, Koster RW, Vreeken J et al., 1997. The clinical value of lactate dehydrogenase in serum: A quantitative review. *Eur J Clin Chem Clin Biochem* **35**:569–579.

31. Rittenhouse HG, Finlay JA, Mikolajczyk SD, and Partin AW, 1998. Human kallikrein 2 (hK2) and prostate-specific antigen (PSA): Two closely related, but distinct, kallikreins in the prostate. *Crit Rev Clin Lab Sci* **35**:275–368

32. Marks LS and Bostwick DG, 2008. Prostate cancer specificity of PCA3 gene testing: Examples from clinical practice. *Rev Urol* **10**:175–181

33. Usuda K, Kono K, Dote T, Nishiura K et al., 1997. Urinary biomarkers monitoring for experimental fluoride nephrotoxicity. *Arch Toxicol* **72**:104–109

34. Petricoin, E F, Rajapaske V, Herman EH, Arekani AM et al., 2004. Toxicoproteomics:serum proteomic pattern diagnostics for early detection of drug induced cardiac toxicities and cardioprotection. *Toxicol Pathol 32*:122–130

35. Hamadeh, HK, Knight BL, Haugen AC, Sieber S et al., 2002. Methapyrilene toxicity:anchorage of pathologic observations to gene expression alterations. *Toxicol Pathol 30*:470–482

36. Lindon JC, Holmes E, Bollard ME, Stanley EG et al., 2004. Metabonomics technologies and their applications in physiological monitoring, drug safety assessment and disease diagnosis. *Biomarkers 9*:1–31

37. Davis JW, Goodsaid FM, Bral CM, Obert LA et al., 2004. Quantitative gene expression analysis in a non-human primate model of antibiotic-induced nephrotoxicity. *Toxicol Appl Pharmacol 200*:16–26

38. Bailey WJ and Ulrich R, 2004. Molecular profiling approaches for identifying novel biomarkers. *Expert Opin. Drug Saf 3*:137–151

39. Huang, Q, Jin X, Gaillard ET, Knight BL et al., 2004. Gene expression profiling reveals multiple toxicity endpoints induced by hepatotoxicants. *Mutat Res 549*:147–167.

40. Fabbrini E, Conte C, and Magkos F, 2009. Methods for assessing intrahepatic fat content and steatosis. *Curr Opin Clin Nutr Metab Care 12*:474–481

41. U.S. Food and Drug Administration, 2006. Critical path opportunities list. http://www.fda.gov/downloads/ScienceResearch/SpecialTopics/CriticalPathInitiative/CriticalPath-OpportunitiesReports/UCM077258.pdf

42. International Conference on Harmonization, 2007. Definitions for genomic biomarkers, pharmacogenomics, pharmacogenetics, genomic data and sample coding categories. http://www.ich.org/LOB/media/MEDIA3383.pdf

43. Shah RR, 2002. The significance of QT interval in drug development. *Br J Clin Pharmacol 54*:188–202

44. Klaassen CD and Hood AM, 2001. Effects of microsomal enzyme inducers on thyroid follicular cell proliferation and thyroidhormone metabolism. *Toxicol Pathol 29*:34–40

45. Jaeschke H, Gores GJ, Cederbaum AI et al., 2002. Mechanisms of hepatotoxicity. *Toxicol Sci 65*:166–176

46. James LP, Mayeux PR, and Hinson JA, 2003. Acetaminophen-induced hepatotoxicity. *Drug Metab Dispos 31*:1499–1506

47. Boelsterli UA, 2007. *Mechanistic Toxicology: The Molecular Basis of How Chemicals Disrupt Biological Targets*, 2nd ed.. London, New York: Taylor & Francis

48. Josephy PD and Mannervik B, 2006. *Molecular Toxicology*. New York: Oxford University Press

49. Timbrell JA, 2008. *Principles of Biochemical Toxicology*, 4th ed.. London: Informa Healthcare

50. Celgene Corporation, 2009. S.T.E.P.S.® http://www.thalomid.com/steps_program.aspx

51. Davies SM, 2006. Pharmacogenetics, pharmacogenomics and personalized medicine: Are we there yet? *Hematology Am Soc Hematol Educ Program* 111–117

52. Guo Y, Shafer S, Weller P, Usuka1 J et al., 2005. Pharmacogenomics and drug development. *Pharmacogenomics 6*:857–864

53. Daly AK and King BP, 2003. Pharmacogenetics of oral anticoagulants. *Pharmacogenomics 13*:247–52

54. Higahi MK, Veenstra DL, Kondo LM, Wittkowsky AK et al., 2002. Association between CYP2C9 genetic variants and anticoagulation-related outcomes during warfarin therapy. *JAMA 287*:1690–1698

55. Tabrizi AR, Zehnbauer BA, Borecki IB, McGrath SD et al., 2002. The frequency and effects of cytochrome P450 (CYP)2C9 polymorphisms in patients receiving warfarin. *J Am Coll Surg 194*:267–273

56. Takahashi H, Kashima T, Nomizo Y, Muramoto N et al., 1998. Metabolism of warfarin enantiomers in Japanese patients with heart disease having different CYP2C9 and CYP2C19 genotypes. *Clin Pharmacol Ther 63*:519–528

57. Scordo MG, Pengo V, Spina E, Dahl ML et al., 2002 Influence of CYP2C9 and CYP2C19 genetic polymorphisms on warfarin maintenance dose and metabolic clearance. *Clin Pharmacol Ther 72*:702–710

58. Lee CR, Goldstein JA, and Pieper JA, 2002. Cytochrome P450 2C9 polymorphisms: A comprehensive review of the in-vitro and human data. *Pharmacogenetics 12*:251–563

59. Ingelman-Sundberg M, 2005. Genetic polymorphisms of cytochrome P450 2D6 (CYP2D6): Clinical consequences, evolutionary aspects and functional diversity. Pharmacogenomics *J 5*:6–13

60. Goetz MP, Rae JM, Suman VJ, Safgren SL et al., 2005. Pharmacogenetics of tamoxifen biotransformation is associated with clinical outcomes of efficacy and hot flashes. *J Clin Oncol 23*:9312–9318.

61. Stearns V, Johnson MD, Rae JM, Morocho A et al., 2003. Active tamoxifen metabolite plasma concentrations after coadministration of tamoxifen and the selective serotonin reuptake inhibitor paroxetine. *J Natl Cancer Inst 95*:1758–1764

62. Desta Z, Ward BA, Soukhova NV, and Flockhart DA, 2004. Comprehensive evaluation of tamoxifen sequential biotransformation by the human cytochrome P450 system in vitro: Prominent roles for CYP3 A and CYP2D6. *J Pharmacol Exp Ther 310*:1062–1075

63. Crewe HK, Notley LM, Wunsch RM, Lennard MS et al., 2002. Metabolism of tamoxifen by recombinant human cytochrome P450 enzymes: Formation of the 4-hydroxy, 4′-hydroxy and N-desmethyl metabolites and isomerization of trans-4-hydroxytamoxifen. *Drug Metab Dispos 30*:869–874

64. Lee KH, Ward BA, Desta Z, Flockhart DA et al., 2003. Quantification of tamoxifen and three metabolites in plasma by high-performance liquid chromatography with fluorescence detection: Application to a clinical trial. *J Chromatogr B Analyt Technol Biomed Life Sci 791*:245–253

65. Lien EA, Solheim E, and Ueland PM, 1991. Distribution of tamoxifen and its metabolites in rat and human tissues during steady-state treatment. *Cancer Res 51*:4837–4844

66. Jin Y, Desta Z, Stearns V, Ward B, Ho H et al., 2005. CYP2D6 genotype, antidepressant use, and tamoxifen metabolism during adjuvant breast cancer treatment. *J Natl Cancer Inst 97*:30–39

67. Stearns V, Beebe KL, Iyengar M, and Dube E, 2003. Paroxetine controlled release in the treatment of menopausal hot flashes: A randomized controlled trial. *JAMA 289*:2827–2834

68. Borgna JL and Rochefort H, 1981. Hydroxylated metabolites of tamoxifen are formed in vivo and bound to estrogen receptor in target tissues. *J Biol Chem 256*:859–868

69. Robertson DW, Katzenellenbogen JA, Long DJ, Rorke EA et al.,1982. Tamoxifen antiestrogens. A comparison of the activity, pharmacokinetics, and metabolic activation of the cis and trans isomers of tamoxifen. *J Steroid Biochem 16*:1–13

70. Borges S, Desta Z, Li L, Skaar TC et al., 2006. Quantitative effect of CYP2D6 genotype and inhibitors on tamoxifen metabolism: Implication for optimization of breast cancer treatment. *Clin Pharmacol Ther* **80**:61–74

71. Goetz MP Goetz MP et al., 2007. The impact of cytochrome P450 2D6 metabolism in women receiving adjuvant tamoxifen. *Breast Cancer Res Treat* **101**:113–121

72. Angelmar R, 2007. The rise and fall of Baycol/Lipobay. *M Med J Med Marketing* **7**:77–88

73. Stancu C and Sima A, 2001. Statins: Mechanism of action and effects. *J Cell Mol Med* **5**:378–387

74. Farmer JA, 2003. Statins and myotoxicity. *Curr Atheroscler Rep* **5**:96–100

75. Chang JT, Staffa JA, Parks M, and Green L, 2004. Rhabdomyolysis with HMG-CoA reductase inhibitors and gemfibrozil combination therapy. *Pharmacoepidemiol Drug Saf* **13**:417–426

76. Madsen CS, Janovitz E, Zhang R et al., 2007. The guinea pig as a preclinical model for demonstrating the efficacy and safety of statins. *J Pharmacol Exp Ther* **324**:576–86

INDEX

Pharmaceutical Toxicology in Practice: A Guide for Non-Clinical Development, Edited by Alberto Lodola and Jeanne Stadler
© 2011 John Wiley & Sons, Inc.